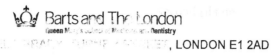

Essential Evidence-Based Medicine

Second Edition

Dan Mayer, MD

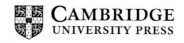

CAMBRIDGE UNIVERSITY PRESS
Cambridge, New York, Melbourne, Madrid, Cape Town, Singapore, São Paulo, Delhi

Cambridge University Press
The Edinburgh Building, Cambridge CB2 8RU, UK

Published in the United States of America by Cambridge University Press, New York

www.cambridge.org
Information on this title: www.cambridge.org/9780521712415

First edition © D. Mayer 2004
Second edition © D. Mayer 2010

First published 2010

Printed in the United Kingdom at the University Press, Cambridge

A catalog record for this publication is available from the British Library

Library of Congress Cataloging in Publication data
Mayer, Dan.
Essential evidence-based medicine / Dan Mayer. – 2nd ed.
   p. ;   cm.
Includes bibliographical references and index.
ISBN 978-0-521-71241-5 (pbk.)
1. Evidence-Based Medicine.   I. Title.
[DNLM: 1. Evidence-Based Medicine.   WB 102.5 M468 2010]
R723.7.M396   2010
616 – dc22   2009024641
ISBN 978-0-521-71241-5 Paperback

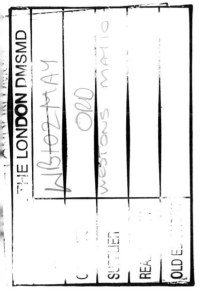

Contents

List of contributors   *page* vii

Preface   ix

Foreword by Sir Muir Gray   xi

Acknowledgments   xiii

1   A brief history of medicine and statistics   1

2   What is evidence-based medicine?   9

3   Causation   19

4   The medical literature: an overview   24

5   Searching the medical literature   33
Sandi Pirozzo and Elizabeth Irish

6   Study design and strength of evidence   56

7   Instruments and measurements: precision and validity   67

8   Sources of bias   80

9   Review of basic statistics   93

10   Hypothesis testing   109

11   Type I errors and number needed to treat   120

12   Negative studies and Type II errors   130

13   Risk assessment   141

14   Adjustment and multivariate analysis   156

15   Randomized clinical trials   164

16   Scientific integrity and the responsible conduct of research   179
John E. Kaplan

17	Applicability and strength of evidence	187
18	Communicating evidence to patients	199
	Laura J. Zakowski, Shobhina G. Chheda, Christine S. Seibert	
19	Critical appraisal of qualitative research studies	208
	Steven R. Simon	
20	An overview of decision making in medicine	215
21	Sources of error in the clinical encounter	233
22	The use of diagnostic tests	244
23	Utility and characteristics of diagnostic tests: likelihood ratios, sensitivity, and specificity	249
24	Bayes' theorem, predictive values, post-test probabilities, and interval likelihood ratios	261
25	Comparing tests and using ROC curves	276
26	Incremental gain and the threshold approach to diagnostic testing	282
27	Sources of bias and critical appraisal of studies of diagnostic tests	295
28	Screening tests	310
29	Practice guidelines and clinical prediction rules	320
30	Decision analysis and quantifying patient values	333
31	Cost-effectiveness analysis	350
32	Survival analysis and studies of prognosis	359
33	Meta-analysis and systematic reviews	367
	Appendix 1　Levels of evidence and grades of recommendations	378
	Appendix 2　Overview of critical appraisal	384
	Appendix 3　Commonly used statistical tests	387
	Appendix 4　Formulas	389
	Appendix 5　Proof of Bayes' theorem	392
	Appendix 6　Using balance sheets to calculate thresholds	394
	Glossary	396
	Bibliography	411
	Index	425

Contributors

Shobhina G. Chheda   *University of Wisconsin School of Medicine and Public Health, Madison, Wisconsin, USA*

Elizabeth Irish   *Albany Medical College, New York, USA*

John E. Kaplan   *Albany Medical College, New York, USA*

Sandi Pirozzo   *University of Queensland, Brisbane, Australia*

Christine S. Seibert   *University of Wisconsin School of Medicine and Public Health, Madison, Wisconsin, USA*

Steven R. Simon   *Harvard Medical School, Boston, Massachusetts, USA*

Laura J. Zakowski   *University of Wisconsin School of Medicine and Public Health, Madison, Wisconsin, USA*

In 1992 during a period of innovative restructuring of the medical school curriculum at Albany Medical College, Dr. Henry Pohl, then Associate Dean for Academic Affairs, asked me to develop a course to teach students how to become lifelong learners and how the health-care system works. This charge became the focus of a new longitudinal required 4-year course initially called CCCS, or Comprehensive Care Case Study. In 2000, the name was changed to Evidence-Based Medicine.

During the next 15 years, a formidable course was developed. It concentrates on teaching evidence-based medicine (EBM) and health-care systems operations to all medical students at Albany Medical College. The first syllabus was based on a course in critical appraisal of the medical literature intended for internal medicine residents at Michigan State University. This core has expanded by incorporating medical decision making and informatics. The basis for the organization of the book lies in the concept of the educational prescription proposed by W. Scott Richardson, M.D.

The goal of the text is to allow the reader, whether medical student, resident, allied health-care provider, or practicing physician, to become a critical consumer of the medical literature. This textbook will teach you to read between the lines in a research study and apply that information to your patients.

For reasons I do not clearly understand, many physicians are "allergic" to mathematics. It seems that even the simplest mathematical calculations drive them to distraction. Medicine is mathematics. Although the math content in this book is on a pretty basic level, most daily interaction with patients involves some understanding of mathematical processes. We may want to determine how much better the patient sitting in our office will do with a particular drug, or how to interpret a patient's concern about a new finding on their yearly physical. Far more commonly, we may need to interpret the information from the Internet that our patient brought in. Either way, we are dealing in probability. However, I have endeavored to keep the math as simple as possible.

This book does not require a working knowledge of statistical testing. The math is limited to simple arithmetic, and a handheld calculator is the only computing instrument that is needed. Online calculators are available to do many of the calculations needed in the book and accompanying CD-ROM. They will be referenced and their operations explained.

The need for learning EBM is elucidated in the opening chapters of the book. The layout of the book is an attempt to follow the process outlined in the educational prescription. You will be able to practice your skills with the practice problems on the accompanying CD-ROM. The CD-ROM also contains materials for "journal clubs" (critical appraisal of specific articles from the literature) and PowerPoint slides.

A brief word about the CD-ROM

The attached CD-ROM is designed to help you consolidate your knowledge and apply the material in the book to everyday situations in EBM. There are four types of problems on the CD:

(1) **Multiple choice questions** are also called self-assessment learning exercises. You will be given information about the answer after pressing "submit" if you get the question wrong. You can then go back and select the correct answer. If you are right, you can proceed to the next question. A record will be kept of your answers.

(2) **Short essay questions** are designed for one- to three-sentence answers. When you press "submit," you will be shown the correct or suggested answer for that question and can proceed to the next question. Your answer will be saved to a specified location in your computer.

(3) **Calculation and graphing questions** require you to perform calculations or draw a graph. These must be done off the program. You will be shown the correct answers after pressing the "submit" button. Your answer will not be saved.

(4) **Journal clubs** require you to analyze a real medical study. You will be asked to fill in a worksheet with your answers in short essay form. After finishing, a sample of correct and acceptable answers will be shown for you to compare with your answers.

The impact of evidence-based decision-making on the way in which we work has had an impact on our understanding of the language that is used to make and take decisions. Decisions are made by language and the language includes both words and numbers, but before evidence-based decision-making came along, relatively little consideration was given to the types of statement or proposition being made. Hospital Boards and Chief Executives, managers and clinicians, made statements but it was never clear what type of statement they were making. Was it, for example, a proposition based on evidence, or was it a proposition based on experience, or a proposition based on values? All these different types of propositions are valid but to a different degree of validity.

This language was hard-packed like Arctic ice, and the criteria of evidence-based decision-making smash into this hard-packed ice like an icebreaker with, on one side propositions based on evidence and, on another, propositions based on experience and values. As with icebreakers, the channel may close up when the icebreaker has moved through but usually it stays open long enough for a decision to be made.

We use a simple arrows diagram to illustrate the different components of a decision, each of which is valid but has a different type of validity.

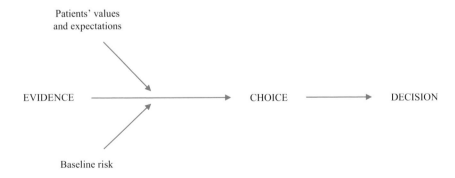

In this book Dan Mayer has demonstrated how to make decisions based on best current evidence while taking into account the knowledge about the particular patient or service under consideration. Evidence-based decision-making is what it says on the tin – it is evidence-based – but it needs to take into account the needs and values of a particular patient, service or population, and this book describes very well how to do that.

Sir Muir Gray, CBE
Former Chief Knowledge Officer
of the National Health Services, UK

Acknowledgments

There are many people who were directly or indirectly responsible for the publication of this book. Foremost, I want to thank my wife, Julia Eddy, without whose insight this book would never have been written and revised. Her encouragement and suggestions at every stage during the development of the course, writing the syllabi, and finally putting them into book form, were the vital link in creating this work. At the University of Vermont, she learned how statistics could be used to develop and evaluate research in psychology and how it should be taught as an applied science. She encouraged me to use the "scientific method approach" to teach medicine to my students, evaluating new research using applied statistics to improve the practice of medicine. She has been my muse for this great project.

Next, I would like to acknowledge the help of all the students and faculty involved in the EBHC Theme Planning Group for the course since the start. This group of committed students and faculty has met monthly since 1993 to make constructive changes in the course. Their suggestions have been incorporated into the book, and this invaluable input has helped me develop it from a rudimentary and disconnected series of lectures and workshops to what I hope is a fully integrated educational text.

I am indebted to the staff of the Office of Medical Education of the Department of Internal Medicine at the Michigan State University for the syllabus material that I purchased from them in 1993. This became the skeleton structure of the course on which this book is based. I think they had a great idea on how to introduce the uninitiated to critical appraisal. The structure of their original course can be seen in this work.

I would like to thank Sandi Pirozzo, B.Sc., M.P.H., John E. Kaplan, Ph.D., Laura J. Zakowski, M.D., Shobhina G. Chheda, M.D., M.P.H., Christine S. Seibert, M.D., and Steven R. Simon, M.D., M.P.H., for their chapters on searching, the ethical conduct of research, communicating evidence to patients, and critical appraisal of qualitative studies, respectively. I would especially like to thank the following faculty and students at Albany Medical College for their review of the manuscript: John Kaplan, Ph.D., Paul Sorum, M.D., Maude Dull, M.D.

(AMC 2000), Kathleen Trapp, B.S., Peter Bernstein, B.S. (AMC 2002), Sue Lahey, M.L.S., Cindy Koman, M.L.S., and Anne Marie L'Hommedieu, M.L.S. Their editorial work over the past several years has helped me refine the ideas in this book. I would also like to thank Chase Echausier, Rachael Levet, and Brian Leneghan for their persistence in putting up with my foibles in the production of the manuscript, and my assistant, Line Callahan, for her Herculean effort in typing the manuscript. For the Second Edition, I also want to thank Abbey Gore (AMC 2009) for her editorial criticism that helped me improve the readability of the text. I also thank the creators of the CD-ROM, which was developed and executed by Tao Nyeu and my son, Noah Mayer and updated by Amanda Hagzan from the Albany Medical College Schaffer Medical Library. I owe a great debt to the staff at the Cambridge University Press for having the faith to publish this book. Specifically, I want to thank Senior Commissioning Editor for Medicine, Peter Silver, for starting the process, and Richard Marley and Katie James for continuing with the Second Edition. Of course, I am very thankful to my original copy-editor, Hugh Brazier, whose expertise and talent made the process of editing the book actually pleasant, and Sally Seehafer, my editor for this second edition, whose efficiency and insight led to the timely publication of this improved effort.

Finally, the First Edition of the book was dedicated to my children: Memphis, Gilah, and Noah. To that list, I want to add my grandchildren: Meira, Chaim, Eliana, Ayelet, Rina, and Talia. Thanks for all of your patience and good cheer.

A brief history of medicine and statistics

History is a pack of lies about events that never happened told by people who weren't there. Those who cannot remember the past are condemned to repeat it.

George Santayana (1863–1952)

Learning objectives

In this chapter, you will learn:

- a brief history of medicine and statistics
- the background to the development of modern evidence-based medicine
- how to put evidence-based medicine into perspective

Introduction

The American health-care system is among the best in the world. Certainly we have the most technologically advanced system. We also spend the most money. Are we getting our money's worth? Are our citizens who have adequate access to health care getting the best possible care? What are the elements of the best possible health care, and who defines it? These questions can be answered by the medical research that is published in the medical literature. When you become an effective and efficient reader of the medical literature, you will be able to answer these questions. It is this process that we will be discussing in this book. This chapter will give you a historical perspective for learning how to find and use the best evidence in the practice of medicine.

Evidence-based medicine (EBM) is a new paradigm for the health-care system involving using the current evidence (results of medical research studies) in the medical literature to provide the best possible care to patients. What follows is a brief history of medicine and statistics, which will give you the historical basis and philosophical underpinnings of EBM. This is the beginning of a process designed to make you a more effective reader of the medical research literature.

Table 1.1. The basis of healing systems in different civilizations

Civilization	Energy	Elements
European	Humors	Earth, air, choler (yellow bile), melancholia (black bile)
East Indian	Chakras	Spirit, phlegm, bile
Chinese	Qi	Earth, metal, fire, water, wood
Native American	Spirits	Earth, air, fire, water

Prehistory and ancient history

Dawn of civilization to about AD 1000

Prehistoric man looked upon illness as a spiritual event. The ill person was seen as having a spiritual failing or being possessed by demons. Medicine practiced during this period and for centuries onward focused on removing these demons and cleansing the body and spirit of the ill person. Trephination, a practice in which holes were made in the skull to vent evil spirits or vapors, and religious rituals were the means to heal. With advances in civilization, healers focused on "treatments" that seemed to work. They used herbal medicines and became more skilled as surgeons.

About 4000 years ago, the Code of Hammurabi listed penalties for bad outcomes in surgery. In some instances, the surgeon lost his hand if the patient died. The prevailing medical theories of this era and the next few millennia involved manipulation of various forms of energy passing through the body. Health required a balance of these energies. The energy had different names depending on where the theory was developed. It was *qi* in China, *chakras* in India, humors in Europe, and natural spirits among Native Americans. The forces achieving the balance of energy also had different names. Each civilization developed a healing method predicated on restoring the correct balance of these energies in the patient, as described in Table 1.1.

The ancient Chinese system of medicine was based upon the duality of the universe. Yin and yang represented the fundamental forces in a dualistic cosmic theory that bound the universe together. The *Nei Ching*, one of the oldest medical textbooks, was written in about the third century BC. According to the *Nei Ching*, medical diagnosis was done by means of "pulse diagnosis" that measured the balance of *qi* (or energy flow) in the body. In addition to pulse diagnosis, traditional Chinese medicine incorporated the five elements, five planets, conditions of the weather, colors, and tones. This system included the 12 channels in which the *qi* flowed. Anatomic knowledge either corroborated the channels or was ignored. Acupuncture as a healing art balanced yin and yang by insertion of needles into the energy channels at different points to manipulate the *qi*. For the

Chinese, the first systematic study of human anatomy didn't occur until the mid eighteenth century and consisted of the inspection of children who had died of plague and had been torn apart by dogs.

Medicine in ancient India was also very complex. Medical theory included seven substances: blood, flesh, fat, bone, marrow, chyle, and semen. From extant records, we know that surgical operations were performed in India as early as 800 BC, including kidney stone removal and plastic surgery, such as the replacement of amputated noses, which were originally removed as punishment for adultery. Diet and hygiene were crucial to curing in Indian medicine, and clinical diagnosis was highly developed, depending as much on the nature of the life of the patient as on his symptoms. Other remedies included herbal medications, surgery, and the "five procedures": emetics, purgatives, water enemas, oil enemas, and sneezing powders. Inhalations, bleeding, cupping, and leeches were also employed. Anatomy was learned from bodies that were soaked in the river for a week and then pulled apart. Indian physicians knew a lot about bones, muscles, ligaments, and joints, but not much about nerves, blood vessels, or internal organs.

The Greeks began to systematize medicine about the same time as the *Nei Ching* appeared in China. Although Hippocratic medical principles are now considered archaic, his principles of the doctor–patient relationship are still followed today. The Greek medical environment consisted of the conflicting schools of the dogmatists, who believed in medical practice based on the theories of health and medicine, and the empiricists, who based their medical therapies on the observation of the effects of their medicines. The dogmatists prevailed and provided the basis for future development of medical theory. In Rome, Galen created popular, albeit incorrect, anatomical descriptions of the human body based primarily on the dissection of animals.

The Middle Ages saw the continued practice of Greek and Roman medicine. Most people turned to folk medicine that was usually performed by village elders who healed using their experiences with local herbs. Other changes in the Middle Ages included the introduction of chemical medications, the study of chemistry, and more extensive surgery by those involved with Arabic medicine.

Renaissance and industrial revolution

The first medical school was started in Salerno, Italy, in the thirteenth century. The Renaissance led to revolutionary changes in the theory of medicine. In the fifteenth century, Vesalius repudiated Galen's incorrect anatomical theories and Paracelsus advocated the use of chemical instead of herbal medicines. In the sixteenth century, the microscope was developed by Janssen and Galileo and popularized by Leeuwenhoek and Hooke. In the seventeenth century, the theory of the circulation of blood was proposed by Harvey and scientists learned about the actual functioning of the human body. The eighteenth century saw the development of modern medicines with the isolation of foxglove to make digitalis by Withering, the use of inoculation against smallpox by Jenner, and the postulation of the existence of vitamin C and antiscorbutic factor by Lind.

During the eighteenth century, medical theories were undergoing rapid and chaotic change. In Scotland, Brown theorized that health represented the conflict between strong and weak forces in the body. He treated imbalances with either opium or alcohol. Cullen preached a strict following of the medical orthodoxy of the time and recommended complex prescriptions to treat illness. Hahnemann was disturbed by the use of strong chemicals to cure, and developed the theory of homeopathy. Based upon the theory that like cures like, he prescribed medications in doses that were so minute that current atomic analysis cannot find even one molecule of the original substance in the solution. Benjamin Rush, the foremost physician of the century, was a strong proponent of bloodletting, a popular therapy of the time. He has the distinction of being the first physician in America who was involved in a malpractice suit, which is a whole other story. He won the case.

The birth of statistics

Prehistoric peoples had no concept of probability, and the first mention is in the Talmud, written between AD 300 and 400. This alluded to the probability of two events being the product of the probability of each, but without explicitly using mathematical calculations. Among the ancients, the Greeks believed that the gods decided all life and, therefore, that probability did not enter into issues of daily life. The Greek creation myth involved a game of dice between Zeus, Poseidon, and Hades, but the Greeks themselves turned to oracles and the stars instead.

The use of Roman numerals made any kind of complex calculation impossible. Numbers as we know them today, using the decimal system and the zero, probably originated around AD 500 in the Hindu culture of India. This was probably the biggest step toward being able to manipulate probabilities and determine statistics. The Arabic mathematician Khowarizmi defined rules for adding, subtracting, multiplying, and dividing in about AD 800. In 1202, the book of the abacus, *Liber abaci* by Leonardo Pisano (more commonly known as Fibonacci), first introduced the numbers discovered by Arabic cultures to European civilization.

In 1494, Luca Paccioli defined basic principles of algebra and multiplication tables up to 60×60 in his book *Summa de arithmetica, geometria, proportioni e proportionalita*. He posed the first serious statistical problem of two men playing a game called balla, which is to end when one of them has won six rounds.

However, when they stop playing A has only won five rounds and B three. How should they divide the wager? It would be another 200 years before this problem was solved.

In 1545, Girolamo Cardano wrote the books *Ars magna* (The Great Art) and *Liber de ludo aleae* (Book on Games of Chance). This was the first attempt to use mathematics to describe statistics and probability, and he accurately described the probabilities of throwing various numbers with dice. Galileo expanded on this by calculating probabilities using two dice. In 1619, a puritan minister named Thomas Gataker, expounded on the meaning of probability by noting that it was natural laws and not divine providence that governed these outcomes.

Other famous scientists of the seventeenth century included Huygens, Leibniz, and Englishman John Graunt, who all wrote further on norms of statistics, including the relation of personal choice and judgment to statistical probability. In 1662, a group of Parisian monks at the Port Royal Monastery wrote an early text on statistics and were the first to use the word probability. Wondering why people were afraid of lightning even though the probability of being struck is very small, they stated that the "fear of harm ought to be proportional not merely to the gravity of the harm but also to the probability of the event."[1] This linked the severity, perception, and probability of the outcome of the risk for the person involved.

In 1660, Blaise Pascal refined the theories of statistics and, with help from Pierre de Fermat, solved the balla problem of Paccioli. All of these theories paved the way for modern statistics, which essentially began with the use of actuarial tables to determine insurance for merchant ships. Edward Lloyd opened his coffee shop in London at which merchant ship captains used to gather, trade their experiences, and announce the arrival of ships from various parts of the world. One hundred years later, this endeavour led to the foundation of Lloyds of London, which began its business of naval insurance in the 1770s.

John Graunt, a British merchant, categorized the cause of death of the London populace using statistical sampling, noting that "considering that it is esteemed an even lay, whether any man lived 10 years longer, I supposed it was the same, that one of any 10 might die within one year." He also noted the reason for doing this: to "set down how many died of each [*notorious disease*]...those persons may better understand the hazard they are in."[2] Graunt's statistics can be compared to recent data from the United States in 1993 in Table 1.2. As a result of this work, the government of the United Kingdom set up the first government-sponsored statistical sampling service.

With the rise in statistical thinking, Jacob Bernoulli devised the law of large numbers, which stated that as the number of observations increased the actual

---

[1] P. L. Bernstein. *Against the Gods: the Remarkable Story of Risk.* New York, NY: Wiley, 1998. p. 71.
[2] *Ibid.*, p. 82.

Table 1.2. Probability of survival: 1660 and 1993

Age, y	Percentage survival to each age	
	1660	1993
0	100%	100%
26	25%	98%
46	10%	95%
76	1%	70%

frequency of an event would approach its theoretical probability. This is the basis of all modern statistical inference. In the 1730s, Jacob's nephew Daniel Bernoulli developed the idea of utility as the mathematical combination of the quantity and perception of risk.

Modern era

Nineteenth century to today

The nineteenth century saw the development of Claude Bernard's modern physiology, William Morton's anesthesia, Joseph Lister and Ignatz Semmelweis' antisepsis, Wilhelm Roentgen's x-rays, Louis Pasteur and Robert Koch's germ theory, and Sigmund Freud's psychiatric theory. Changes in medical practice were illustrated by the empirical analysis done in 1838 by Pierre Charles Alexandre Louis. He showed that blood-letting therapy for typhoid fever was associated with increased mortality and changed this practice as a result. The growth of sanitary engineering and public health preceded this in the seventeenth and eighteenth centuries. This improvement had the greatest impact on human health through improved water supplies, waste removal, and living and working conditions. John Snow performed the first recorded modern epidemiological study in 1854 during a cholera epidemic in London. He found that a particular water pump located on Broad Street was the source of the epidemic and was being contaminated by sewage dumped into the River Thames. At the same time, Florence Nightingale was using statistical graphs to show the need to improve sanitation and hygiene in general for the British troops during the Crimean War. This type of data gathering in medicine was rare up to that time.

The twentieth century saw an explosion of medical technology. Specifics include the discovery of modern medicines by Paul Erlich, antibiotics (specifically sulfanilamide by Domagk and penicillin by Fleming), and modern chemotherapeutic agents to treat ancient scourges such as diabetes (specifically the discovery of insulin by Banting, Best, and McLeod), cancer, and hypertension. The modern era of surgery has led to open-heart surgery, joint replacement, and organ transplantation. Advances in medicine continue at an ever-increasing rate.

Why weren't physicians using statistics in medicine? Before the middle of the twentieth century, advances in medicine and conclusions about human illness occurred mainly through the study of anatomy and physiology. The case study or case series was a common way to prove that a treatment was beneficial or that a certain etiology was the cause of an illness. The use of statistical sampling techniques took a while to develop. There were intense battles between those physicians who wanted to use statistical sampling and those who believed in the power of inductive reasoning from physiological experiments.

This argument between inductive reasoning and statistical sampling continued into the nineteenth century. Pierre Simon Laplace (1814) put forward the idea that essentially all knowledge was uncertain and, therefore, probabilistic in nature. The work of Pierre Charles Alexandre Louis on typhoid and diphtheria (1838) debunking the theory of bleeding used probabilistic principles. On the other side was Francois Double, who felt that treatment of the individual was more important than knowing what happens to groups of patients. The art of medicine was defined as deductions from experience and induction from physiologic mechanisms. These were felt to be more important than the "calculus of probability." This debate continued for over 100 years in France, Germany, Britain, and the United States.

The rise of modern biomedical research

Most research done before the twentieth century was more anecdotal than systematic, consisting of descriptions of patients or pathological findings. James Lind, a Royal Navy surgeon, carried out the first recorded clinical trial in 1747. In looking for a cure for scurvy, he fed sailors afflicted with scurvy six different treatments and determined that a factor in limes and oranges cured the disease while other foods did not. His study was not blinded, but as a result, 40 years later limes were stocked on all ships of the Royal Navy, and scurvy among sailors became a problem of the past.

Research studies of physiology and other basic science research topics began to appear in large numbers in the nineteenth century. By the start of the twentieth century, medicine had moved from the empirical observation of cases to the scientific application of basic sciences to determine the best therapies and catalog diagnoses. Although there were some epidemiological studies that looked at populations, it was uncommon to have any kind of longitudinal study of large groups of patients. There was a 200-year gap from Lind's studies before the controlled clinical trial became the standard study for new medical innovations. It was only in the 1950s that the randomized clinical trial became the standard for excellent research.

There are three more British men who made great contributions to the early development of the current movement in EBM. Sir Ronald Fisher was the father of statistics. Beginning in the early 1900s, he developed the basis for most theories of modern statistical testing. Austin Bradford Hill was another statistician, who, in 1937, published a series of articles in the *Lancet* on the use of statistical methodology in medical research. In 1947, he published a simple commentary in the *British Medical Journal* calling for the introduction of statistics in the medical curriculum.[3] He called for physicians to be well versed in basic statistics and research study design in order to avoid the biases that were then so prevalent in what passed for medical research. Bradford Hill went on to direct the first true modern randomized clinical trial. He showed that streptomycin therapy was superior to standard therapy for the treatment of pulmonary tuberculosis.

Finally, Archie Cochrane was particularly important in the development of the current movement to perform systematic reviews of medical topics. He was a British general practitioner who did a lot of epidemiological work on respiratory diseases. In the late 1970s, he published an epic work on the evidence for medical therapies in perinatal care. This was the first quality-rated systematic review of the literature on a particular topic in medicine. His book *Effectiveness and Efficiency* set out a rational argument for studying and applying EBM to the clinical situation.[4] Subsequently, groups working on systematic reviews spread through the United Kingdom and now form a network in cyberspace throughout the world. In his honor, this network has been named the Cochrane Collaboration.

As Santayana said, it is important to learn from history so as not to repeat the mistakes that civilization has made in the past. The improper application of tainted evidence has resulted in poor medicine and increased cost without improving on human suffering. This book will give physicians the tools to evaluate the medical literature and pave the way for improved health for all. In the next chapter, we will begin where we left off in our history of medicine and statistics and enter the current era of evidence-based medicine.

---

[3] A. Bradford Hill. Statistics in the medical curriculum? *Br. Med. J.* 1947; ii: 366.
[4] A. L. Cochrane. *Effectiveness & Efficiency: Random Reflections on Health Services.* London: Royal Society of Medicine, 1971.

2

What is evidence-based medicine?

The most savage controversies are those about matters as to which there is no good evidence either way.

Bertrand Russell (1872–1970)

Learning objectives

In this chapter, you will learn:
- why you need to study evidence-based medicine
- the elements of evidence-based medicine
- how a good clinical question is constructed

The importance of evidence

In the 1980s, there were several studies looking at the utilization of various surgeries in the northeastern United States. These studies showed that there were large variations in the amount of care delivered to similar populations. They found variations in rates of prostate surgery and hysterectomy of up to 300% between similar counties. The variation rate in the performance of cataract surgery was 2000%. The researchers concluded that physicians were using very different standards to decide which patients required surgery. Why were physicians using such different rules? Weren't they all reading the same textbooks and journal articles? In that case, shouldn't their practice be more uniform?

"Daily, clinicians confront questions about the interpretation of diagnostic tests, the harm associated with exposure to an agent, the prognosis of disease in a specific patient, the effectiveness of a preventive or therapeutic intervention, and the costs and clinical consequences of many other clinical decisions. Both clinicians and policy makers need to know whether the

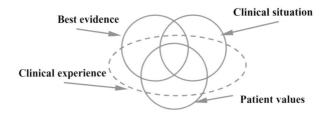

conclusions of a systematic review are valid, and whether recommendations in practice guidelines are sound."[1]

This is where Evidence-Based Medicine comes in.

Evidence-based medicine (EBM) has been defined as "the conscientious, explicit, and judicious use of the best evidence in making decisions about the care of individual patients" (http://ebm.mcmaster.ca/documents/how_to_teach_ebcp_workshop_brochure_2009.pdf).[2] The EBM stems from the physician's need to have *proven* therapies to offer patients. This is a paradigm shift that represents both a breakdown of the traditional hierarchical system of medical practice and the acceptance of the scientific method as the governing force in advancing the field of medicine. Simply stated, EBM is applying the best evidence that can be found in the medical literature to the patient with a medical problem, resulting in the best possible care for each patient. Evidence-based clinical practice (EBCP) is a definition of an approach to medical practice in which you the clinician are able to evaluate the strength of that evidence and use it in the best clinical practice for the patient sitting in your office.

Evidence-based medicine can be seen as a combination of three skills by which practitioners become aware of, critically analyze, and then apply the best available evidence from the medical research literature for the care of individual patients. The first of these is Information Mastery (IM), the skill of searching the medical literature in the most efficient manner to find the best available evidence. This skill will be the focus of Chapter 5. The majority of the chapters in this book will focus on the skill of Critical Appraisal (CA) of the literature. This set of skills will help you to develop critical thinking about the content of the medical literature. Finally, the results of the information found and critically appraised must be applied to patient care in the process of Knowledge Translation (KT), which is the subject of Chapter 17. The application of research results is a blend of the available evidence, the patient's preferences, the clinical situation, and the practitioner's clinical experience (Fig. 2.1).

---

[1] McMaster University Department of Clinical Epidemiology and Biostatistics. Evidence-based clinical practice (EBCP) course, 1999.

[2] D. L. Sackett, W. M. Rosenberg, J. A. Gray, R. B. Haynes & W. S. Richardson. Evidence based medicine: what it is and what it isn't. *BMJ* 1996; 312: 71–72.

Medical decision making: expert vs. evidence-based

Because of the scientific basis of medical research, the essence of evidence-based medical practice has been around for centuries. Its explicit application as EBM to problem solving in clinical medicine began simultaneously in the late 1980s at McMaster University in Canada and at Oxford University in the United Kingdom. In response to the high variability of medical practice and increasing costs and complexity of medical care, systems were needed to define the best and, if possible, the cheapest treatments. Individuals trained in both clinical medicine and epidemiology collaborated to develop strategies to assist in the critical appraisal of clinical data from the biomedical journals.

In the past, a physician faced with a clinical predicament would turn to an expert physician for the definitive answer to the problem. This could take the form of an informal discussion on rounds with the senior attending (or consultant) physician, or the referral of a patient to a specialist. The answer would come from the more experienced and usually older physician, and would be taken at face value by the younger and more inexperienced physician. That clinical answer was usually based upon the many years of experience of the older physician, but was not necessarily ever empirically tested. Evidence-based medicine has changed the culture of health-care delivery by encouraging the rapid and transparent translation of the latest scientific knowledge to improve patient care. This new knowledge translation begins at the time of its discovery until its general acceptance in the care of patients with clinical problems for which that knowledge is valid, relevant, and crucial.

Health-care workers will practice EBM on several levels. Most practitioners have to keep up by regularly reading relevant scientific journals and need to decide whether to accept what they read. This requires having a critical approach to the science presented in the literature, a process called "doing" EBM and the activity is done by "doers." Some of these "doers" are also the people who create critically appraised sources of evidence and systematic reviews or meta-analyses.

Most health-care workers will spend a greater part of their time functioning as "users" of the medical evidence. They will have the skills to search for the best available evidence in the most efficient way. They will be good at looking for pre-appraised sources of evidence that will help them care for their patients in the most effective way. Finally, there is one last group of health-care workers that can be called the "replicators," who simply accept the word of experts about the best available evidence for care of their patients. The goal of this book is to teach you, the clinician, to be a "doer."

With the rise of EBM, various groups have developed ways to package evidence to make it more useful to individual practitioners. These sources allow health-care professionals to practice EBM in a more efficient manner at the point of patient care. Information Mastery will help you to expedite your searches for information when needed during the patient care process. Ideally, you'd like to find and use critical evaluations of clinically important questions done by authors other than those who wrote the study. Various online databases around the world serve as repositories for these summaries of evidence. To date, most of the major centers for the dissemination of these have been in the United Kingdom.

The National Health Service sponsors the Centre for Evidence-Based Medicine based at Oxford University. This center is the home of various EBM resources, one in particular is called the *Bandolier*. *Bandolier* is a summary of recent interesting evidence evaluated by the center and is published monthly. It is found at www.jr2.ox.ac.uk/bandolier and is a wonderful blend of interesting medical information and uniquely British humor in an easy-to-read format. It is excellent for student use and free to browse. The center also has various other free and easily accessible features on its main site found at www.cebm.net. Other useful EBM websites are listed in the Bibliography and additional IM sites, and processes will be discussed in Chapter 6.

Alphabet soup of critical appraisal of the medical literature

Several commonly used forms of critical appraisal are the Critically Appraised Topic (CAT), Disease Oriented Evidence (DOE), the Patient-Oriented Evidence that Matters (POEM), and the Journal Club Bank (JCB). The CAT format is developed by the Centre for Evidence-Based Medicine, and many CATs are available online at the center's website. They use the User's Guide to the Medical Literature format (see Bibliography) to catalog reviews of clinical studies. In a similar format DOEs and POEMs are developed for use by family physicians by the American Academy of Family Practice. The JCB is the format for critical appraisal used by the Evidence-Based Interest Group of the American College of Physicians (ACP) and the Evidence-Based Emergency Medicine group (www.ebem.org) working through the New York Academy of Medicine. Other organizations are beginning to use these formats to disseminate critical reviews on the World Wide Web.

A DOE is a critical review of a study that shows that there is a change in a particular disease marker when a particular intervention is applied. However, this disease-specific outcome may not make a difference to an individual patient. For example, it is clear that statins lower cholesterol. However, it is not necessarily true that the same drugs reduce mortality from heart disease. This is where POEMs come in. A POEM would be that the studies for some of these statin drugs have shown the correlation between statin use and decreased mortality from heart disease, an outcome that matters to the patient rather than simply a disease-oriented outcome. Another example is the prostate-specific antigen (PSA) test for detecting prostate cancer. There is no question that the test can detect prostate cancer most of the time at a stage that is earlier than would be detected by a physician examination, so it is a positive DOE. However, it has yet to be shown that early detection using the PSA results in a longer life span or an improved quality of life; thus, it is not a positive POEM.

Other compiled sources of evidence are the American Society of Internal Medicine and the American College of Physicians' *ACP Journal Club*, published by the journal *Annals of Internal Medicine*, and the Cochrane Library, sponsored by the National Health Service in the United Kingdom. Both are available by subscription. The next step for the future use of EBM in the medical decision-making process is making the evidence easily available at the patient's bedside. This has been tried using an "evidence cart" containing a computer loaded with evidence-based resources during rounds.[3] Currently, personal digital assistants (PDAs) and other handheld devices with evidence-based databases downloaded onto them are being used at the bedside to fulfil this mission.

How to put EBM into use

For many physicians, the most complex part of the process of EBM is the critical appraisal of the medical literature. Part of the perceived complexity with this process is a fear of statistics and consequent lack of understanding of statistical processes. The book will teach this in several steps. Each step will be reinforced on the CD-ROM with a series of practice problems and self-assessment learning exercises (SALEs) in which examples from the medical literature will be presented. This will also help you develop your skills of formulating clinical questions, and in time, you will become a competent evaluator of the medical literature. This skill will serve you well for the rest of your career.

The clinical question: background vs. foreground

You can classify clinical questions into two basic types. **Background** questions are those which have been answered in the past and are now part of the "fiber of medicine." Answers to these questions are usually found in medical textbooks. The learner must beware, since the answers to these questions may be inaccurate and not based upon any credible evidence. Typical background questions relate to the nature of a disease or the usual cause, diagnosis, or treatment of illnesses.

---

[3] D. L. Sackett & S. E. Straus. Finding and applying evidence during clinical rounds: the "evidence cart". *JAMA* 1998; 280: 1336–1338.

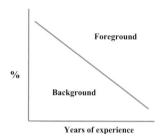

Fig. 2.2 The relationship between foreground and background questions and the clinician's experience.

Foreground questions are those usually found at the cutting edge of medicine. They are questions about the most recent therapies, diagnostic tests, or current theories of illness causation. These are the questions that are the heart of the practice of EBM. A four-part clinical question called a PICO question is designed to easily search for this evidence.

The determination of whether a question is foreground or background depends upon your level of experience. The experienced clinician will have very few background questions that need to be researched. On the other hand, the novice has so many unanswered questions that most are of a background nature. The graph in Fig. 2.2 shows the relationship between foreground and background questions and the clinician's experience.

When do you want to get the most current evidence? How often is access to EBM needed each day for the average clinician? Most physician work is based upon knowledge gained by answering background questions. There are some situations for which current evidence is more helpful. These include questions that are going to make a major impact for your patient. Will the disease kill them, and if so, how long will it take and what will their death be like? These are typical questions that a cancer patient would ask. Other reasons for searching for the best current evidence include problems that recur commonly in your practice, those in which you are especially interested, or those for which answers are easily found. The case in which you are confronted with a patient whose problem you cannot solve and for which there is no good background information would lead you to search for the most current foreground evidence.

Steps in practicing EBM

There are six steps in the complete process of EBM. It is best to start learning EBM by learning and practicing these steps. As you become more familiar with the process, you can start taking short cuts and limiting the steps. Using a patient scenario as a starting point, the first step is recognizing that there is an educational need for more current information. This step leads to the "educational prescription,"[4] which can be prepared by the learner or given to them by the teacher. The steps then taken are as follows:

(1) Craft a clinical question. Often called the PICO or PICOT formulation, this is the most important step since it sets the stage for a successful answer to the clinical predicament. It includes four or sometimes five parts:
  • the patient
  • the intervention
  • the comparison

___

[4] Based on: W. S. Richardson. *Educational prescription: the five elements.* University of Rochester.

- the **outcome** of interest
- the time frame

(2) Search the medical literature for those studies that are most likely to give the best evidence. This step requires good searching skills using medical informatics.

(3) Find the study that is most able to answer this question. Determine the magnitude and precision of the final results.

(4) Perform a critical appraisal of the study to determine the validity of the results. Look for sources of bias that may represent a fatal flaw in the study.

(5) Determine how the results will help you in caring for your patient.

(6) Finally, you should evaluate the results of applying the evidence to your patient or patient population.

The clinical question: structure of the question

The first and most critical part of the EBM process is to ask the right question. We are all familiar with the computer analogy, "garbage in, garbage out." The clinical question (or query) should have a defined structure. The **PICO** model has become the standard for stating a searchable question. A good question involves **Patient**, **Intervention**, **Comparison**, and **Outcome**. A fifth element, **Time**, is often added to this list. These must be clearly stated in order to search the question accurately.

The **Patient** refers to the population group to which you want to apply the information. This is the patient sitting in your office, clinic, or surgery. If you are too specific with the population, you will have trouble finding any evidence for that person. Therefore, you must initially be general in your specification of this group. If your patient is a middle-aged man with hypertension, there may be many studies of the current best treatment of hypertension in this group. However, if you had a middle-aged African-American woman in front of you, you may not find studies that are limited to this population. In this case, asking about treatment of hypertension in general will turn up the most evidence. You can then look through these studies to find those applicable to that patient.

The **Intervention** is the therapy, etiology, or diagnostic test that you are interested in applying to your patient. A therapy could simply be a new drug. If you are answering a question about the causes of diseases, the exposure to a potentially harmful process, or risk factors leading to premature mortality, you will be looking for etiology. We will discuss studies of diagnostic tests in more detail in Chapters 20–26.

The **Comparison** is the intervention (therapy, etiology, or diagnostic test) against which the intervention is measured. A reasonable comparison group is one that would be commonly encountered in clinical practice. Testing a new drug against one that is never used in current practice is not going to help the practitioner. The comparison group ought to be a real alternative and not just a "straw man." Currently, the use of placebo for comparison in many studies is no longer considered ethical since there are acceptable treatments for the problem being studied.

The **Outcome** is the endpoint of interest to you or your patient. The most important outcomes are the ones that matter to the patient. These are most often death, disability, or full recovery. Surprisingly, not all outcomes are important to the patient. One specific type of outcome is referred to as the surrogate outcome. This refers to disease markers that ought to cause changes in the disease process. However, the expected changes to the disease process may not actually happen. Studies of heart-attack patients done in the 1960s showed that some died suddenly from irregular heart rhythms. These patients were identified before death by the presence of premature ventricular contractions (PVCs) on the electrocardiogram. Physicians thereafter began treating all patients with heart attacks with drugs to suppress PVCs and noted that there was a lower rate of death of patients with PVCs. Physicians thought this would reduce deaths in all patients with heart attacks, but a large study found that the death rate actually increased when all patients were given these drugs. While they prevented death in a small number of patients who had PVCs, they increased death rates in a majority of patients.

The **Time** relates to the period over which the intervention is being studied. This element is usually omitted from the searching process. However, it may be considered when deciding if the study was carried out for a sufficient amount of time.

Putting EBM into context in the current practice of medicine: the science and art of medicine

Evidence-based medicine should be part of the everyday practice of all physicians. It has been only slightly more than 50 years since statistics was first felt to be an important part of the medical curriculum. In a 1947 commentary in the *British Medical Journal* entitled "Statistics in the medical curriculum?",[5] Sir Austin Bradford Hill lamented that most physicians would interpret this as "What! Statistics in the medical curriculum?" We are now in a more enlightened era. We recognize the need for physicians to be able to understand the nature of statistical processes and to be able to interpret these for their patients. This

[5] A. Bradford Hill. Statistics in the medical curriculum? *Br. Med. J.* 1947; ii: 366.

goes to the heart of the science and art of medicine. The science is in the medical literature and in the ability of the clinician to interpret that literature. Students learn the clinical and basic sciences that are the foundation of medicine during the first 2 years of medical school. These sciences are the building blocks for a physician's career. The learning doesn't stop there. Having a critical understanding of new advances in medicine by using EBM is an important part of medical practice.

The art of medicine is in determining to which patients the literature will apply and then communicating the results to the patients. Students learn to perform an adequate history and physical examination of patients to extract the maximum amount of evidence to use for good medical decision making. Students must also learn to give patients information about their illnesses and empower them to act appropriately to effect a cure or control and moderate the illness. Finally, as praciticioners, physicians must be able to know when to apply the results of the most current literature to patients, and when other approaches should be used for their patients.

Although most practicing physicians these days believe that they practice EBM all the time, the observed variation in practice suggests otherwise. Evidence-based medicine can be viewed as an attempt to standardize the practice of medicine, but at the same time, it is not "cookbook" medicine. The application of EBM may suggest the best approach to a specific clinical problem. However, it is still up to the clinician to determine whether the individual patient will benefit from that approach. If your patient is very different from those for whom there is evidence, you may be justified in taking another approach to solve the problem. These decisions ought to be based upon sound clinical evidence, scientific knowledge, and pathophysiological information.

Evidence-based medicine is not cookbook medicine. Accused of being "micro-fascist" by some, EBM can be used to create clinical practice guidelines for a common medical problem that has led to a large variation in practice and has several best practices that ought to be standardized. Evidence-based medicine is not a way for managed care (or anyone else) to simply save money. Evidence-based practices can be more or less expensive than current practices, but they should be better.

Evidence-based medicine is the application of good science to the practice of health care, leading to reproducibility and transparency in the science supporting health-care practice. Evidence-based medicine is the way to maximize the benefits of science in the practice of health care.

Finally, Fig. 2.3 is a reprint from the *BMJ* (the journal formerly known as the *British Medical Journal*) and is a humorous look at alternatives to EBM.

Departments of
Education and
Medicine, New
Children's Hospital,
Westmead,
NSW 2145,
Australia
David Isaacs
clinical professor
Dominic Fitzgerald
staff physician

Correspondence to:
D Isaacs
davidi@nch.edu.au

BMJ 1999;319:1618

Clinical decisions should, as far as possible, be evidence based. So runs the current clinical dogma.[1][2] We are urged to lump all the relevant randomised controlled trials into one giant meta-analysis and come out with a combined odds ratio for all decisions. Physicians, surgeons, nurses are doing it[3-5]; soon even the lawyers will be using evidence based practice.[6] But what if there is no evidence on which to base a clinical decision?

Participants, methods, and results

We, two humble clinicians ever ready for advice and guidance, asked our colleagues what they would do if faced with a clinical problem for which there are no randomised controlled trials and no good evidence. We found ourselves faced with several personality based opinions, as would be expected in a teaching hospital. The personalities transcend the disciplines, with the exception of surgery, in which discipline transcends personality. We categorised their replies, on the basis of no evidence whatsoever, as follows.

Eminence based medicine—The more senior the colleague, the less importance he or she placed on the need for anything as mundane as evidence. Experience, it seems, is worth any amount of evidence. These colleagues have a touching faith in clinical experience, which has been defined as "making the same mistakes with increasing confidence over an impressive number of years."[7] The eminent physician's white hair and balding pate are called the "halo" effect.

Vehemence based medicine—The substitution of volume for evidence is an effective technique for brow beating your more timorous colleagues and for convincing relatives of your ability.

Eloquence based medicine—The year round suntan, carnation in the button hole, silk tie, Armani suit, and tongue should all be equally smooth. Sartorial elegance and verbal eloquence are powerful substitutes for evidence.

Providence based medicine—If the caring practitioner has no idea of what to do next, the decision may be best left in the hands of the Almighty. Too many clinicians, unfortunately, are unable to resist giving God a hand with the decision making.

Diffidence based medicine—Some doctors see a problem and look for an answer. Others merely see a problem. The diffident doctor may do nothing from a sense of despair. This, of course, may be better than doing

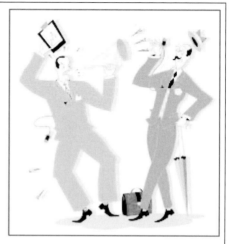

something merely because it hurts the doctor's pride to do nothing.

Nervousness based medicine—Fear of litigation is a powerful stimulus to overinvestigation and overtreatment. In an atmosphere of litigation phobia, the only bad test is the test you didn't think of ordering.

Confidence based medicine—This is restricted to surgeons (table).

Comment

There are plenty of alternatives for the practising physician in the absence of evidence. This is what makes medicine an art as well as a science.

Contributors: DI and DF each contributed half the jokes and will both act as guarantors.
Funding: None.
Competing interests: None declared.

1   Evidence Based Medicine Working Group. Evidence-based medicine: a new approach to teaching the practice of medicine. *JAMA* 1992;268:2420-5.
2   Rosenberg W, Donald A. Evidence based medicine: an approach to clinical problem solving. *BMJ* 1995;310:1122-6.
3   Sackett DL, Rosenberg WM, Gray JAM, Haynes RB, Richardson WS. Evidence based medicine: what it is and what it isn't. *BMJ* 1996;312:71-2.
4   Solomon MJ, McLeod RS. Surgery and the randomised controlled trial: past, present and future. *Med J Aust* 1998;169:380-3.
5   McClarey M. Implementing clinical effectiveness. *Nursing Management* 1998;5:16-9.
6   EBM and the IMF. *J Exponential Salaries* 1999;99:1-9.
7   O'Donnell M. *A sceptic's medical dictionary.* London: BMJ Books, 1997.

Basis of clinical practice

Basis for clinical decisions	Marker	Measuring device	Unit of measurement
Evidence	Randomised controlled trial	Meta-analysis	Odds ratio
Eminence	Radiance of white hair	Luminometer	Optical density
Vehemence	Level of stridency	Audiometer	Decibels
Eloquence (or elegance)	Smoothness of tongue or nap of suit	Teflometer	Adhesin score
Providence	Level of religious fervour	Sextant to measure angle of genuflection	International units of piety
Diffidence	Level of gloom	Nihilometer	Sighs
Nervousness	Litigation phobia level	Every conceivable test	Bark balance
Confidence*	Bravado	Sweat test	No sweat

*Applies only to surgeons.

Fig. 2.3 Isaacs, D. & Fitzgerald, D. Seven alternatives to evidence based medicine. BMJ 1999; 319: 1618. Reprinted with permission.

3

Causation

Heavier than air flying machines are impossible.

Lord Kelvin, President of the Royal Society, 1895

Learning objectives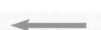

In this chapter you will learn:

- cause-and-effect relationships
- Koch's principles
- the concept of contributory cause
- the relationship of the clinical question to the type of study

The ultimate goal of medical research is to increase our knowledge about the interaction between a particular agent (cause) and the health or disease in our patient (effect). Causation is the relationship between an exposure or cause and an outcome or effect such that the exposure resulted in the outcome. However, a strong association between an exposure and outcome may not be equivalent to proving a cause-and-effect relationship. In this chapter, we will discuss the theories of causation. By the end of this chapter, you will be able to determine the type of causation in a study.

Cause-and-effect relationships

Most biomedical research studies try to prove a relationship between a particular cause and a specified effect. The **cause** may be a risk factor resulting in a disease, an exposure, a diagnostic test, or a treatment helping alleviate suffering. The **effect** is a particular outcome that we want to measure. The stronger the design of a study, the more likely it is to prove a relationship between cause and effect. Not all study designs are capable of proving a cause-and-effect relationship, and these study designs will be discussed in a later chapter.

The cause is also called the **independent variable** and is set by the researcher or the environment. In some studies relating to the prognosis of disease, time is the independent variable. The effect is called the **dependent variable**. It is dependent upon the action of the independent variable. It can be an outcome such as death or survival, the degree of improvement on a clinical score or the detection of disease by a diagnostic test. You ought to be able to identify the cause and effect easily in the study you are evaluating if the structure of the study is of good quality. If not, there are problems with the study design.

Types of causation

It's not always easy to establish a link between a disease and its suspected cause. For example, we think that hyperlipidemia (elevated levels of lipids or fats in the blood) is a cause of cardiovascular disease. But how can we be sure that this is a cause and not just a related factor? Perhaps hyperlipidemia is caused by inactivity or a sedentary lifestyle and the lack of exercise actually causes both cardiovascular disease and hyperlipidemia.

This may even be true with acute infections. *Streptococcus viridans* is a bacterium that can cause infection of the heart valves. However, it takes more than the presence of the bacterium in the blood to cause the infection. We cannot say that the presence of the bacterium in the blood is sufficient to cause this infection. There must be other factors such as local deformity of the valve or immunocompromise that make the valve prone to infection.

In a more mundane example, it has been noted that the more churches a town has, the more robberies occur. Does this mean that clergy are robbing people? No – it simply means that a third variable, population, explains the number both of churches and of muggings. The number or churches is a **surrogate marker** for population, the true cause. Likewise, we know that *Streptococcus viridans* is a cause of subacute endocarditis. But it is neither the only cause, nor does it always lead to the result of an infected heart valve. How are we to be sure then, of cause-and-effect?

In medical science, there are two types of cause-and-effect relationships: **Koch's postulates** and **contributory cause**. Robert Koch, a nineteenth-century microbiologist, developed his famous postulates as criteria to determine if a certain microbiologic agent was the cause of an illness. Acute infectious diseases were the scourge of mankind before the mid twentieth century. As a result of better public health measures such as water treatment and sewage disposal, and antibiotics, these are less of a problem today. Dr. Koch studied the anthrax bacillus as a cause of habitual abortion in cattle. He created the following postulates in an attempt to determine the relationship between the agent causing the illness and the illness itself.

Koch's postulates stated four basic steps to prove causation. First, the infectious agent must be found in all cases of the illness. Second, when found it must be able to be isolated from the diseased host and grown in a pure culture. Next, the agent from the culture when introduced into a healthy host must cause the illness. Finally, the infectious agent must again be recovered from the new host and grown in a pure culture. This entire cascade must be met in order to prove causation.

While this model may work well in the study of acute infectious diseases, most modern illnesses are chronic and degenerative in nature. Illnesses such as diabetes, heart disease, and cancer tend to be multifactorial in their etiology and usually have multiple treatments that can alleviate the illness. For these diseases, it is virtually impossible to pinpoint a single cause or the effect of a single treatment from a single research study. Stronger studies of these diseases are more likely to point to useful clinical information relating one particular cause with an effect on the illness.

Applying **contributory cause** helps prove causation in these complex and multifactorial diseases. The requirements for proof are less stringent than Koch's postulates. However, since the disease-related factors are multifactorial, it is more difficult to prove that any one factor is decisive in either causing or curing the disease. Contributory cause recognizes that there is a large gray zone in which some of the many causes and treatments of a disease overlap.

First, the cause and effect must be seen together more often than would be expected to occur by chance alone. This means that the cause and effect are associated more often than would be expected by chance if the concurrence of those two factors was a random event. Second, the cause must always be noted to precede the effect. If there were situations for which the effect was noted before the occurrence of the cause, that would negate this relationship in time. Finally and ideally, it should be shown that changing the cause changes the effect. This last factor is the most difficult to prove and requires an intervention study be performed. Overall, contributory cause to prove the nature of a chronic and multifactorial illness must minimally show association and temporality. However, to strengthen the causation, the change of the effect by a changing cause must also be shown. Table 3.1 compares Koch's postulates and contributory cause.

Causation and the clinical question

The two main components of causation are also parts of the clinical question. Since the clinical question is the first step in EBM, it is useful to put the clinical question into the context of causation. The **intervention** is the cause that is being investigated. In most studies, this is compared to another cause, named the **comparison**. The **outcome** of interest is the effect. You will learn to use good

Table 3.1. Koch's postulates vs. contributory cause

Koch's postulates (most stringent)
(1) **Sufficient**: if the agent (cause) is present, the disease (effect) is present
(2) **Necessary**: if the agent (cause) is absent, the disease (effect) is absent
(3) **Specific**: the agent (cause) is associated with only one disease (effect)

Contributory cause (most clinically relevant)
(1) Not all patients with the particular cause will develop the effect (disease): the cause is **not sufficient**
(2) Not all patients with the specific effect (disease) were exposed to the particular cause: the cause is **not necessary**
(3) The cause may be associated with several diseases (effects) and is therefore **non-specific**

Table 3.2. Cause and effect relationship for most common types of studies

Type of study	Cause	Effect
Etiology, harm, or risk	Medication, environmental, or genetic agent	Disease, complication, or mortality
Therapy or prevention	Medication, other therapy, or preventive modality	Improvement of symptoms or mortality
Prognosis	Disease or therapy	Time to outcome
Diagnosis	Diagnostic test	Accuracy of diagnosis

searching techniques so that you find the study that answers this query in the best manner possible. The intervention, comparison, and outcome all relate to the patient **population** being studied.

Primary clinical research studies can be roughly divided into four main types, determined by the elements of cause and effect. They are studies of **etiology** (or harm or risk), **therapy**, **prognosis**, and **diagnosis**. There are numerous secondary study types that will be covered later in the book. The nomenclature used for describing the cause and effect in these studies can be somewhat confusing and is shown in Table 3.2.

- Studies of etiology, harm, or risk compare groups of patients that do or don't have the outcome of interest and look to see if they do or don't have the risk factor. They can also go in the other direction, starting from the presence or absence of the risk factor and finding out who went on to have or not have the outcome. Also, the direction of the study can be either forward or backward in time. Useful ways of looking at this category of studies is to look for **cohort**, case–control, or cross-sectional studies. These will be defined in more detail in Chapter 6. In studies of etiology, the risk factor for a disease is the cause and the presence of disease is the outcome. In other studies, the cause could be a therapy for a disease and the effect could be the improvement in disease.

- Studies of therapy or prevention tend to be **randomized clinical trials**, in which some patients get the therapy or preventive modality being tested and others do not. The outcome is compared between the two groups.
- Studies of prognosis look at disease progression over time. They can be either **cohort** studies or **randomized clinical trials**. There are special elements to studies of prognosis that will be discussed in Chapter 33.
- Studies of diagnosis are unique in that we are looking for some diagnostic maneuver that will separate those with a disease from those who may have a similar presentation and yet do not have the disease. Usually these are **cohort**, **case–control**, or **cross-sectional studies**. These will be discussed in more detail in Chapter 28.

There is a relationship between the clinical question and the study type. In general the clinical question can be written as: among patients with a particular disease (population), does the presence of a therapy or risk factor (intervention), compared with no presence of the therapy or risk factor (comparison), change the probability of an adverse event (outcome)? For a study of risk or harm, we can write this as: among patients with a disease, does the presence of a risk factor, compared with the absence of a risk factor, worsen the outcome? We can also write it as: among patients with exposure or non-exposure to a risk factor, are they more likely to have the outcome of interest? For therapy, the question is: among patients with a disease, does the presence of an exposure to therapy, compared with the use of placebo or standard therapy, improve the outcome? The form of the question can help you perform better searches, as we will see in Chapter 5. Through regular practice, you will learn to write better questions and in turn, find better answers.

4

The medical literature: an overview

It is astonishing with how little reading a doctor can practice medicine, but it is not astonishing how badly he may do it.

Sir William Osler (1849–1919)

Learning objectives

In this chapter you will learn:
- the scope and function of the articles you will find in the medical literature
- the function of the main parts of a research article

The medical literature is the source of most of our current information on the best medical practices. This literature consists of many types of articles, the most important of which for our purposes are research studies. In order to evaluate the results of a research study, you must understand what clinical research articles are designed to do and what they are capable of accomplishing. Each part of a study contributes to the final results of the published research. To be an intelligent reader of the medical literature, you then must understand which types of articles will provide the information you are seeking.

Where is clinical research found?

In your medical career, you will read and perhaps also write, many research papers. All medical specialties have at least one primary peer-reviewed journal and most have several. There are also many general-interest medical journals. One important observation you will make is that not all journals are created equal. For example, peer-reviewed journals are "better" than non–peer-reviewed journals since their articles are more carefully screened and contain fewer "problems." Many of these peer-reviewed journals have a statistician on staff to ensure that the statistical tests used are correct. This is just one example of differences between journals and journal quality.

The *New England Journal of Medicine* and the *Journal of the American Medical Association (JAMA)* are the most widely read and prestigious general medical journals in the United States. The *Lancet* and the *British Medical Journal (BMJ)* are the other top English-language journals in the world. However, even these excellent journals print imperfect studies. As the consumer of this literature, you are responsible for determining how to use the results of clinical research. You will also have to translate the results of these research studies to your patients. Many patients these days will read about medical studies in the lay press or hear about them on television, and may even base their decisions about health care upon what the magazine writers or journalists say. Your job as a physician is to help your patient make a more informed medical decision rather than just taking the media's word for it. In order to do this, you will need to have a healthy skepticism of the content of the medical literature as well as a working knowledge of critical appraisal. Other physicians, journal reviewers, and even editors may not be as well trained as you.

Non–peer-reviewed and minor journals may still have articles and studies that give good information. Many of the articles in these journals tend to be expert reviews or case reports. All studies have some degree of useful information, and the aforementioned articles are useful for reviewing and relearning background information. Bear in mind that no matter how prestigious the journal, no study is perfect. But, all studies have some degree of useful information. A partial list of common and important medical journals is included in the Bibliography.

What are the important types of articles?

Usually, when asked about articles in the medical literature, one thinks of clinical research studies. These include such epidemiological studies as case–control, cohort or cross-sectional studies, and randomized clinical trials. These are not the only types of articles that are important for the reader of the medical literature. There are several other broad types of articles with which you should be familiar, and each has its own strengths and weaknesses. We will discuss studies other than clinical research in this chapter, and will address the common types of clinical research studies in Chapter 6.

Basic science research

Animal or **basic science research** studies are usually considered pure research. They may be of questionable usefulness in your patients since people clearly are not laboratory rats and in vitro does not always equal in vivo. Because of this, they may not pass the "so what?" test. However, they are useful preliminary studies, and they may justify human clinical studies. It is only through these types of studies that medicine will continue to push the envelope of our knowledge of physiological and biochemical mechanisms of disease.

Animal or other bench research is sometimes used to rationalize certain treatments. This leap of faith may result in unhelpful, and potentially harmful, treatments being given to patients. An example of potentially useful basic science research is the discovery of angiostatin, a chemical that stops the growth of blood vessels into tumors. The publication of research done in mice showing that infusion of this chemical caused regression of tumors resulted in a sudden increase in inquiries to physicians from family members of cancer patients. These family members were hoping that they would be able to obtain the drug and get a cure for their loved ones. Unfortunately, this was not going to happen. When the drug was given to patients in a clinical trial, the results were much less dramatic. This is not the only clinical trial that diplayed less dramatic results in humans. In another example, there were similar outcomes when bone-marrow transplant therapy was used to treat breast cancer.

The discovery of two forms of the enzyme cyclo-oxygenase (COX 1 and 2) occurred in animal research and subsequently was identified using research in humans. Cyclo-oxygenase 2 is the primary enzyme in the inflammatory process, while COX 1 is the primary enzyme in the maintenance of the mucosal protection of the stomach. Inhibition of both enzymes is the primary action of most non-steroidal anti-inflammatory drugs (NSAIDs). With the discovery of these two enzymes, drugs selective for inhibition of the COX 2 enzyme were developed. These had anti-inflammatory action without causing gastric mucosal irritation and gastrointestinal bleeding. At first glance, this development appeared to be a real advance in medicine. However, extending the use of this class of drug to routine pain management was not warranted. Clinical studies have since demonstrated equivalence in pain control with other NSAIDs with only modest reductions in side effects at a very large increase in cost. Finally, more recently, the drugs were found to actually increase the rate of heart attacks.

Basic science research is important for increasing the content of biomedical knowledge. For instance, recent basic science research has demonstrated the plasticity of the nervous system. Prior to this discovery, it was standard teaching that nervous system cells were permanent and not able to regenerate. Current research now shows that new brain and nerve cells can be grown, in both animals and in humans. While not clinically useful at this time, it is promising research for the future treatment of degenerative nerve disorders such as Alzheimer's disease.

Because these basic science studies seem to be more reliable given that they measure basic physiologic processes, the results of these studies are sometimes accepted without question. Doing this could be an error. A recent study by Bogardus *et al.* found that there were significant methodological problems in many clinical studies of molecular genetics. These studies used basic science techniques in clinical settings.[1] Thus, while this book focuses on clinical studies, the principles discussed also apply to your critical appraisal of basic science research studies.

Editorials

Editorials are opinion pieces written by a recognized expert on a given topic. Most often they are published in response to a study in the same journal issue. Editorials are the vehicle that puts a study into perspective and shows its usefulness in clinical practice. They give contextual commentary to the study, but, because they are written by an expert who is giving an opinion, the piece incorporates that expert's biases. Editorials should be well referenced and they should be read with a skeptical eye and not be the only article that you use to form your opinion.

Clinical review

A **clinical review** article seeks to review all the important studies on a given subject to date. It is written by an expert or someone with a special interest in the topic and is more up to date than a textbook. Clinical reviews are most useful for new learners updating their background information. Because a clinical review is written by a single author, it is subject to the writer's biases in reporting the results of the referenced studies. Due to this, it should not be accepted uncritically. However, if you are familiar with the background literature and can determine the accuracy of the citations and subsequent recommendations, a review can help to put clinical problems into perspective. The overall strength of the review depends upon the strength (validity and impact) of each individual study.

Meta-analysis or systematic review

Meta-analysis or systematic review is a relatively new technique to provide a comprehensive and objective analysis of all clinical studies on a given topic. It attempts to combine many studies and is more objective in reviewing these studies than a clinical review. The authors apply statistical techniques to quantitatively combine the results of the selected studies. We will discuss the details on evaluating these types of article in Chapter 33.

Components of a clinical research study

Clinical studies should be reported upon in a standardized manner. The most important reporting style is referred to as the IMRAD style. This stands for

---

[1] S. T. Bogardus, Jr., J. Concato & A. R. Feinstein. Clinical epidemiological quality in molecular genetic research: the need for methodological standards. *JAMA* 1999; 281: 1919–1926.

Table 4.1. Components of reported clinical studies

---

(1) Abstract
(2) Introduction
(3) Methods
(4) Results
(5) Discussion
(6) Conclusion
(7) References/bibliography

Introduction, Methods, Results, and Discussion. First proposed by Day in 1989, it is now the standard for all clinical studies reported in the English-language literature.[2] Structured abstracts proposed by the SORT (Standards of Reporting Trials) group are now required by most medical journals. The structure of the abstract follows the structure of the full article (Table 4.1).

Abstract

The **abstract** is a summary of the study. It should accurately reflect what actually happened in the study. Its purpose is to give you an overview of the research and let you decide if you want to read the full article. The abstract includes a sentence or two on each of the elements of the article. These include the introduction, study design, population studied, interventions and comparisons, outcomes measured, primary or most important results, and conclusions. The abstract may not completely or accurately represent the actual findings of the article and often does not contain important information found only in the article. Therefore it should never be used as the sole source of information about the study.

Introduction

The **introduction** is a brief statement of the problem to be solved and the purpose of the research. It describes the importance of the study by either giving the reader a brief overview of previous research on the same or related topics or giving the scientific justification for doing the study. The hypotheses being tested should be *explicitly* stated. Too often, the hypothesis is only implied, potentially leaving the study open to misinterpretation. As we will learn later, only the **null hypothesis** can be directly tested. Therefore, the null hypothesis should either be explicitly stated or obvious from the statement of the expected outcome of the research, which is also called the **alternative hypothesis**.

---

[2] R. A. Day. The origins of the scientific paper: the IMRAD format. *AMWAJ* 1989; 4: 16–18.

Methods

The **methods** section is the most important part of a research study and should be the first part of a study that you read. Unfortunately, in practice, it is often the least frequently read. It includes a detailed description of the research design, the population sample, the process of the research, and the statistical methods. There should be enough details to allow anyone reading the study to replicate the experiment. Careful reading of this section will suggest potential biases and threats to the validity of the study.

(1) The **sample** is the population being studied. It should also be the population to which the study is intended to pertain. The processes of **sample selection** and/or **assignment** must be adequately described. This includes the **eligibility requirements** or **inclusion criteria** (who could be entered into the experiment) and **exclusion criteria** (who is not allowed to be in the study and why). It also includes a description of the **setting** in which the study is being done. The site of research such as a community outpatient clinic, specialty practice, hospital, or others may influence the types of patients enrolled in the study thus these settings should be stated in the methods section.

(2) The **procedure** describes both the experimental processes and the outcome measures. It includes **data acquisition, randomization,** and **blinding** conditions. Randomization refers to how the research subjects were allocated to different groups. The blinding information should include whether the treating professionals, observers, or participants were aware of the nature of the study and if the study is **single-, double-,** or **triple-blinded.** All of the important outcome measures should be examined and the process by which they are measured and the quality of these measures should all be explicitly described. These are known as the **instruments** and **measurements** of a study. In studies that depend on patient record review, the process by which that review was carried out should be explicitly described.

(3) The **statistical analysis** section includes types of data such as nominal, ordinal, interval, ratio, continuous, or dichotomous data; how the data are described, including the measures of central tendency and dispersion of data; and what analytic statistical tests will be used to assess statistical relationships between two or more variables. It should also note the levels of α and β **error** and the **power.**

Results

The **results** section should summarize all the data pertinent to the purpose of the study. It should also give an explanation of the statistical significance of the data. This part of the article is not a place for commentary or opinions – "just the facts!"[3] All important sample and subgroup characteristics, and the results of all important research outcomes, should be included. The description of the measurements should include the **measures of central tendency** and **dispersion** (e.g., standard deviations or standard error of the mean) and the *P* **values** or **confidence intervals**. These values should be given so that readers may determine for themselves if the results are statistically and/or clinically significant. In addition, the tables and graphs should be clearly and accurately labeled.

Discussion

The **discussion** includes an interpretation of the data and a discussion of the clinical importance of the results. It should flow logically from the data shown and incorporate other research about the topic, explaining why this study did or did not corroborate the results of those studies. Unfortunately, this section is often used to spin the results of a study in a particular direction and will over- or under-emphasize certain results. This is why the reader's critical appraisal is so important. The discussion section should include a discussion of the statistical and clinical significance of the results, the non-significant results, and the potential biases in the study.

(1) The **statistical significance** is a mathematical phenomenon depending only on the **sample size**, the **precision** of the data, and the magnitude of the difference found between groups, also known as **effect size**. As the sample size increases, the power of the study will increase, and a smaller effect size will become statistically significant.

(2) The **clinical significance** means that the results are important and will be useful in clinical practice. If a small effect size is found, that treatment may not be clinically important. Also, a study with enough subjects may find statistical significance if even a tiny difference in outcomes of the groups is found. In these cases, the study result may make no clinical difference for your patient. What is important is a change in disease status that matters to the patient sitting in your office.

(3) Interpretation of results that are **not statistically significant** must be included in the discussion section. A study result that is not statistically significant does not conclusively mean that no relationship or association exists. It is possible that the study may not have had adequate **power** to find those results to be statistically significant. This is often true in studies with small sample sizes. On the whole, absence of evidence of an effect is not the same thing as evidence of absence of an effect.

---

[3] Sargent Friday (played by Jack Webb) in the 1960s television show *Dragnet.*

(4) Finally, the discussion should address all **potential biases** in the study and hypothesize on their effects on the study conclusions. The directions for future research in this area should then be addressed.

Conclusion

The study results should be accurately reflected in the **conclusion** section, a one-paragraph summary of the final outcome. There are numerous points that should be addressed in this section. Notably, important sources of bias should be mentioned as disclaimers. The reader should be aware that pitfalls in the interpretations of study conclusions include the use of biased language and incorrect interpretation of results not supported by the data. Studies sponsored by drug companies or written by authors with other conflicts of interest may be more prone to these biases and should be regarded with caution. All sources of conflict of interest should be listed either at the start or at the end of the article.

Bibliography

The **references/bibliography** section demonstrates how much work from other writers the author has acknowledged. This includes a comprehensive reference list including all important studies of the same or similar problem. You will be better at interpreting the completeness of the bibliography when you have immersed yourself in a specialty area for some time and are able to evaluate this author's use of the literature. Be wary if there are multiple citations of works by just one or two authors, especially if by the author(s) of the current study.

How can you get started?

You have to decide which journals to read. The *New England Journal of Medicine* is a great place for medical students to start. It publishes important and high quality studies and includes a lot of correlation with basic sciences. There are also excellent case discussions, review articles, and basic-science articles. In general, begin by reading the abstract. This will tell you if you really want to read this study in the first place. If you don't care about this topic, go on to the next article. Remember, that what you read in the abstract should not be used to apply the results of the study to a clinical scenario. You still need to read and evaluate the article, especially the methods section. *JAMA* (*Journal of the American Medical Association*) is another excellent journal with many studies regarding medical education and the operation of the health-care system. For readers in the United Kingdom, the *Lancet* and the *BMJ* (*British Medical Journal*) are equivalent journals for the student to begin reading.

The rest of this book will present a set of useful skills that will assist you in evaluating clinical research studies. Initially, we will focus on learning how to critically evaluate the most common clinical studies. Specifically, these are studies of therapy, risk, harm, and etiology. These skills will help you to grade the quality of the studies using a schema outlined in Appendix 1. Appendix 2 is a useful outline of steps to help you to do this. Later the book will focus on studies of diagnostic tests, clinical decision making, cost analyses, prognosis, and meta-analyses or systematic reviews.

5

Searching the medical literature

Sandi Pirozzo, B.Sc., M.P.H.
Updated by Elizabeth Irish, M.L.S.

Through seeking we may learn and know things better. But as for certain truth, no man has known it, for all is but a woven web of guesses.

Xenophanes (sixth century BC)

Learning objectives

In this chapter you will learn how to:

- use a clinical question to initiate a medical literature search
- formulate an effective search strategy to answer specific clinical questions
- select the most appropriate database to use to answer a specific clinical question
- use Boolean operators in developing a search strategy
- identify the types and uses of various evidence-based review databases

To become a lifelong learner, the physician must be a competent searcher of the medical literature. This requires one to develop an effective search strategy for a clinical question. By the end of this chapter you will understand how to write a clinical question and formulate a search of the literature. Once an answerable clinical question is written and the best study design that could answer the question is decided upon, the next task is to search the literature to find the best available evidence. This might appear an easy task, but, unless one is sure of which database to use and has good searching skills, it can be time-consuming, frustrating, and wholly unproductive. This chapter will go through some common databases and provide the information to make the search for evidence both efficient and rewarding.

Introduction

Finding all relevant studies that have addressed a single question is not an easy task. The exponential growth of medical literature necessitates a systematic searching approach in order to identify the best evidence available to answer a clinical question. While many people have a favorite database or website, it is important to consult more than one resource to ensure that all relevant information is retrieved.

Use of different databases

Of all the databases that index medical and health-related literature, **MEDLINE** is probably the best known. Developed by the National Library of Medicine at the National Institutes of Health in the United States, it is the world's largest general biomedical database and indexes approximately one-third of all biomedical articles. Since it was the first medical literature database available for electronic searching, most clinicians are familiar with its use. Due to its size and breadth, it is sometimes a challenge to get exactly what one wants from it. This will be the first database discussed, after a discussion of some basic principles of searching.

In addition to MEDLINE, there are other, more specialized databases that may yield more clinically useful information, depending on the nature of the clinical query. The database selected depends on the content area and the type of question being asked. The database for nursing and allied health studies is called **CINAHL**, and the one for psychological studies is called **PsycINFO**. If searching for the answer to a question of therapy or intervention, then the **Cochrane Library** might be a particularly useful resource. It provides systematic reviews of trials of health-care interventions and a registry of controlled clinical trials. The **TRIP database** will do a systematic search of over 100 critically appraised evidence-based websites and databases, including MEDLINE via PubMed and the Cochrane Library, to provide a synopsis of results in one place. It is free and can be found at www.tripdatabase.com.

For information at the point of care, **DynaMed Essential Evidence Plus** and **Ganfyd** at www.ganfyd.org are designed to provide quick synopses of topics that are meant to be accessed at the bedside using a hand-held device, such as a PDA or Smart Phone. Many would consider these to be essentially on-line textbooks and only provide background information. They may have explicit levels of evidence and the most current evidence, but are works in progress. To broaden your search to the life sciences as well as conference information and cited articles, the search engines **Scopus** or **Web of Science** should be consulted. It is easy to surmise that not only is the medical literature growing exponentially, but that the available databases and websites to retrieve this literature are also increasing. In addition to the resources covered in this chapter, an additional list of relevant databases and other online resources is provided in the Bibliography.

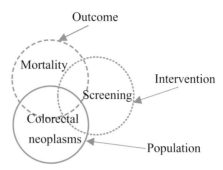

Fig. 5.1 Venn diagram for colorectal screening search. Comparison is frequently omitted in search strategies.

Developing effective information retrieval strategies

Having selected the most appropriate database one must develop an effective search strategy to retrieve the best available evidence on the topic of interest. This section will give a general searching framework that can be applied to any database. Databases often vary in terms of software used, internal structure, indexing terms, and amount of information that they give. However, the principles behind developing a search strategy remain the same.

The first step is to identify the key words or concepts in the study question. This leads to a systematic approach of breaking down the question into its individual components. The most useful way of dividing a question into its components is to use the PICO format that was introduced in Chapter 2. To review: P stands for the population of interest; I is the intervention, whether a therapy, diagnostic test, or risk factor; C is the comparison to the intervention; and O is the outcome of interest.

A PICO question can be represented pictorially using a Venn diagram. As an example, we will use the following question: *What is the mortality reduction in colorectal cancer as a result of performing hemoccult testing of the stool (fecal occult blood test, FOBT) screening in well-appearing adults?* Using the PICO format, we recognize that mortality is the **outcome**, screening with the hemoccult is the **intervention**, not screening is the **comparison**, and adults who appear well but do and don't have colorectal neoplasms is the **population**. The Venn diagram for that question is shown in Fig. 5.1.

Once the study question has been broken into its components, they can be combined using Boolean logic. This consists of using the terms **AND, OR,** and **NOT** as part of the search. The AND operator is used when you wish to retrieve those records containing both terms. Using the AND operator serves to narrow your search and reduces the number of citations recovered. The OR operator is used when at least one of the terms must appear in the record. It broadens the search, should be used to connect synonyms or related concepts, and will increase the number of citations recovered. Finally, the NOT operator is used to

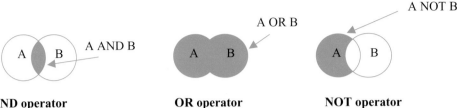

AND operator   **OR operator**   **NOT operator**

Fig. 5.2 Boolean operators (AND, OR, and NOT). Blue areas represent the search results in each case.

retrieve records containing one term and not the other. This also reduces the number of citations recovered and is useful to eliminate documents relating to potentially irrelevant topics. Be careful using this operator as it can eliminate useful references too. It can be used to narrow initially wide-ranging searches or to remove duplicate records from a previously viewed set. The use of these operators is illustrated in Fig. 5.2.

Using the example of the question about the effect of hemoccult screening on colon cancer mortality, the combination of the initial search terms *colorectal neoplasms AND screening* represents the overlap between these two terms and retrieves only articles that use both terms. This will give us a larger number of articles from our search than if we used all three terms in one search: *screening AND colorectal neoplasms AND mortality*. That combination represents a smaller area, the one where all three terms overlap, and will retrieve only articles with all three terms.

Although the overlap of all three parts may have the highest concentration of relevant articles, the other areas may still contain many relevant and important articles. We call this a high-specificity search. The set we retrieve will contain a high proportion of articles that are useful, but many others may be missed. This means that the search lacks sensitivity in that it will not identify some studies that are relevant to the question being asked. Hence, if the *disease AND study factor* combination (*colorectal neoplasms AND screening*) yields a manageable number of citations, it is best to work with this and not further restrict the search by using the outcomes (*screening AND colorectal neoplasms AND mortality*).

Everyone searches differently! Most people will start big (most hits possible) and then begin limiting the results. Look at these results along the way to make sure you are on the right track. My preference is to start with the smallest number of search terms that gives a reasonable number of citations and then add others (in a Boolean fashion) as a means of either increasing (OR operator) or limiting (AND or NOT operators) the search. Usually, for most searches, anything less than about 50 to 100 citations to look through by hand is reasonable. Remember that these terms are entered into the database by hand and errors of classification will occur. The more that searches are limited, the more likely they are to miss important citations. In general, both the outcome and study design terms are options usually needed only when the search results are very large and unmanageable.

You can use nested Boolean search to form more complex combinations that will capture all the overlap areas between all three circles. For our search, these are: *(mortality AND screening) OR (mortality AND colorectal neoplasms) OR (screening AND colorectal neoplasms).* This strategy will yield a higher number of hits, but will still find less than all three terms with OR function connecting them. However, it may not be appropriate if you are looking for a quick answer to a clinical question since you will then have to hand-search more citations. Whatever strategy you choose to start with, try it. You never know a priori what results you are going to get.

Use of synonyms and wildcard symbol

When the general structure of the question is developed and only a small number of citations are recovered, it may be worthwhile to look for synonyms for each component of the search. For our question about mortality reduction in colorectal cancer due to fecal occult blood screening in adults, we can use several synonyms. Screening can be *screen* or *early detection,* colorectal cancer can be *bowel cancer,* and mortality can be *death* or *survival.* Since these terms are entered into the database by coders they may vary greatly from study to study for the same ultimate question. What you miss with one synonym, you may pick up with another.

Truncation or the "wildcard" symbol can be used to find all the words with the same stem in order to increase the scope of successful searching. Thus our search string can become *(screen* OR early detection) AND (colorectal cancer OR bowel cancer) AND (mortality OR death* OR survival).* The term *screen** is shorthand for words beginning with "screen." It will turn up screen, screened, screening, etc. The wildcard is extremely useful but should be used with caution. If you were searching for information about hearing problems and you used *hear** as one of your search terms you would retrieve not only articles with the word "hear" and "hearing" but also all those articles with the word "heart." Note that the wildcard symbol varies between systems but, most commonly it will be an asterisk (*) or dollar sign (\$). It is important to check the database's help documentation to determine not only the correct symbol, but to also ensure that the database supports truncation. For instance, if a database automatically truncates then the use of a wildcard symbol could inadvertently result in a smaller retrieval rather than a broader one.

MEDLINE via PubMed

MEDLINE is available online for free using the PubMed website at www.pubmed. gov. It is often assumed that MEDLINE and PubMed are one and the same.

But, PubMed is actually a very user-friendly interface for searching MEDLINE as well as several other data bases. These are: OLDMEDLINE, in-process citations that are not yet included in MEDLINE, selected life science journals beyond the scope of MEDLINE, and citations to author manuscripts for NIH-funded researchers' publications. PubMed also provides time-saving search services such as Clinical Queries and the MeSH database, which help the user to search more efficiently. The best way to get to know PubMed is to use it, explore its capabilities, and experiment with some searches. Rather than provide a comprehensive tutorial on searching PubMed, this chapter will focus on a few of the features that are most helpful in the context of EBM. Remember that all databases are continually being updated and upgraded, so that it is important to consult the help documentation or your health sciences librarian for searching guidance.

PUBMED Clinical Queries: searching using methodological filters

Within PubMed there is a special feature called **Clinical Queries**, which can be found in the left-hand side bar of the PubMed home page. It uses a set of built-in search filters that are based on methodological search techniques developed by Haynes in 1994 and which search for the best evidence on clinical questions in four study categories: diagnosis, therapy, etiology, and prognosis. In turn each of these categories may be searched with an emphasis on **specificity** for which most of the articles retrieved will be relevant, but many articles may be missed or **sensitivity** for which, the proportion of relevant articles will decrease, but many more articles will be retrieved and fewer missed. It is also possible to limit the search to a systematic review of the search topic by clicking on the "systematic review" option. Figure 5.3 shows the PubMed clinical queries page. In order to continue searching in clinical queries, click on the "clinical queries" link in the left-hand side bar each time a search is conducted. If this is not done, searches will be conducted in general PubMed. Clicking on the "filter table" option within clinical queries shows how each filter is interpreted in PubMed query language.

It is best to start with the specificity emphasis when initiating a new search and then add terms to the search if not enough articles are found. Once search terms are entered into the query box on PubMed and "go" is clicked, the search engine will display your search results. This search is then displayed with the search terms that were entered combined with the methodological filter terms that were applied by the search engine. Below the query box is the features bar, which provides access to additional search options. The PubMed query box and features bar are available from every screen except the Clinical Queries home page. Return to the Clinical Queries homepage each time a new Clinical Queries search is desired.

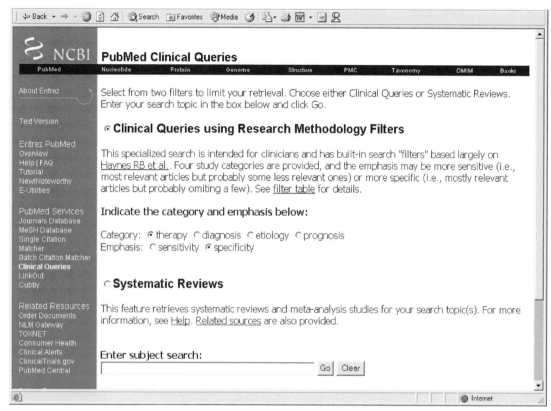

Fig. 5.3 PubMed "clinical queries." (National Library of Medicine. Used with permission.)

Entering search terms can be done in a few ways. Terms are searched in various fields of the record when one or more terms are entered (e.g., *vitamin c AND common cold*) in the query box. The Boolean operators AND, OR, NOT must be in upper-case (e.g., *vitamin c OR zinc*). The truncation or wildcard symbol (*) tells PubMed to search for the first 600 variations of the truncated term. If a truncated term (e.g., *staph**) produces more than 600 variations, PubMed displays a warning message such as "*Wildcard search for 'staph*' used only the first 600 variations. Lengthen the root word to search for all endings*". Use caution when applying truncation in PubMed, because it turns off the automatic term mapping and the automatic explosion of a MeSH term features, resulting in an incomplete search retrieval. As a rule of thumb, it is better to use the wildcard symbol as a last resort in PubMed.

Limits

The features bar consists of **limits**, **preview/index**, **history**, **clipboard**, and **details**. To limit a search, click "limits" from the features bar, which opens the

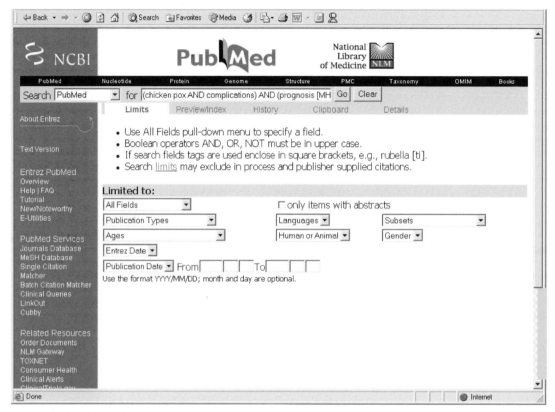

Fig. 5.4 The "limits" window in PubMed. (National Library of Medicine. Used with permission.)

Limits window shown in Fig. 5.4. This offers a number of useful ways of reducing the number of retrieved articles. A search can be restricted to words in a particular field within a citation, a specific age group or gender, human or animal studies, articles published with abstracts or in a specific language, or a specific publication type (e.g., meta-analysis or RCT). Limiting by publication type is especially useful when searching for evidence-based studies.

Another method of limiting searches is by either the Entrez or publication date of a study. The "Entrez date" is the date that the citation was entered into the Medline system and the publication date is the month and year it was published. Finally, the subset pull-down menu allows retrieval to be limited to a specific subset of citations within PubMed, such as AIDS-related or other citations. Applying limits to a search results in a check-box next to the "limits" space and a listing of the limit selections will be displayed. To turn off the existing limits remove the check before running the next search.

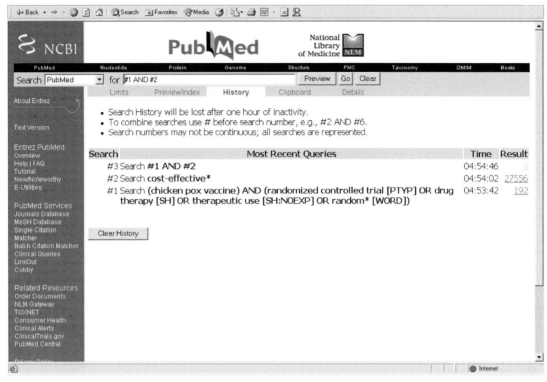

Fig. 5.5 The history of a search in PubMed. (National Library of Medicine. Used with permission.)

History

PubMed will retain an entire search strategy with the results, which can be viewed by clicking on "history" function on the features bar. This is only available after running a search and it will list and number the searches in the order in which they were run. As shown in Fig. 5.5, the history displays the search number, search query, the time of search, and the number of citations in the results. Searches can be combined or additional terms added to an existing search by using the number (#) sign before the search number: e.g., *#1 AND #2, or #1 AND (drug therapy OR diet therapy)*. Once a revised search strategy has been entered in the query box, clicking "go" will view the search results. Clicking "clear history" will remove all searches from the history and preview/index screens. The maximum number of queries held in the history is 100 and once that number is reached, PubMed will remove the oldest search from the history to add the most recent search. The search history will be lost after 1 hour of inactivity on PubMed. PubMed will move a search statement number to the top of the history if that new search is the same as a previous search. The preview/index allows search terms to be entered one at a time using pre-selected search fields, making it useful for finding specific references.

Clipboard

The clipboard is a place to collect selected citations from one or several searches to print or save for future use. Up to 500 items can be placed in the clipboard at any time. After adding items to the clipboard, click on "clipboard" from the features bar to view the saved selections. Citations in the clipboard are displayed in the order they were added. To place an item in the clipboard, click on the check-box to the left of the citation, go to the send menu and select "clipboard," and then click "send." Once a citation has been added to the clipboard, the record-number color will change to green. By sending to the clipboard without selecting citations, PubMed will add up to 500 citations of the search results to the clipboard. Clipboard items are automatically removed after eight hours of inactivity.

Printing and saving

When ready to save or print clipboard items it is best to change them to ordinary text to simplify the printout and save paper so it will not print all the PubMed motifs and icons. To do this, click on "clipboard" on the features bar, which will show only the articles placed on the clipboard. From the send menu select "text" and a new page will be displayed which resembles an ordinary text document for printing. This "send to text" option can also be used for single references and will omit all the graphics. To save the entire set of search results click the display pull-down menu to select the desired format and then select "send to file" from the send menu. To save specific citations click on the check-box to the left of each citation, including other pages in the retrieval process, and when finished making all of the desired selections, select "send to file."

To save the entire search to review or update at a later time, it is best to create a free, "My NCBI account." "My NCBI" is a place where current searches can be saved, reviewed, and updated. It can also be used to send e-mail alerts, apply filters, and other customization features. Unlike the Clipboard, searches on "My NCBI" are permanently saved and will not be removed unless chosen to be deleted.

General searching in PubMed

The general search page in PubMed is useful to find evidence that is not coming up on the Clinical Queries search, or when looking for multiple papers by a single author who has written extensively in a single area of interest. Begin by clicking on the PubMed symbol in the top left-hand corner of the screen to display the general search screen (Fig. 5.6). Simply type the search terms in the query box and your search results will be displayed as before. If there are too many articles found, apply limits and if too few, add other search terms using the OR function.

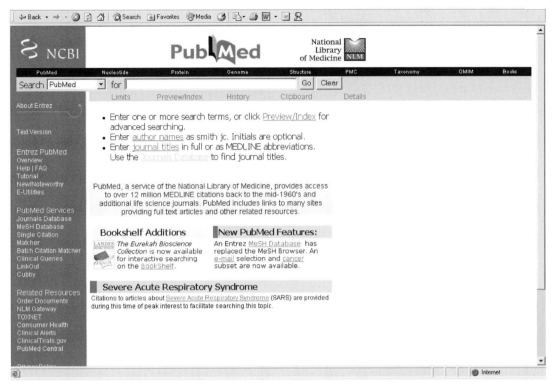

Fig. 5.6 General search screen in PubMed. (National Library of Medicine. Used with permission.)

MeSH terms to assist in searching

In looking for synonyms to broaden or improve a search consider using both text words and keywords (index terms) in the database. One of MEDLINE's great strengths is its MeSH (Medical Subject Headings) system. By default, PubMed automatically "maps" the search terms to the appropriate MeSH terms. A specific MeSH search can also be performed by clicking on the "MeSH database" link in the left-hand side bar. Typing in "colorectal cancer" will lead to the MeSH term *colorectal neoplasms* (Fig. 5.7). The search can then be refined by clicking on the term to bring up the detailed display (Fig. 5.8). This allows the selection of subheadings (*diagnosis*, *etiology*, *therapy*, etc.) to narrow the search, and also get access to the MeSH tree structure.

The "explode" (exp) feature will capture an entire subtree of MeSH terms with a single word. For the search term *colorectal neoplasms,* the "explode" incorporates the entire MeSH tree below *colorectal neoplasms* (Table 5.1). Click on any specific terms in the tree to search that term and the program will get all the descriptors for that MeSH term and all those under it. Select the appropriate MeSH term, with or without subheadings, and with or without explosion, and use the send menu to "send to search box." These search terms will appear in

Table 5.1. A MeSH tree containing the term colorectal neoplasms

Neoplasms
    Neoplasms by Site
        Digestive System Neoplasms
            Gastrointestinal Neoplasms
                Intestinal Neoplasms
                    Colorectal Neoplasms
                        Colonic Neoplasms
                            Colonic Polyps +
                            Sigmoid Neoplasms
                      Colorectal Neoplasms, Hereditary
                    Nonpolyposis
                    Rectal Neoplasms
                      Anus Neoplasms +

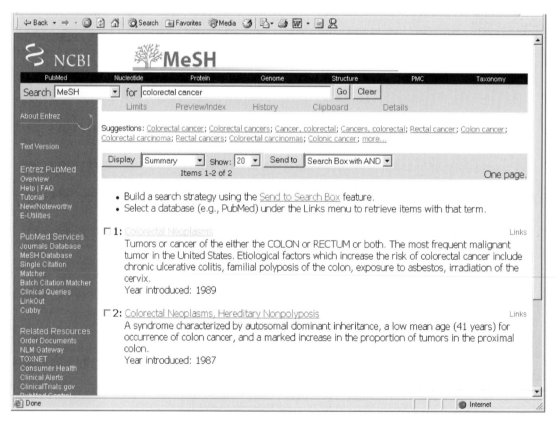

Fig. 5.7 PubMed MeSH database. (National Library of Medicine. Used with permission.)

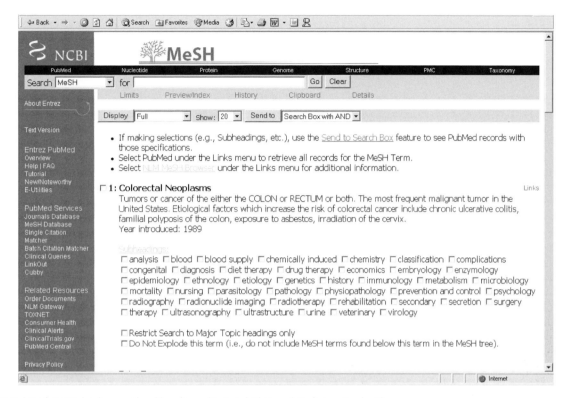

Fig. 5.8 PubMed MeSH database with subheadings. (National Library of Medicine. Used with permission.)

the query box at the top of the screen. Clicking "search PubMed" will execute the search, which will automatically explode the term unless restricted by selecting the "do not explode this term" box. Every article has been indexed by at least one of the MeSH keywords from the tree. To see the difference that exploding a MeSH term makes, repeat the search using the term *colorectal neoplasms* in the search window without exploding. This will probably result in retrieval of about one-quarter of the articles retrieved in the previous search.

Novice users of PubMed often ask "how do I find out the MeSH keywords that have been used to categorize a paper?" Knowing the relevant MeSH keywords will help to focus and/or refine the search. A simple way to do this is that once a relevant citation has been found, click on the author link to view the abstract and then go to the "display" box and open it as shown in Fig. 5.9. Select MEDLINE and click "display." The record is now displayed as it is indexed and by scrolling down the MeSH terms for this paper will be listed. The initials MH precede each of the MeSH terms. Linking to "related articles" will find other relevant citations, but the selected limits are not applied to this retrieval. If there was a search limited

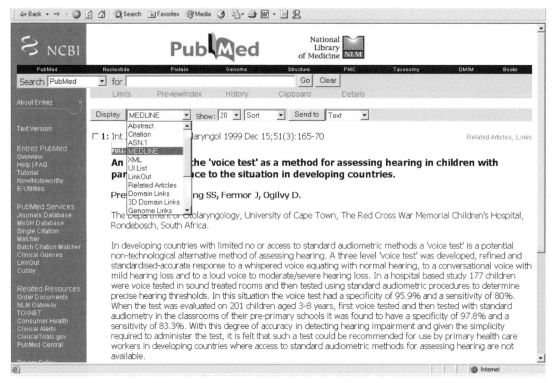

Fig. 5.9 The "display" menu in PubMed. (National Library of Medicine. Used with permission.)

to English language only then selecting the related articles link will get articles that appear in other languages.

While the MeSH system is useful, it should supplement rather than usurp the use of textwords so that incompletely coded articles are not missed. PubMed is a compilation of a number of databases not just MEDLINE and includes newer articles that have not been indexed for MEDLINE yet.

Methodological terms and filters

MeSH terms cover not only subject content but also a number of useful terms on study methodology. For example, looking for the answer to a question of therapy, many randomized trials are tagged in MEDLINE by the specific methodological term *randomized controlled trial* or *clinical trial*. These can be selected by limiting the search to one study design type in PubMed under the limit feature for publication types in the pull-down menu.

An appropriate methodological filter may help confine the retrieved studies to primary research. For example, if searching whether a screening intervention reduces mortality from colorectal cancer, confine the retrieved studies to controlled trials. The idea of methodological terms as filters may be extended to multiple terms that attempt to identify particular study types. Such terms are used extensively in the Clinical Queries search functions.

Note that many studies do not have the appropriate methodological tag. The Cochrane Collaboration and the US National Library of Medicine (NLM) are working on correctly retagging all the controlled trials, but this is not being done for other study types.

Field searching

It is possible to shorten the search time by searching in a specific field. This works well if there is a recent article by a particular author renowned for work in the area of interest or if a relevant study in a particular journal in the library has recently been published on the same topic. Searching in specific fields will prove to be invaluable in these circumstances. To search for an article with "colorectal cancer" in the title using PubMed, select the title field in the limits option using the fields pull-down menu in the "Tag Term" default tag for the selected search term. Another option is to simply type "colorectal cancer[ti]" in the query box. As with truncation this turns off the automatic mapping and exploding features and will not get articles with the words "colorectal neoplasms" in the article title.

The field-label abbreviations can be found by accessing the help menu. The most commonly used field labels are abstract (ab), title (ti), source (so), journal (jn), and author (au). The difference between source and journal is that "source" is the abbreviated version of the journal title, while "journal" is the full journal title. In PubMed the journal or the author can be selected simply by using the journals database located on the left-hand side bar or by typing in the author's last name and initials in the query box. Remember, when searching using "text words," the program searches for those words in any of the available fields. For example, if "death" is one search term then articles where "death" is an author's name as well as those in which it occurs in the title or abstract will be retrieved. Normally this isn't a problem but once again could be a problem when using "wildcard" searches.

The Cochrane Library

The Cochrane Library owes it genesis to an astute British epidemiologist and doctor, Archie Cochrane, who is best known for his influential book *Effectiveness and Efficiency: Random Reflections on Health Services,* published in 1971. In the book, he suggested that because resources would always be limited they should be used to provide equitably those forms of health care which had been shown in properly designed evaluations to be effective. In particular, he stressed the importance of using evidence from randomized controlled trials (RCTs) because these were likely to provide much more reliable information than other sources of evidence. Cochrane's simple propositions were soon widely recognized as seminally important – by lay people as well as by health professionals. In his 1971 book he wrote: "It is surely a great criticism of our profession that we have not organized a critical summary, by specialty or subspecialty, adapted periodically, of all relevant randomised controlled trials."[1]

His challenge led to the establishment of an international collaboration to develop the Oxford Database of Perinatal Trials. In 1987, the year before Cochrane died, he referred to a systematic review of randomized controlled trials (RCTs) of care during pregnancy and childbirth as "a real milestone in the history of randomized trials and in the evaluation of care" and suggested that other specialties should copy the methods used.

The Cochrane Collaboration was developed in response to Archie Cochrane's call for systematic and up-to-date reviews of all health care-related RCTs. His suggestion that the methods used to prepare and maintain reviews of controlled trials in pregnancy and childbirth should be applied more widely was taken up by the Research and Development Programme, initiated to support the United Kingdom's National Health Service. Funds were provided to establish a "Cochrane Centre," to collaborate with others, in the United Kingdom and elsewhere, to facilitate systematic reviews of randomized controlled trials across all areas of health care. When the Cochrane Centre was opened in Oxford in October 1992, those involved expressed the hope that there would be a collaborative international response to Cochrane's agenda. This idea was outlined at a meeting organized six months later by the New York Academy of Sciences. In October 1993 – at what was to become the first in a series of annual Cochrane Colloquia – 77 people from 11 countries co-founded the **Cochrane Collaboration**. It is an international organization that aims to help people make well-informed decisions about health care by preparing, maintaining, and ensuring the accessibility of systematic reviews of the effects of health-care interventions.

The Cochrane Library comprises several databases. Each database focuses on a specific type of information and can be searched individually or as a whole. Current databases are:

The Cochrane Database of Systematic Reviews (CDSR) contains systematic reviews of the effects of health care prepared by the Cochrane Collaboration. In addition to complete reviews, the database contains protocols for reviews currently being prepared.

The Database of Abstracts of Reviews of Effects (DARE) includes structured abstracts of systematic reviews which have been critically appraised

---

[1] A. L. Cochrane. *Effectiveness & Efficiency: Random Reflections on Health Services.* London: Royal Society of Medicine, 1971.

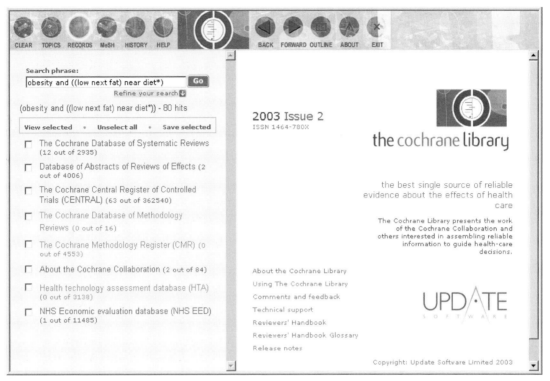

Fig. 5.10 The opening page of the Cochrane Collaboration.

by reviewers at the NHS Centre for Reviews and Dissemination in York and by other people. DARE is meant to complement the CDSR.

The Cochrane Central Register of Controlled Trials (CENTRAL) is a bibliographic database of controlled trials identified by contributors to the Cochrane Collaboration and others.

Cochrane Methodology Register focuses on articles, books, and conference proceedings that report on methods used in controlled trials. Bibliographic in nature, the register's contents is culled from both MEDLINE and hand searches.

Health Technology Assessment Database is a centralized location to find completed and ongoing health technology assessments that study the implications of health-care interventions around the world. Medical, social, ethical, and economic factors are considered for inclusion.

NHS Economic Evaluation Database identifies and summarizes economic evaluations throughout the world that impact health care decision making.

As with MEDLINE, there are various interfaces for searching the Cochrane Library. The interface that is linked directly from the Cochrane Collaborations homepage (http://www.cochrane.org) is the Wiley InterScience interface (Fig. 5.10). While it is subscription based, it is possible to view the abstracts without a subscription. Some countries or regions have subsidized full-text access to the Cochrane Library for their health-care professionals. Consult the homepage to see if you live in one of these areas.

The Cochrane Library supports various search techniques. The searcher can opt to search all text or just the record title, author, abstract, keywords, tables, or publication type. The default for a quick search is a combination of title, abstract, or keyword. The advanced search feature allows you to search multiple fields using Boolean operators. You can also restrict by product, record status, or date. You can also opt to search using MeSH terms since MeSH descriptors and qualifiers are supported by the search engine as the explode feature. The Cochrane Library also supports wildcard searching using the asterisk*. Once a search is complete, you can opt to save your searches. The "My Profile" feature is similar to "My NCBI" as it allows you to store titles, articles, and searches and to set up journal and search e-mail update alerts. There is no cost to register, although some services are fee-based, such as purchasing individual documents online through Pay-Per-View. Always check with your health sciences library first prior to purchasing any information to ensure that it's not available by another method.

TRIP database

Sometimes when conducting a search, it is helpful to start in a database with an interface that can search numerous resources at once from one search query while at the same time providing the results in one convenient location. The TRIP database (http://www.tripdatabase.com) was created in 1997 with the intended purpose of providing an evidence-based method of answering clinical questions in a quick and timely manner by reducing the amount of search time needed. Freely available on the Web since 2004, TRIP had developed a systematic, federated searching approach to retrieving information from such resources as various clinical practice guideline databases, Bandolier, InfoPOEMS, Cochrane, Clinical Evidence, and core medical journals. Additionally, each search is performed within PubMed's Clinical Queries service. All potential information sources are reviewed by an in-house team of information experts and clinicians and external experts to assess quality and clinical usefulness prior to being included.

The TRIP database has a very straightforward searching interface that supports both basic and advanced techniques. For basic searching the search terms are entered into a search box. TRIP supports Boolean searching as well as the asterisk* for truncation. Phrase searching is supported by using quotation marks, such as, "myocardial infarction." There is also a mis-spelling function that will automatically activate if no results are found. The advance search allows for title or title and text searching. These results are assigned search numbers (#1) and can be combined using Boolean operators (#1 AND #2). Results can be sorted by relevance or year prior to conducting the search. Once the search has been run, the results can further be sorted by selecting more specialized filters such as systematic reviews, evidenced-based synopses, core primary research, and subject specialty. The PubMed Clinical Query results are also provided separately by therapy, diagnosis, etiology, prognosis, and systematic reviews. With a "My Trip" account, a keyword auto-search function can be set up that will provide one with regular clinical updates. These will automatically be e-mailed with any new records that have the selected keyword in the title.

The advantage of the TRIP database is that more than one evidence-based resource can be searched at a time. The main disadvantage is that although Trip uses carefully selected filters to ensure quality retrievals, you lose some of the searching control that you would have searching the original database. However, in many cases the time saved outweighs this consideration.

Specific point of care databases

For information at the point of care, DynaMed, Clinical Evidence, and Essential Evidence Plus are fee-based databases designed to be provide quick, evidence-based answers to clinical questions that commonly arise at the bedside. The information is delivered in a compact format that highlights the pertinent information while at the same time providing enough background information for further research if required.

Developed by a family physician, DynaMed (http://www.ebscohost.com/dynamed/) has grown to provide clinically organized summaries for nearly 2000 medical topics covering basic information such as etiology, diagnosis and history, complications, prognosis, treatment, prevention and screening, references and guidelines, and patient information. DynaMed uses a seven-step evidence-based methodology to create topic summaries that are organized both alphabetically and by category. The selection process includes daily monitoring of the content of over 500 medical journals and systematic review databases. This includes a systematic search using such resources as PubMed's Clinical Queries feature, the Cochrane Library databases, and the National Guidelines Clearinghouse. Once this step is complete, relevance and validity are determined and the information is critically appraised. DynaMed uses the Users' Guides to Evidence-Based Practice from the Evidence-Based Medicine Working Group, Centre for Health Evidence as a basis for determining the level of evidence. DynaMed ranks information into three levels: Level 1 (likely reliable), Level 2 (mid-level), and Level 3 (lacking direction). All authors and reviewers of DynaMed topics are required to have some clinical practice experience.

Formally known as InfoPOEMS with InfoRetriever, Essential Evidence Plus (http://essentialevidenceplus.com/) provides filtered, synopsized, evidence-based information, including EBM guidelines, topic reviews, POEMs, Derm Expert, decision support tools and calculators, and ICD-9 codes, that has also been developed by physicians. Individual topics can be searched or can be browsed by subject, database, and tools. At the bedside POEMS can be invaluable as they summarize articles by beginning with the "clinical question," followed by the "bottom line" and rounded out with the complete reference, the study design, the setting, and the article synopsis. The bottom line provides the conclusion arrived at to answer the clinical question and provides a level of evidence ranking based on the five levels of evidence ranking from the Centre for Evidence-Based Medicine in Oxford. Sources used to find information for Essential Evidence Plus include EBM Guidelines and Abstracts of Cochrane Systematic Reviews.

Clinical Evidence, published by the *British Medical Journal* is available on their website at www.clinicalevidence.org. Clinical Evidence is a decision-support tool sponsored by the *British Medical Journal*, the *BMJ*. An international group of peer reviewers publish summaries of systematic reviews of important clinical questions. These are regularly updated and integrated with various EBM resources to summarize the current state of knowledge and uncertainty about various clinical conditions. It is primarily focused on conditions in internal medicine and surgery and does cover many newer technologies. The evidence provided is rated as definitely beneficial, probably beneficial, uncertain, probably not beneficial, or definitely not beneficial.

Created in 1999, it has been redesigned and revised by an international advisory board, clinicians, patient support groups, and contributors. They aim for sources that have high relevance and validity and require low time and effort by the user. Their reviews are transparent and explicit. Their reviews try to show when uncertainty stems from gaps in the best available evidence. Clinical Evidence is currently available in print, using a PDA interface and online. It is free in the UK National Health Services in Scotland and Wales, to most clinicians in the United States through the United Health Foundation and in several other countries. The complete list is available on their website. It has been translated into Italian, Spanish, Russian, German, Hungarian, and Portuguese. It is available for free to people in developing countries through an initiative sponsored by the *BMJ* and the World Health Organization.

Efficient searching at the point of care databases

The searching techniques described in this chapter are designed to find primary studies of medical research. These comprehensive searching processes will

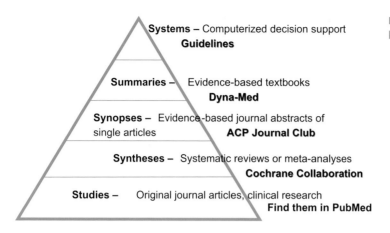

Systems – Computerized decision support
          Guidelines

Summaries – Evidence-based textbooks
                    Dyna-Med

Synopses – Evidence-based journal abstracts of
single articles   **ACP Journal Club**

Syntheses – Systematic reviews or meta-analyses
                    Cochrane Collaboration

Studies –   Original journal articles, clinical research
                    Find them in PubMed

Fig. 5.11 The Haynes 5S knowledge acquisition pyramid

best serve the doer in answering clinical questions for the purpose of critically reviewing the most current available evidence for that question. The practice-based learner must find primary sources at the point of care and will not perform comprehensive PubMed searches on a regular basis. They will be looking for pre-appraised sources and well done meta-analyses such as those done by the Cochrane Collaboration. Most clinicians will want to do the most efficient searching at the point of care possible to aid the patient sitting in front of them. An increasing number of sites on the Internet are available for doing this point of care searching.

David Slawson and Allen Shaughnessy proposed an equation to determine the usefulness of evidence (or information) to practicing clinicians. They described the usefulness as equal to the relevance times validity divided by effort (to obtain). Always turning to primary sources of evidence whenever a clinical question comes up is very inefficient at best and impossible for most busy practitioners. The busy clinician in need of rapid access to the most current literature requires quick access to high quality pre-appraised and summarized sources of evidence that can be accessed during a patient visit.

For the "users," the 5S schema of Haynes is a construct to help focus the skills of Information Mastery. This is a process of helping to find the best evidence at the point of care. The sources that are higher up on the appraisal pyramid (Fig. 5.11) are the ones easiest to use and needing the least amount of critical appraisal by the user.

The highest level is that of systems, which are decision support tools integrated into the daily practice of medicine through mechanisms such as computerized order entry systems or electronic medical records. The system links directly to the high quality information needed at the point of care and seamlessly integrated into the care process. There are very few systems that have been developed and most of the current ones are standalone applications set up by an institution within its electronic medical record or IT system.

The next level is synthesis, which are critically appraised topics and guidelines. Many of these are through publishing enterprises such as Clinical Evidence published by the *British Medical Journal*. This print-based resource summarizes the best available evidence of prevention and treatment interventions for commonly eoncountered clinical problems in internal medicine. Evidence is presented as being beneficial, equivocal, or not beneficial.

The third level is synopses of critically appraised individual studies. These might be found in CAT banks such as Best Bets and Evidence Based On Call. Finding your answer here is a matter of trial and error.

The fourth level is summaries, which is synonymous with systematic reviews. The primary ones in the category are from the Cochrane Database of Systematic Reviews, described earlier in the book as a database of systematic reviews authored and updated by the worldwide Cochrane Collaboration. The Database of Abstracts of Reviews of Effects (DARE) is a database of non-Cochrane systematic reviews catalogued by the Centre for Reviews and Dissemination at the University of York in the United Kingdom and presented with critical reviews.

The fifth level is individual studies, which are original research studies found through Ovid MEDLINE or PubMed. The Cochrane Central Register of Controlled Trials repository of randomized controlled trials is a more comprehensive source for RCTs than MEDLINE, including meeting abstracts and unique EMBASE records. Finally, the lowest level is "Expert Opinion" or Replication level, which is not considered bona fide evidence, but only anecdote or unsubstantiated evidence. Included in this level are textbooks that are not explicitly evidence based.

Final thoughts

Conducting a thorough search can be a daunting task. The process of identifying papers is an iterative one. It is best initially to devise a strategy on paper. No matter how thorough a search strategy is, inevitably some resources will be missed and the process will need to be repeated and refined. Use the results of an initial search to retrieve relevant papers which can then be used to further refine the searches by searching the bibliographies of the relevant papers for articles missed by the initial search and by performing a citation search using either Scopus or Web of Science databases. These identify papers that have cited the identified relevant studies, some of which may be subsequent primary research. These "missed" papers are invaluable and provide clues on how the search may be broadened to capture further papers by studying the MeSH terms that have been used. Google, Google Scholar, and PogoFrog (www.pogofrog.com) can also be used as a resource to not only find information but to help design a strategy to use in other databases such as PubMed and Cochrane. These records can be used to design a strategy that can be executed within a more specialized database. The whole procedure may then be repeated using the new terms identified. This iterative process is sometimes referred to as "snowballing."

Searching for EBM can be time consuming, but more and more database providers are developing search engines and features that are designed to find reliable, valid, and relevant information quickly and efficiently. Podcasts, RSS feeds, and alerts are just a few of the advances that demonstrate how technology is continually advancing to improve access and delivery of information to the office as well as the bedside. Always remember that, if the information isn't found in the first source consulted, there are a myriad of options available to the searcher. Finally, the new reliance on electronic searching methods has increased the role of the health sciences librarian who can provide guidance and assistance in the searching process and should be consulted early in the process. Databases and websites are updated frequently and it is the librarian's role to maintain a competency in expert searching techniques to help with the most difficult searching challenge.

6

Study design and strength of evidence

Louis Pasteur's theory of germs is ridiculous fiction.

Pierre Pachet, Professor of Physiology, Toulouse University, 1872

 Learning objectives

In this chapter you will learn:

- the unique characteristics, strengths, and weaknesses of common clinical research study designs
  - descriptive – cross-sectional, case reports, case series
  - timed – prospective, retrospective
  - longitudinal – observational (case–control, cohort, non-concurrent cohort), interventional (clinical trial)
- the levels of evidence and how study design affects the strength of evidence.

There are many types of research studies. Since various research study designs can accomplish different goals, not all studies will be able to show the same thing. Therefore, the first step in assessing the validity of a research study is to determine the study design. Each study design has inherent strengths and weaknesses. The ability to prove causation and expected potential biases will largely be determined by the design of the study.

Identify the study design

When critically appraising a research study, you must first understand what different research study designs are able to accomplish. The design of the study will suggest potential biases you can expect. There are two basic categories of studies that are easily recognizable. These are **descriptive** and **longitudinal** studies. We will discuss each type and its subtypes.

One classification commonly used to characterize longitudinal clinical research studies is by the direction of the study in time. Characterizations in this manner, or so-called timed studies, have traditionally been divided into **prospective** and **retrospective** study designs. Prospective studies begin at a time in the past and subjects are followed to the present time. Retrospective studies begin at the present time and look back on the behavior or other characteristics of those subjects in the past. These are terms which can easily be used incorrectly and misapplied, and because of this, they should not be referred to except as generalizations. As we will see later in this chapter, "retrospective" studies can be of several types and should be identified by the specific type of study rather than the general term.

Descriptive studies

Descriptive studies are records of events which include studies that look at a series of cases or a cross-section of a population to look for particular characteristics. These are often used after several cases are reported in which a novel treatment of several patients yields promising results, and the authors publishing the data want other physicians to know about the therapy. **Case reports** describe individual patients and **case series** describe accounts of an illness or treatment in a small group of patients. In **cross-sectional studies** the interesting aspects of a group of patients, including potential causes and effects, are all observed at the same time.

Case reports and case series

Case reports or small numbers of cases are often the first description of a new disease, clinical sign, symptom, treatment, or diagnostic test. They can also be a description of a curriculum, operation, patient-care strategy, or other health-care process. Some case reports can alert physicians to a new disease that is about to become very important. For example, AIDS was initially identified when the first cases were reported in two case series in 1981. One series consisted of two groups of previously healthy homosexual men with *Pneumocystis carinii* pneumonia, a rare type of pneumonia. The other was a series of men with Kaposi's sarcoma, a rare cancer. These diseases had previously only been reported in people who were known to be immunocompromised. This was the start of the AIDS epidemic, a fact that was not evident from these first two reports. It quickly became evident as more clinicians noticed cases of these rare diseases.

Since most case reports are descriptions of rare diseases or rare presentations of common diseases, they are unlikely to occur again very soon, if ever.

A recent case series reported on two cases of stroke in young people related to illicit methamphetamine use. To date, physicians have not been deluged with a rash of young methamphetamine users with strokes. Although it makes patho-physiological sense, the association may only be a fluke. Therefore, case reports are a useful venue to report unusual symptoms of a common illness, but have limited value. New treatments or tests described in a study without any control group also fall under this category of case reports and case series. At best, these descriptive studies can suggest future directions for research on the treatment or test being reported.

Case studies and cross-sectional studies have certain strengths. They are cheap, relatively easy to do with existing medical records, and potential clinical material is plentiful. If you see new presentations of disease or interesting cases, you can easily write a case report. However, their weaknesses outweigh their strengths. These studies do not provide explanations and cannot show association between cause and effect. Therefore, they do not provide much useful evidence! Since no comparison is made to any control group, contributory cause cannot be proven. A good general rule for case studies is to "take them seriously and then ignore them." By this it is meant that you should never change your practice based solely on a single case study or series since the probability of seeing the same rare presentation or rare disease is quite remote.

There is one situation in which a case series may be useful. Called the "all-or-none case series," this occurs when there is a *very dramatic* change in the outcome of patients reported in a case series. There are two ways this can occur. First, *all* patients died before the treatment became available and *some* in the case series with the treatment survive. Second, *some* patients died before the treatment became available, but *none* in the case series with the treatment die. This all-or-none idea is roughly what happened when penicillin was first introduced. Prior to this time, most patients with pneumonia died of their illness. When penicillin was first given to patients with pneumonia, most of them lived. The credibility of these all-or-none case reports depends on the numbers of cases reported, the relative severity of the illness, and the accuracy and detail of the case descriptions given in the report.

The case series can be abused. It can be likened to a popular commercial for Life cereal from the 1970s. In the scene, two children are unsure if they will like the new cereal Life, so they ask their little brother, Mikey, to try it. He liked it and they both decided that since "Mikey liked it!" they would like it too. Too often, a series of cases is presented showing apparent improvement in the condition of several patients that is then attributed to a particular therapy. The authors conclude that this means it should be used as a new standard of care. The fact that everyone got better is not proof that the therapy or intervention in question is causative. This is called the "Mikey liked it" phenomenon.[1]

---

[1] This construct is attributed to J. Hoffman, *Emergency Medical Abstracts*, 2000.

Cross-sectional studies

Cross-sectional studies are descriptive studies that look at a sample of a population to see how many people in that population are afflicted with a particular disease and how many have a particular risk factor. Cross-sectional studies record events and observations and describe diseases, causes, outcomes, effects, or risk factors in a single population at a single instant in time.

The strengths of cross-sectional studies are that they are relatively cheap, easy, and quick to do. The data are usually available through medical records or statistical databases. They are useful *initial exploratory studies* especially to screen or classify aspects of disease. They are only capable of demonstrating an *association* between the cause and effect. They have no ability to determine the other elements of contributory cause. In order to draw conclusions from this study, patient exposure to the risk factor being studied must continue until the outcome occurs. If the exposure began long before the outcome occurs and is intermittent, it will be more difficult to associate the two. If done properly, cross-sectional studies are capable of calculating the prevalence of disease in the population. **Prevalence** is the percentage of people in the population with the outcome of interest at any point in time. Since all the cases are looked at in one instant of time, cross-sectional studies cannot calculate **incidence**, the rate of appearance of new cases over time. Another strength of cross-sectional studies is that they are ideal study designs for studying the operating characteristics of diagnostic tests. We compare the test being studied to the "gold standard" test in a cross-section of patients for whom the test might be used.

The trade-off to the ease of this type of study is that the rules of cause and effect for contributory cause cannot be fulfilled. Since the risk factor and outcome are measured at the same time, you cannot be certain which is the cause and which the effect. A cross-sectional study found that teenagers who smoked early in life were more likely to become anxious and depressed as adults than those who began smoking at a later age. Does teenage smoking cause anxiety and depression in later years, or are those who have subclinical anxiety or depression more likely to smoke at an early age? It is impossible to tell if the cause preceded the effect, the effect was responsible for the cause, or both are related to an unknown third factor called a **confounding** or **surrogate variable**. Confounding or surrogate variables are more likely to apply if the time from the cause to the effect is short. For example, it is very common for people to visit their doctor just before their death. The visit to the doctor is not a risk factor for death but is a "surrogate" marker for severe and potentially life-threatening illness. These patients visit their doctors for symptoms associated with their impending deaths.

Cross-sectional studies are subject to prevalence–incidence bias. **Prevalence–incidence bias** is defined as a situation when the element that seems to cause an outcome is really an effect of or associated with that cause. This occurs when a risk factor is strongly associated with a disease and is thought to occur before the disease occurs. Thus the risk factor appears to cause the disease when in reality it simply affects the duration or prognosis of the disease. An association was noted between HLA-A2 antigen and the presence of acute lymphocytic leukemia in children in a cross-sectional study. It was assumed to be a risk factor for occurrence of the disease. Subsequent studies found that long-term survivors had the HLA-A2 antigen and its absence was associated with early mortality. The antigen was not a risk factor for the disease but an indicator of good prognosis.

Longitudinal studies

Longitudinal study is a catchall term describing either observations or interventions made over a given period of time. There are three basic longitudinal study designs: **case–control** studies, **cohort** studies, and **clinical trials**. These are **analytic** or **inferential** studies, meaning that they look for a statistical association between risk factors and outcomes.

Case–control studies

These studies were previously called retrospective studies, but looking at data in hindsight is not the only attribute of a case–control study. There is another unique feature that should be used to identify a case–control study. The subjects are initially selected because they either have the outcome of interest – **cases** – or do not have the outcome of interest – **controls**. They are grouped at the start of the study by the presence or absence of the outcome, or in other words, are grouped as either cases or controls. This type of study is good to screen for potential risk factors of disease by reviewing elements that occurred in the past and comparing the outcomes. The ratio between cases and controls is arbitrarily set rather than reflecting their true ratio in the general population.. The study then examines the odds of exposure to the risk factor among the cases and compares this to the odds of exposure among the controls. Figure 6.1 is a schematic description of a case–control study.

The strengths of case–control studies are that they are relatively easy, cheap, and quick to do from previously available data. They can be done using current patients and asking them about events that occurred in the past. They are well suited for studying rare diseases since the study begins with subjects who already have the outcome. Each case patient may then be matched up with one or more suitable control patients. Ideally the controls are as similar to the cases as possible except for the outcome and then their degree of exposure to the risk factor of interest can be calculated. Case–controls are good exploratory studies and can look at many risk factors for one outcome. The results can then be used to

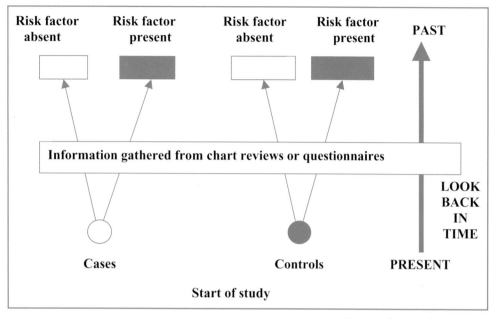

Fig. 6.1 Schematic diagram of a case–control study.

suggest new hypotheses for a later study with stronger research study design, such as a cohort study or clinical trial.

Unfortunately, there are many potentially serious weaknesses in case–control studies, which in general, make them only fair sources of evidence. Since the data are collected retrospectively, data quality may be poor. Data often come from a careful search of the medical records of the cases and controls. The advantage of these records being easily available is counteracted by their questionable reliability. These studies rely on subjective descriptions to determine exposure and outcome, and the subjective standards of the record reviewers to determine the presence of the cause and effect. This is called **implicit review** of the medical records. Implicit review of charts introduces the researcher's bias in interpreting the measurements or outcomes. Stronger case–control studies will use explicit reviews. An **explicit review** only uses clearly objective measures in reviews of medical charts, or the chart material is reviewed in a blinded manner using previously determined outcome descriptors. These chart reviews are better but are more difficult to perform.

When a patient is asked to remember something about a medical condition that occurred in the past, their memory is subject to recall or reporting bias. **Recall** or **reporting bias** occurs because those with the disease are more likely to recall exposure to many risk factors simply because they have the disease. Another problem is that subjects in the sample may not be representative of all patients with the outcome. This is called **sampling** or **referral bias** and commonly occurs in studies done at specialized referral centers. These referred patients may be different from those seen in a primary-care practice and often in referral centers, only the most severe cases of a given disorder will be seen, thus limiting the generalizability of the findings.

When determining which of many potential risk factors is associated with an outcome using a case–control study a derivation set is developed. A **derivation set** is the initial series of results of a study. The results of the derivation set should be used cautiously since any association discovered may have turned up by chance alone. The study can then be repeated using a cohort study design to look at those factors that have the highest correlation with the outcome in question to see if the association still holds. This is called a **validation set** and has greater generalizability to the population.

Other factors to be aware of when dealing with case–control studies are that case–controls can only study one disease or outcome at a given time. Also, prevalence or incidence cannot be calculated since the ratio of cases to controls is preselected by the researchers. In addition, they cannot prove contributory cause since they cannot show that altering the cause will alter the effect and the study itself cannot show that the cause preceded the effect. Often times, researchers and clinicians can extrapolate the cause and effect from knowledge of biology or physiology.

Cohort studies

These were previously called prospective studies since they are usually done from past to present in time. The name comes from the Latin *cohors*, meaning a tenth of a legion marching together in time. However, they can be and are now as frequently done retrospectively and called **non-concurrent cohort studies**. The cohort is a group of patients who are selected based on the presence or absence of the *risk factor* (Fig. 6.2). They are followed in time to determine which of them will develop the outcome or disease. The probability of developing the outcome is the incidence or risk, and can be calculated for each group. The degree of risk can then be compared between the two groups.

The cohort study can be one of the strongest research study designs. They can be powerful studies that can determine the incidence of disease and are able to show that the cause is associated with the effect more often than by chance alone. They can also show that the cause preceded the effect. They do not attempt to manipulate the cause and cannot prove that altering the cause alters the effect. Cohort studies are an ideal study design for answering questions of etiology, harm, or prognosis as they collect the data in an objective and uniform fashion. The investigators can predetermine the entry criteria, what measurements are to be made, and how they are best made. As a result, there is usually no recall bias,

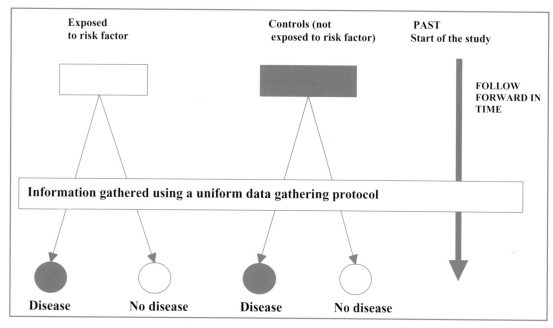

Fig. 6.2 Schematic diagram of a cohort study.

except as a possibility in non-concurrent cohort studies where the researchers are asking for subjective information from the study subjects.

The main weakness of cohort studies is that they are expensive in time and money. The startup and ongoing monitoring costs may be prohibitive. This is a greater problem when studying rare or uncommon diseases as it may be difficult to get enough patients to find clinically or statistically significant differences between the patients who are exposed and those not exposed to the risk factor. Since the cohort must be set up prospectively by the presence or absence of the risk factor, they are not good studies to uncover new risk factors.

Confounding variables are factors affecting both the risk factor and the outcome. They may affect the exposed and unexposed groups differently and lead to a bias in the conclusions. There are often reasons why patients are exposed to the risk factor that may lead to differences in the outcome. For example, patients may be selected for a particular therapy, the risk factor in this case, because they are sicker or less sick, which then cause differences in outcomes that result.

Patients who leave the study, called **patient attrition**, can cause loss of data about the outcomes. The cause of their attrition from the study may be directly related to some conditions of the study. Therefore, it is imperative for researchers to account for all patients. In practice an acceptable level of attrition is less than 20%. However, this should be used as a guide rather than an absolute value. A value of attrition lower than 20% may bias the study if the reason patients were lost from the study is related to the risk factor. In long-running studies, patients may change some aspect of their behavior or exposure to the risk factor after the initial grouping of subjects, leading to **misclassification bias**. Safeguards to prevent these issues should be clearly outlined in the methods section of the study.

A special case of the cohort study, the **non-concurrent cohort study** is also called a **database study**. It is essentially a cohort study that begins in the present and utilizes data on events that took place in the past. The cohort is still separated by the presence or absence of the risk factor that is being studied, although this risk factor is usually not the original reason that patients were entered into the study. Non-concurrent cohort studies are not retrospective studies, but have been called "retrospective cohort studies" in the past. They have essentially the same strengths and weaknesses as cohort studies, but are more dependent on the quality of the recorded data from the past.

In a typical non-concurrent cohort study design, a cohort is put together in the past and many baseline measurements are made. The follow-up measurements and determination of the original outcomes are made when the data are finally analyzed at the end of the study. The data will then be used for another, later study and analyzed for a new risk factor other than the one for which the original study was done. For example, a cohort of patients with trauma due to motor-vehicle-accident is collected to look at the relationship of wearing seat belts to death. After the data are collected, the same group of patients is looked at to see if there is any relationship between severe head injury and the wearing of seat belts. Both data elements were collected as part of the original study.

In general, for a non-concurrent cohort study, the data are available from databases that have already been set up. The data should be gathered in an objective manner or at least without regard for the association which is being sought. Data gatherers are ideally blinded to the outcomes. Since non-concurrent cohort studies rely on historical data, they may suffer some of the weaknesses associated with case–control studies regarding recall bias, the lack of uniformity of data recorded in the data base, and subjective interpretation of records.

To review

> Subjects in case–control studies are initially grouped according to the presence or absence of the *outcome* and the ratio between cases and controls is arbitrary and not reflective of their true ratio in the population.
> Subjects in cohort studies are initially grouped according to the presence or absence of *risk factors* regardless of whether the group was assembled in the past or the present.

Clinical trials

A **clinical trial** is a cohort study in which the investigator intervenes by manipulating the presence or absence of the risk factor, usually a therapeutic maneuver.

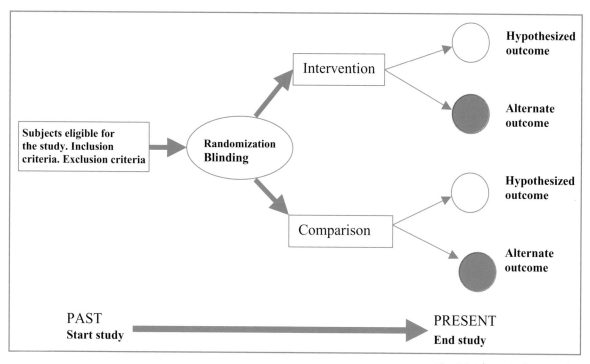

Fig. 6.3 Schematic diagram of a randomized clinical trial.

Clinical trials are human experiments, also called **interventional studies**. Traditional cohort and case–control studies are **observational studies** in which there is no intentional intervention. An example of a clinical trial is a study in which a high-soy-protein diet and a normal diet were given to middle-aged male smokers to determine if it reduced their risk of developing diabetes. The diet is the intervention. A cohort study of the same 'risk factor' would look at a group of middle-aged male smokers and see which of them ate a high-soy-protein diet and then follow them for a period of time to determine their rates of developing diabetes. Figure 6.3 is a schematic diagram of a randomized clinical trial.

Clinical trials are characterized by the presence of a control group identical to the experimental patients in every way except for their exposure to the intervention being studied. Patients entering controlled clinical trials should be **randomized**, meaning that all patients signed up for the trial should have an equal chance of being placed in either the control group (also called the comparison group, placebo group, or standardized therapy group) or the experimental group, which gets the intervention being tested. Subjects and experimenters should ideally be **blinded** to the therapy and group assignment during the study, such that the experimenters and subjects are unaware if the patient is in the control or experimental group, and are thus unaware whether they are receiving the experimental treatment or the comparison treatment.

Clinical trials are the only study design that can fulfill all the rules of contributory cause. They can show that the cause and effect are associated more than by chance alone, that the cause precedes the effect, and that altering the cause alters the effect. When properly carried out they will have fewer methodological biases than any other study design.

However, they are far from perfect. The most common weakness of controlled clinical trials is that they are very expensive. Because of the high costs, multi-center trials that utilize cooperation between many research centers and are funded by industry or government are becoming more common. Unfortunately, the high cost of these studies has resulted in more of them being paid for by large biomedical (pharmaceutical or technology) companies and as a result, the design of these studies could favor the outcome that is desired by the sponsoring agency. This could represent a conflict of interest for the researcher, whose salary and research support is dependent on the largess of the company providing the money. Other factors that may compromise the research results are patient attrition and patient compliance.

There may be ethical problems when the study involves giving potentially harmful, or withholding potentially beneficial, therapy. The Institutional Review Boards (IRB) of the institutions doing the research should address these. A poorly designed study should not be considered ethical by the IRB. However, just because the IRB approves the study doesn't mean that the reader should not critcally read the study. It is still the reader's responsibility to determine how valid a study is based upon the methodology. In addition, the fact that a study is a randomized controlled trial does not in itself guarantee validity, and there can still be serious methodological problems that will bias the results.

7

Instruments and measurements: precision and validity

Not everything that can be counted counts, and not everything that counts can be counted.

Albert Einstein (1879–1955)

Learning objectives

In this chapter you will learn:
- different types of data as basic elements of descriptive statistics
- instrumentation and measurement
- precision, accuracy, reliability, and validity
- how researchers should optimize these factors

All clinical research studies involve observations and measurements of the phenomena of interest. Observations and measurements are the desired output of a study. The instruments used to make them are subject to error, which may bias the results of a study. The first thing we will discuss is the type of data that can be generated from clinical research. This chapter will then introduce concepts related to instruments and measurements.

Types of data and variables

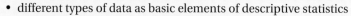

There are several different ways of classifying data. They can be classified by their function as independent or dependent variables, their nature as nominal, ordinal, interval, or ratio variables, and whether they are continuous, discrete, or dichotomous variables.

When classifying variables by function we want to know what the variable does in the experiment. Is it the cause or the effect? In most clinical trials one variable is held constant relative to the other. The **independent** variable is under the control of or can be manipulated by the investigator. Generally this is the cause we are interested in, such as a drug, a treatment, a risk factor, or a diagnostic test. The **dependent** variable changes as a result of or as an effect of the action of the independent variable. It is usually the outcome of exposure to the treatment or risk factor, or the presence of a particular diagnosis. We want to find out if changing the independent variable will produce a change in the dependent variable. The nature of each variable should be evident from the study design or there is a serious problem in the way the study was conducted.

When classifying variables by their nature, we mean the hierarchy that describes the mathematical characteristics of the value generated for that variable. The choice of variables becomes very important in the application of statistical tests to the data. **Nominal** data are simply named categories. One can assign a number to each of these categories, but it would have no intrinsic significance and cannot be used to compare one piece of the data set to another. Changing the number assignment has no effect on the interpretation of the data. Examples of nominal data are classification of physicians by specialty or of patients by the type of cancer from which they suffer. There is no relationship between the various types of specialty physicians except that they are all physicians and went to medical school. There is certainly no mathematical relationship between them.

Ordinal data are nominal data for which the order of the variables has importance and intrinsic meaning. However, there is still no mathematical relationship between data points. Typical examples of ordinal data include certain pain scores that are measured by scales called Likert scales, severity of injury scores as reflected in a score such as the Trauma Score where lower numbers are predictive of worse survival than higher ones, or the grading and staging of a tumor where higher number stages are worse than lower ones. Common questionnaires asking the participant to state whether they agree, are neutral, or disagree with a statement are also examples of an ordinal scale. Although there is a directional value to each of these answers, there is no numerical or mathematical relationship between them.

Interval data are ordinal data for which the interval between each number is also a meaningful real number. However, interval data have only an arbitrary zero point and, therefore, there is no proportionality ratio relationship between two points. One example is temperature in degrees Celsius where $64°C$ is $32°C$ hotter than $32°C$ but not twice as hot. Another example is the common IQ score where 100 is average, but someone with a score of 200 is not twice as smart since a score of 200 is super-genius, and less than 0.01% the population has a score this high.

Ratio data are interval data that have an absolute zero value. This makes the results take on meaning for both absolute and relative changes in the variable. Examples of ratio variables are the temperature in degrees Kelvin where $100°$ Kelvin is $50°K$ hotter than $50°K$ and is twice as hot, age where a 10-year-old is twice as old as a 5-year-old, and common biological measurements such as pulse, blood pressure, respiratory rate, blood chemistry measurements, and weight.

Data can also be described as either having or lacking continuity. **Continuous** data may take any value within a defined range. For most purposes we choose to round off to an easily usable number of digits. This is called the number of significant places, which is taught in high school and college, although it is often forgotten by students quickly thereafter. Height is an example of a continuous measure since a person can be 172 cm or 173 cm or 172.58763248 ... cm tall. The practical useful value would be 172.6 or 173 cm.

Values for **discrete** data can only be represented by whole numbers. For example, a piano is an instrument with only discrete values in that there are only 88 keys, therefore, only 88 possible notes. Scoring systems like the Glasgow Coma Score for measuring neurological deficits, the Likert scales mentioned above, and other ordinal scales contain only discrete variables and mathematically can have only integer values.

We commonly use **dichotomous** data to describe binomial outcomes, which are those variables that can have only two possible values. Obvious examples are alive or dead, yes or no, normal or abnormal, and better or worse. Sometimes researchers convert continuous variables to dichotomous ones. Selecting a single cutoff as the division between two states does this. For example, serum sodium is defined as normal if between 135 and 145 mEq/dL. Values over 145 define hypernatremia, and values below this don't. This has the effect of dichotomizing the value of the serum sodium into either hypernatremic or not hypernatremic.

Measurement in clinical research

All natural phenomena can be measured, but it is important to realize that errors may occur in the process. These errors can be classified into two categories: random and systematic. **Random error** is characteristically unpredictable in direction or amount. Random error leads to a lack of precision due to the innate variability of the biological or sociological system being studied. This biological variation occurs for most bodily functions. For example, in a given population, there will be a more or less random variation in the pulse or blood pressure. Many of these random events can be described by the normal distribution, which we will discuss in Chapter 9. Random error can also be due to a lack of precision of the measuring instrument. An imprecise instrument will get slightly different results each time the same event is measured. In addition, certain measurements are inherently more precise than others. For example, serum sodium measured inside rat muscle cells will show less random error than the degree of depression in humans. There can also be innate variability in the way that different researchers or practicing physicians interpret various data on certain patients.

Systematic error represents a consistent distortion in direction or magnitude of the results. Systematic or systemic error is a function of the person making the measurement or the calibration of the instrument. For example, researchers could consistently measure blood pressure using a blood-pressure cuff that always reads high by 10 mmHg. More commonly, a measurement can be influenced by knowledge of other aspects of the patient's situation leading to researchers responding differently to some patients in the study. In a study of asthma, the researcher may consistently coach some research subjects differently in performing the peak expiratory flow rate (PEFR), an effort-dependent test. Another source of systematic error can occur when there is non-random assignment of subjects to one group in a study. For instance, researchers could preferentially assign patients with bronchitis to the placebo group when studying the effect of antibiotics on bronchitis and pneumonia. This would be problematic since bronchitis almost always gets better on its own and pneumonia sometimes gets better on its own, but it is less likely and occurs more slowly. Then, if the patients assigned to placebo get better as often as those taking antibiotics, the cause of the improvement is uncertain since it may have occurred because the placebo patients were going to get better more quickly anyway.

Both types of errors may lead to incorrect results. The researcher's job is to minimize the error in the study to minimize the bias in the study. Researchers are usually more successful at reducing systematic error than random error. Overall, it is the reader's job to determine if bias exists, and if so to what extent and in what direction that bias is likely to change the study results.

Instruments and how they are chosen

Common instruments include objective instruments like the thermometer or sphygmomanometer (blood-pressure cuff and manometer) and subjective instruments such as questionnaires or pain scales. By their nature, objective measurements made by physical instruments such as automated blood-cell counters tend to be very precise. However, these instruments may also be affected by random variation of biological systems in the body. An example of this is hemodynamic pressure measurements such as arterial or venous pressure, oxygen saturation, and airway pressures taken by transducers. The actual measurement may be very precise, but there can be lots of random variation around the true measurement result. Subjective instruments include questions that must be answered either yes or no or with an ordinal scale (0, 1, 2, 3, 4, or 5) or by placing an x on a pre-measured line. Measures of pain or anxiety are common examples and these are commonly known to be unreliable, inaccurate, and often imprecise.

Overall, **measurements**, the data that instruments give us, are the final goals of research. They are the result of applying an instrument to the process of systematically collecting data. Common instruments used in medicine measure the temperature, blood pressure, number of yes or no answers, or level of pain. The quality of the measurements is only as good as the quality of the instrument used to make them.

Good instrument selection is a vital part of the research study design. The researcher must select instruments that will measure the phenomena of interest. If the researcher wishes to measure blood pressure accurately and precisely, a standard blood-pressure cuff would be a reasonable tool. The researcher could also measure blood pressure using an intra-arterial catheter attached to a pressure transducer. This will give a more precise result, but the additional precision may not help in the ultimate care of the patient. If survival is the desired outcome, a simple record of the presence or absence of death is the best measure. For measuring the cause of death, the death certificate can also be the instrument of choice but has been shown to be inaccurate.

When subjective outcomes like pain, anxiety, quality of life, or patient satisfaction are measured, the selection of an instrument becomes more difficult. Pain, a very subjective measure, is appreciated differently by different people. Some patients will react more strongly and show more emotion than others in response to the same levels of pain. There are standardized pain scores available that have been validated in research trials. The most commonly used pain scale is the Visual Analog Scale (VAS). A 10-cm line is placed on the paper with one end labeled "no pain at all," and the other end "worst pain ever." The patient puts a mark on the scale corresponding to the pain level. If this exercise is repeated and the patient reports the same level of pain, then the scale is validated. The best outcome measure when using this scale becomes the change in the pain score and not the absolute score. Since pain is quantified differently in different patients, it is only the difference in scores that is likely to be similar between patients. In fact, when this was studied, it was found that patients would use consistently similar differences for the same degree of pain difference.[1] This study found that a difference in pain scores of 1.5 cm is a clinically important difference in degree of pain.

Another type of pain score is the Likert Scale, which is a five- or six-point ordinal scale in which each of the points represents a different level of pain. A sample Likert Scale begins with 0 = no pain, continues with 1 = minimal pain, and ends

---

[1] K. H. Todd & J. P. Funk. The minimum clinically important difference in physician-assigned visual analog pain scores. *Acad. Emerg. Med.* 1996; 3: 142–146; and K. H. Todd, K. G. Funk, J. P. Funk & R. Bonacci. Clinical significance of reported changes in pain severity. *Ann. Emerg. Med.* 1996; 27: 485–489.

with 5 = worst pain ever. The reader must be careful when interpreting studies using this type of scoring system. Like the VAS for pain, personal differences in the quantification may result in large differences in the score. A patient who puts a 3 for their pain is counted very differently from a patient who puts a 4 for the same level of pain. The differences in pain level have not been quantified in the same way as the VAS, and as it is an ordinal scale, the results may not be used the same way. The VAS score behaves like a continuous variable while Likert scales should be treated as ordinal variables. Because of this, Likert scales are very useful for measuring opinions about a given question. For example, when evaluating a course, you are given several graded choices such as strongly agree, agree, neutral, disagree, or strongly disagree.

Similar problems will result with other questionnaires and scales. The reader must become familiar with the commonly used survey instruments in their specialty. Commonly used scores in studies of depression are the Beck Depression Inventory or the Hamilton Depression Scale. In the study of alcoholism, the commonly used scores are the CAGE score, Michigan Alcohol Screening Test (MAST), and the Alcohol Use Disorders Identification Test (AUDIT). The reader is responsible for understanding the limitations of each of these scores when reviewing the literature. This will require the reader to look further into the use of these tests when first reviewing the medical literature. Be aware that sometimes scores are developed specifically for a study, and in that case, they should be independently validated before use.

A common problem in selecting instruments is the practice of measuring **surrogate markers**. These are markers that may or may not be related to or be predictive of the outcome of interest. For example, the degree of blood flow through a coronary artery as measured by "TIMI grade" of flow is a good measure of the flow of blood through the artery. But, it may not predict the ultimate survival of a patient. The measure of TIMI grade flow is called a **disease-oriented outcome** while overall survival is a **patient-oriented outcome**. **Composite outcomes** are multiple outcomes put together in the hope that the combination will more often achieve statistical significance. This is done when each individual outcome is too infrequent to expect that it will demonstrate statistical significance. Only consider using composite outcomes if all the outcomes are more or less equally important to your patient. One example is the use of death and recurrent transient ischemic attack (TIA) as an outcome. Death is important to all patients, but recurrent TIA may not have the same level of importance, and should not be considered equal when measuring outcome events. We'll discuss composite outcomes and how to evaluate them in a future chapter.

Attributes of measurements

Measurements should be precise, reliable, accurate, and valid. **Precision** simply means that the measurement is nearly the same value each time it is measured.

This is a measure of random variation, noise, or random error. Statistically it states that for a precise measurement, there is only a small amount of variation around the true value of the variable being measured. In statistical terminology this is equivalent to a small standard deviation or range around the central value of multiple measurements. For example, if each time a physician takes a blood pressure, the same measurement is obtained, then we can say that the measurement is precise. The same measurement can become imprecise if not repeated the same way, for example if different blood-pressure cuffs are used.

Reliability has been used loosely as a synonym of precision but it also incorporates durability or reproducibility of the measurement in its definition. It tells you that no matter how often you repeat the measurement you will get the same or similar result. It can be precise, in which case the results of repeated measurements are almost exactly the same. We are looking for instruments that will give precise, consistent, reproducible, and dependable data.

Accuracy is a measure of the trueness of the result. This tells you how close the measured value is to the actual value. Statistically, it is equivalent to saying that the mean or arithmetic average of all measurements taken is the actual and true value of the thing being measured. For example, if indirect blood-pressure measurements use a manometer and blood-pressure cuff that correlate closely to direct intra-arterial measurements in healthy, young volunteers using a pressure transducer, it means that the blood pressure measured using the manometer and blood-pressure cuff is accurate. The measurement will be inaccurate if the manometer is not calibrated properly or if an incorrect cuff size is used. Accuracy doesn't mean the same thing as precision. It is possible for a measurement to be accurate but not precise if the average measured result is the true value of the thing being measured but the spread around that measure is very great.

Precision and accuracy are direct functions of the instruments chosen to make a particular measurement. **Validity** tells us that the measurement actually represents what we want to measure. We may have accurate and precise measurements that are not valid. For example, weight is a less valid measure for obesity than skin fold thickness or body mass index. Blood pressure measured with a standard blood-pressure cuff is a valid measure of the intra-arterial pressure. However, a single blood-sugar measurement is not a valid measure of overall diabetic control. A test called glycosylated hemoglobin is a valid measure of this.

Types of validity

There are several definitions of validity. The first set of definitions defines validity by the process with which it is determined. This includes criterion-based, predictive, and face validity. The second definition defines where validity is found in a clinical study and includes internal and external validity.

Criterion-based or **construct validity** is a description of how close the measurement of the phenomenon of interest is to other measurements of the same thing using different instruments. This means that there is a study showing that the measurement of interest agrees with other accepted measures of the same thing. For example, the score of patients on the CAGE questionnaire for alcoholism screening correlates with the results on the more complex and previously validated Michigan Alcohol Screening Test (MAST) for the diagnosis of alcoholism. Similarly, blood-pressure cuff readings correlate with intra-arterial blood pressure as recorded by an electrical pressure transducer.

Predictive validity is a type of criterion-based validity that describes how well the measurement predicts an outcome event. This could be the result of another measurement or the presence or absence of a particular outcome. For example, lack of fever in an elderly patient with pneumonia predicts a higher mortality than in the same group of patients with fever. This was determined from studies of factors related to the specific outcome of mortality in elderly patients with pneumonia. We would say that lack of fever in elderly pneumonia patients gives predictive validity to the outcome of increased mortality.

Finally, **face validity** is how much common sense the measurement has. It is a statement of the fact that the instrument measures the phenomenon of interest and that it makes sense. For example, the measured performance of a student on one multiple-choice examination should predict that student's performance on another multiple-choice examination. Performance on an observed examination of a standardized patient accurately measures the student's ability to accurately perform a history and physical examination on any patient. However, having face validity doesn't mean that the measure can be accepted without verification. In this example, it must be validated because the testing situation may cause some students to freeze up, which they wouldn't do when face-to-face with a real patient, thus decreasing its face validity.

Validity can also be classified by the potential effect of bias or error on the results of a study. Internal and external validity are the terms used to describe this and are the most common ways to classify validity. You should use this schema when you assess any research study. **Internal validity** exists when precision and accuracy are not distorted by bias introduced into a study. An internally valid study precisely and accurately measures what is intended. Internal validity is threatened by problems in the way a study is designed or carried out, or with the instruments used to make the measurements. **External validity** exists when the measurement can be generalized and the results extrapolated to other clinical situations or populations. External validity is threatened when the population studied is too restrictive and you cannot apply the results to another and usually larger, population.

Schematically, truth in the study is a function of internal validity. The results of an internally valid study are true if there is no serious source of bias that can produce a fatal flaw and invalidate the study. Truth in the universe relating to all other patients with this problem is only present if the study is externally valid. The process by which this occurs will be discussed in a later chapter.

Improving precision and accuracy

In the process of designing a study, the researcher should maximize precision, accuracy, and validity. The methods section detailing the protocol used in the study should enable the reader to determine if enough safeguards have been taken to ensure a valid study. The protocol should be explicit and given in enough detail to be reproduced easily by anyone reading the study.

There are four possible error patterns that can occur in the process of measuring data.

(1) Both precision and accuracy can be good: the result is equal to the true value and there is only a small degree of variation around that true value, or the standard deviation is small.

(2) The results may be precise but not accurate: the result is not equal to the true value, but there is only a small degree of variation around that value; this pattern is characteristic of systematic error or bias.

(3) Results that are accurate but not precise: the result is equal to the true value but there is a large amount of variation around that value, or the standard deviation is large. This is typical of random error, a statistical phenomenon.

(4) The result may be neither accurate nor precise: this is due to both random and systematic error and in this case the result of the study is not equal to the true value and there is a large amount of variability around that value.

Look for these patterns of error or potential error when reviewing a study.

Using exactly reproducible and objective measurements, standardizing the performance of the measurements and intensively training the observers will increase precision. Automated instruments can give more reliable measurements, assuming that they are regularly calibrated. The number of trained observers should be kept to a minimum to increase precision, since having more observers increases the likelihood that one will make a serious error.

Making unobtrusive measurements reduces subject bias. **Unobtrusive measurements** are those which cannot be detected by the subject. For example, taking a blood pressure is obtrusive while simply observing a patient for an outcome like death or living is usually non-obtrusive. Watching someone work and recording his or her efficiency is obtrusive since it could result in a change in behavior, called the **Hawthorne effect**. Therefore, unobtrusive measurements are best made in a blinded manner. If the observer is unaware of the group to which the patient is assigned, there is less risk that the measurement will be biased. Blinding creates the climate for consistency and fairness in the measurements, and results in reduced systematic error. Non-blinded measurements can lead to differential treatment being given to one of the groups being studied. This can lead to **contamination** or **confounding** of the results. In **single blinding**, either the researcher or the patient doesn't know who is in each group. In **double blinding**, neither the researchers nor subject knows who is in each group. **Triple blinding** occurs if the patient, person treating the patient, and the researcher measuring the outcome are all blind to the treatment being rendered.

Tests of inter- and intra-rater reliability

Different observers can obtain different results when they make a measurement. Several observers may measure the temperature of a child using slightly different techniques when using the thermometer like varying the time the thermometer is left in the patient or reading the mercury level in different ways.

Precision is improved when inter- or intra-observer variation is minimized. The researcher should account for variability between observers and between measurements made by the same observer. Variability between two observers or between multiple observations by a single observer can introduce bias into the results. Therefore a subset of all the measurements should be repeated and the variability of the results measured. This is referred to as inter-observer and intra-observer variability. **Inter-observer variability** occurs when two or more observers obtain different results when measuring the same phenomenon. **Intra-observer variability** occurs when the same observer obtains different results when measuring the same phenomenon on two or more occasions. Tests for inter-observer and intra-observer variability should be done before any study is completed.

Both the inter-observer and intra-observer reliability are measured by the kappa statistic. The **kappa statistic** is a quantitative measure of the degree of agreement between measurements. It measures the degree of agreement beyond chance between two observers, called the inter-rater agreement, or between multiple measurements made by a single observer, called the intra-rater agreement.

The kappa statistic applies because physicians and researchers often assume that all diagnostic tests are precise. However, many studies have demonstrated that most non-automated tests have a degree of subjectivity in their interpretation. This has been seen in commonly used radiologic tests such as CT scan, mammography, and angiography. It is also present in tests commonly considered to be the gold standard such as the interpretation of tissue samples from autopsy, biopsy, or surgery.

	Resident 1: Normal	Resident 1: Abnormal	
Resident 2: Normal	90	0	90
Abnormal	10	0	10
	100	0	

Fig. 7.1 Observed agreement between two residents when one (no. 1) reads them all as normal and the other (no. 2) reads 90 as normal and 10 as abnormal.

Here is a clinical example of how the kappa statistic applies. One morning, two radiology residents were reading mammograms. There were 100 mammograms to be read. The first resident, Number 1, had been on night call and was pretty tired. He didn't really feel like reading these and knew that all of his readings would be reviewed by the attending. He also reasoned that since this was a screening clinic for young women with an average age of 32, there would be very few positive studies. This particular radiology department had a computerized reading system where the resident pushes either the "normal" or the "cancer" button on a console and that reading would be entered into the file. After reading the first three as negative, he fell asleep on the "negative" button, making all one hundred readings negative.

The second resident, Number 2, was really interested in mammography and had slept all night, since she was not on call. She carefully read each study and pushed the appropriate button. She read 90 films as normal and 10 as suspicious for early breast cancer. The two residents' readings are tabulated in the 2 × 2 table in Fig. 7.1.

The level of agreement that was observed was 90/100 or 90%. Is this agreement of 90% very good? What would the agreement be if they read the mammograms by chance alone? Assuming that there are 90% normals and 10% abnormals, we can assume that each read their films with that proportion of each result and do the same 2 × 2 table (Fig. 7.2). Agreement by chance would be (81 + 1)/100 or 82%.

Kappa is the ratio of the actual agreement beyond chance and the potential agreement beyond chance. The actual agreement beyond chance is the difference between the actual agreement found and that expected by chance. In our example it is 90 – 82 = 8% (0.08). The potential agreement beyond chance is the difference between the highest possible agreement (100%) and that expected by chance alone. In our example, 100 – 82 = 18% (0.18). This makes Kappa = (0.90 – 0.82)/(1.00 – 0.82) = 0.08/0.18 = 0.44.

Table 7.1. Interpretation of the kappa statistic

$$\text{Kappa} = \frac{\text{Actual agreement between measurements beyond chance}}{\text{Potential agreement between measurements beyond chance}}$$

Range: 0–1 (0 = no agreement; 1 = complete agreement)

Numerical level of kappa Qualitative significance

0.0–0.2	slight
0.2–0.4	fair
0.4–0.6	moderate
0.6–0.8	substantial
0.8–1.0	almost perfect

Fig. 7.2 Observed agreement between two residents when both (no. 1 and no. 2) read 90 as normal and 10 as abnormal, but there is no relationship between their readings. The 90% read normal by no. 1 are not the same as the 90% read as normal by no. 2.

	Resident 1 Normal	Resident 1 Abnormal	
Resident 2 Normal	81	9	90
Resident 2 Abnormal	9	1	10
	90	10	

	Resident 1 Normal	Resident 1 Abnormal	
Resident 2 Normal	25	25	50
Resident 2 Abnormal	25	25	50
	50	50	A

	Resident 1 Normal	Resident 1 Abnormal	
Resident 2 Normal	50	0	50
Resident 2 Abnormal	0	50	50
	50	50	B

Fig. 7.3 Kappa for chance agreement only (A, $\kappa = 0.0$) and for perfect agreement (B, $\kappa = 1.0$).

Overview of kappa statistic

You should use the kappa statistic when you want to know the **precision** of a measurement or the **inter-observer** or **intra-observer** consistency. This gives a reasonable estimate of how "easily" the measurement is made. The "easier" it is to make a measurement, the more likely that two different observers will agree on the result and that agreement is not just due to chance. Some experts have related the value of kappa to qualitative descriptors, which are given in Table 7.1. In general, look for a kappa higher than 0.6 before you consider the agreement to be reasonably acceptable.

Kappa ranges from 0 to 1 where 0 means that there is no agreement and 1 means there is complete agreement beyond that expected by chance alone. You can see from making a 2×2 table that if there is an equal number in each cell the agreement occurs purely by chance (Fig. 7.3). Similarly if there is perfect agreement, it is very unlikely that the agreement occurred completely by chance. However, it is still possible: if there are only a few readings in each cell, 100% agreement could occur by chance, even though the chance of this happening is very small. Confidence intervals, which we will discuss later in the book, should be calculated to determine the statistically feasible range within which 95% of possible kappa values will be found.

There are other statistics that more or less measure the same thing as the kappa statistic. These are the standard deviation of repeated measurements, coefficient of variation, correlation coefficient of paired measurements, intraclass correlation coefficient and Cronbach's alpha.[2]

---

[2] A more detailed discussion of kappa can be found in D. L. Sackett, R. B. Haynes, P. Tugwell & G. H. Guyatt *Clinical Epidemiology: a Basic Science for Clinical Medicine.* 2nd edn. Boston: Little Brown, 1991.

8

Sources of bias

Of all the causes which conspire to blind
Man's erring judgment, and misguide the mind;
What the weak head with strongest bias rules, –
Is pride, the never-failing vice of fools.

Alexander Pope (1688–1744): Essay on Criticism

Learning objectives

In this chapter you will learn:
- sources of bias
- threats to internal and external validity
- how to tell when bias threatens the conclusions of a study

All studies involve observations and measurements of phenomena of interest, but the observations and instruments used to make these measurements are subject to error. Bias introduced into a study can result in systematic error which may then affect the results of the study and could invalidate the conclusions. Since there is no such thing as a perfect study, in reading the medical literature you should be familiar with common sources of bias in clinical studies. By understanding how these biases could affect the results of the study, it is possible to detect bias and predict the potential effect on the conclusions. You can then determine if this will invalidate the study conclusions enough to deter you from using the results in your patients' care. This chapter will give you a schema for looking for bias, and present some common sources of bias.

Overview of bias in clinical studies

Bias was a semilegendary Greek statesman who tried to make peace between two city-states by lying about the warlike intention of the enemy state. His ploy failed and ultimately he told the truth, allowing his city to win the war. His name became forever associated with slanting the truth as a means to accomplish an end.

Bias is defined as the systematic introduction of error into a study that can distort the results in a non-random way. It is almost impossible to eliminate all sources of bias, even in the most carefully designed study. It is the job of the researcher to attempt to remove as much bias as possible and to identify potential sources of bias for the reader. It is the job of the reader to find any sources of bias and assess the importance and potential effects of bias on the results of the study. Virtually no study is 100% bias-free and not all bias will result in an invalid study and in fact, some bias may actually increase the validity of a study.

After identifying a source of bias, you must determine the likely effect of that bias on the results of the study. If this effect is likely to be great and potentially decrease the results found by the research, internal validity and the conclusions of the study are threatened. If it could completely reverse the results of the study, it is called a "fatal" flaw. The results of a study with a fatal flaw should generally not be applied to your current patients. If the bias could have only small potential effects, then the results of these studies can be accepted and used with caution. Bias can be broken down into three areas according to its source: the population being studied, the measurement of the outcome, and miscellaneous sources.

Bias in the population being studied

Selection bias

Selection **bias** or **sampling bias** occurs when patients are selected in a manner that will systematically influence the outcome of the study. There are several ways that this type of bias can occur. Subjects who are volunteers or paid to be in the study may have different characteristics than the "average person" with the disease in question. Another form of selection bias occurs when patients are chosen to be in a study based upon certain physical or social characteristics. These characteristics may then change the outcome of the study. Commonly, selection bias exists in studies of therapy when patients chosen to be one arm of the study are 'selected' by some characteristics determined by the physicians enrolling them in the study. A few examples will help demonstrate the effects of this bias.

An investigator offered free psychiatric counseling to women who had just had an abortion if they took a free psychological test. He found the incidence of depression was higher in these women than in the general population. He concluded that having an abortion caused depression. It is very likely that women who had an abortion and were depressed, therefore needing counseling, would preferentially sign up to be in the study. Women who had an abortion and were not depressed would be less likely to sign up for the study and take the free psychological test. This is a potentially fatal flaw of this study, and therefore, the conclusion is very likely to be biased.

Patients with suspected pulmonary embolism (PE, blood clot in the lung), were studied with angiograms, an x-ray of the blood vessels in the lung capable of showing a blood clot. It was found that those patients with an angiogram positive for pulmonary embolus were less likely to have a deep vein thrombosis (DVT, blood clot in a leg vein) than those patients with an angiogram negative for pulmonary embolus. The authors concluded that DVT was not a risk factor for PE. This study did not include all patients in whom a physician would suspect a possible PE but instead only included those with a high enough clinical suspicion of a PE to be referred for an angiogram. This is a form of selection bias. The presence of a DVT is a well known risk factor for a PE, and if diagnosed, could lead to direct treatment for a PE rather than an angiogram to make the diagnosis more certain. Therefore, patients suspected of having PE and who didn't have clinical signs of a DVT were more likely to be selected for the angiogram. Similarly, those DVT patients with no signs or symptoms of PE who were entered into the study only because they had a DVT wouldn't have a PE. This is a fatal flaw and would seriously skew the results, so the results of this study should not change a physician's approach to these patients.

Referral bias

Referral bias is a special form of selection bias. Studies performed in tertiary care or referral centers often use only patients referred for specialty care as subjects. This eliminates cases that are milder and more easily treated or those diagnosed at an earlier stage and who are more likely to be seen in a primary care provider's office. Overall, the subjects in the study are not like those patients with similar complaints seen in the primary care office, who will be much less likely to have unusual causes for their symptoms. This limits the external validity of the study and the results should not be generalized to all patients with the same complaint.

An example will help to understand referral bias. Patients presenting to a neurology clinic with headaches occurring days to weeks after apparently minor head traumas were given a battery of tests: CT scan of the head, EEG, MRI of the brain, and various psychological tests. Most of these tests were normal, but some of the MRIs showed minor abnormalities. Most of the patients with the abnormalities on the MRI had a brief loss of consciousness at the time of injury. The authors concluded that all patients with any loss of consciousness after minor head trauma should have immediate MRI scans done. This is an incorrect conclusion. The study patients reflected only those who were referred to the neurologist, who therefore had persistent problems from their head injury. The researchers did not measure the percentage of all patients with head injuries who had loss of consciousness for a brief period of time and who had the reported MRI abnormalities. The results, even if significant in this selected population, would not apply to the general population of all head-injured patients.

Spectrum bias

Spectrum bias occurs when only patients with classical or severe symptoms are selected for a study. This makes the expected outcomes more or less likely than for the population as a whole. For example, patients with definite subarachnoid hemorrhages (bleeding in or around the brain) who have the worst headache of their life and present with coma or a severe alteration of their mental status will almost all have a positive CT of their head showing the bleed. Those patients who have similar headaches but no neurological symptoms are much less likely to have a positive CT of the head. Selecting only those patients with severe symptoms will bias the study and make the results inapplicable to those with less severe symptoms.

Detection bias

Detection bias is a form of selection bias that preferentially includes patients in a study if they have been exposed to a particular risk factor. In these cases, exposure causes a sign or symptom that precipitates a search for the disease and then is blamed for causing the disease. Estrogen therapy was thought to be a risk factor for the development of endometrial cancer. Patients in a tumor registry who had cancer were compared to a similar group of women who were referred for dilatation and curettage (D&C) (diagnostic scraping of the uterine lining) or hysterectomy (removal of the uterus). The proportion of women taking estrogen was the same in both groups, suggesting no relationship between estrogen use and cancer of the uterus. However, many of the women in the D&C or hysterectomy group who were taking estrogen turned out to have uterine cancer. Did estrogen cause cancer? Estrogen caused the bleeding, which led to a search for a cause of the bleeding. This led to the use of a D&C, which subsequently detected uterine cancer in these patients. This and subsequent studies showed that there was a relationship between postmenopausal estrogen therapy and the development of this cancer.

Recall bias

Recall or **reporting bias** occurs most often in a retrospective study, either a case–control or non-concurrent cohort study. When asked about certain exposures, subjects with the outcome in the study are more likely than controls to recall the factors to which they were exposed. It is human nature to search for a reason for an illness, and patients with an illness will be much more aware of their exposures than those without an illness. This is a potential problem whenever subjective information is used to determine exposure and is less likely to occur when objective information is used. This is illustrated by a study that was performed looking for the connection of childhood leukemia to living under high-tension wires. Mothers of children with leukemia were more likely to remember living anywhere near a high-tension power line than were mothers who did not have a leukemic child. **Exposure suspicion bias** is a type of recall bias that occurs on the part of the researcher. When asking subject patients about exposure, researchers might phrase the question in ways that encourage recall bias in the study subjects. The control subjects similarly might be asked in subtly different ways that could make them less likely to recall the exposure.

Non-respondent bias

Non-respondent bias is a bias in the results of a study because of patients who don't respond to a survey or who drop out of a study. It occurs because those people who don't respond to a survey may be different in some fundamental way from those who do respond. The reasons for not responding are numerous, but may be related to the study. Past studies have noted that smokers are less likely than non-smokers to respond to a survey when it contains questions about smoking. This will lead to bias in the results of such a survey. It is also true that healthy people are more likely to participate in these surveys than unhealthy ones. In this case, the bias of having more healthy people in the study group will underestimate the apparent ill effects of smoking.

Membership bias

Membership bias occurs because the health of some group members differs in a systematic way from the general population. This is obvious when one group of subjects is chosen from members of a health club, has higher average education, or is from other groups that might intrinsically be more health-conscious than the average person. It is a problem with studies that look at nurses or physicians and attempt to extrapolate the results to the general population. Higher socio-economic status and generally more healthy living are factors that may distinguish these groups and limit generalizability to others in the population.

A recent review of all studies of thrombolytic therapy, the use of clot-dissolving medication to treat acute myocardial infarction, AMI or heart attacks, was conducted. The reviewers found that on average, patients who were eligible for the studies were younger and healthier than patients who either were ineligible for inclusion or not enrolled in the study but treated with these drugs anyway. Over-all, study patients got more intensive therapy for their AMI in many ways. The mortality for study patients was less than half that of ineligible patients and about two thirds that of non-study patients.

Berkerson's bias is a specific bias that occurs when patients in the control group are selected because they are patients in a selected ward of the hospital. These patients may share group characteristics that separate them from the normal population. This difference in baseline characteristics will affect the outcome of the study.

Bias in the measurements of the outcome

Subject bias

Subject bias is a constant distortion of the measurement by the subject. In general, patients try to please their doctors and will tell them what they think the doctor wants to hear. They also may consciously change their behavior or responses in order to please their physicians. They may not report some side effects, may overestimate the amount of medications taken and may report more improvement if they know they were given a therapy approved of by their doctor rather than the placebo or control therapy. Only effective blinding of subjects and ideally, also of observers, can prevent this bias from occurring.

Observer bias

Observer bias is the conscious or unconscious distortion in perception of reporting the measurement by an observer. It may occur when physicians treat patients differently because of the group to which they are assigned. Physicians in a study may give more intensive adjunctive treatment to the patients who are assigned to the intervention group rather than to the placebo or comparison group. They may interpret the answers to questions on a survey differently in patients known to be in the active treatment rather than control group. An observer not blinded to patient selection may report the results of one group of patients differently from those of the other group. One form of this bias occurs when patients who are the sickest may be either preferentially included or excluded from the sample because of bias on the part of the observer making the assignment to each group. This is known as **filtering** and is a form of selection bias.

Data collected retrospectively by reviewing the medical records may have poor data quality. The records used to collect data may contain inadequate detail and possess questionable reliability. They may also use varying and subjective standards to judge symptoms, signs of disease severity, or outcomes.

This is a common occurrence in chart review or retrospective case–control or non-concurrent cohort studies. The implicit review of charts introduces the researcher's bias in interpreting both measurements and outcomes. If there are no objective and explicit criteria for evaluating the medical records, the information contained in them is open to misinterpretation from the observer. It has been shown that when performing implicit chart reviews, researchers subconsciously fit the response that best matched their hypothesis. Researchers came up with different results if they performed a blinded chart review as opposed to an unblinded review. Explicit reviews are better and can occur when only clearly objective outcome measures are reviewed. Even when the outcomes are more objective it is better to have the chart material reviewed in a blinded manner.

The **Hawthorne effect** was first noticed during a study of work habits of employees in a light bulb factory in Illinois during the 1920s. It occurs because being observed during the process of making measurements changes the behavior of the subject. In the physical sciences, this is known as the Heisenberg Uncertainty Principle. If subjects change their behavior when being observed, the outcome will be biased. One study was done to see if physicians would prescribe less expensive antibiotics more often than expensive new ones for strep throat. In this case, the physicians knew that they were being studied and in fact, they prescribed many more of the low-price antibiotics during the course of the study. After the study was over, their behavior returned to baseline, thus they acted differently and changed their clinical practices when being observed. This and other observer biases can be prevented through the use of unobtrusive, blinded, or objective measurements.

Misclassification bias

Misclassification bias occurs when the status of patients or their outcomes is incorrectly classified. If a subject is given an inaccurate diagnosis, they will be counted with the wrong group, and may even be treated inappropriately due to their misclassifaction. This bias could then change the outcome of the study. For instance, in a study of antibiotic treatment of pneumonia, patients with bronchitis were misclassified as having pneumonia. Those patients were more likely to get better with or without antibiotics, making it harder to find a difference in the outcomes of the two treatment groups. Patients may also change their behaviors or risk factors after the initial grouping of subjects, resulting in misclassification bias on the basis of exposure. This bias is common in cohort studies.

Misclassification of outcomes in case control studies can result in failure to correctly distinguish cases from controls and lead to a biased conclusion. One must know how accurately the cases and controls are being identified in order to avoid this bias. If the disorder is relatively common, some of the control patients may be affected but not have the symptoms yet. One way of compensating for this bias is to dilute the control group with extra patients. This will reduce the extent to which misclassification of cases incorrectly counted as controls will affect the data.

Let's say that a researcher wanted to find out if people who killed themselves by playing Russian Roulette were more likely to have used alcohol than those who committed suicide by shooting themselves in the head. The researcher would look at death investigations and find those that were classified as suicides and those that were classified as Russian Roulette. However, the researcher suspects that some of the Russian Roulette cases may have been misclassified as suicides to "protect the victim." To compensate for this, or dilute the effect of the bias, the researcher decides that the control group will include three suicide deaths for every one Russian Roulette death. Obviously if Russian Roulette deaths are routinely misclassified, this strategy will not result in any change in the bias. This is called **outcome misclassification**. Outcome classification based upon subjective data including death certificates, is more likely to exhibit this misclassification. This will most likely result in an outcome that is of smaller size than the actual effect. This bias can be prevented with objective standards for classification of patients, which should be clearly outlined in the methods section of a study.

Miscellaneous sources of bias

Confounding

Confounding refers to the presence of several variables that could explain the apparent connection between the cause and effect. If a particular variable is present more often in one group of patients than in another, it may be responsible for causing a significant effect. For example, a study was done to look for the effect of antioxidant vitamin E intake on the outcome of cardiovascular disease. It turned out that the group with high vitamin E intake also had a lower rate of smoking, a higher socioeconomic status, and higher educational level than the groups with lower vitamin E intake. It is much more likely that those other variables are responsible for all or part of the decrease in observed cases of cardiovascular disease. There are statistical ways of dealing with confounding variables called **multivariate analyses**. The rules governing the application of these types of analyses are somewhat complex and will be discussed in greater detail in Chapter 14. When looking at studies always look for the potential presence of confounding variables and at least make certain that the authors have adjusted for those variables. However, no matter how well the authors have adjusted, it can be very difficult to completely remove the effects of confounding from a study.

Contamination and cointervention

Contamination occurs when the control group receives the same therapy as the experimental group. Contimination is more commonly seen in randomized clinical trials, but can also exist in observational studies. In an observational study, it occurs if the control group is exposed to the same risk factor as the study group. However, there may be an environmental situation by which those classified as not exposed to the risk factor are actually exposed. For example, a study is done to look at the effect of living near high-tension wires on the incidence of leukemia. Those patients who live within 30 miles of a high-tension wire are considered the exposed group and those who live more than 30 miles away are considered the unexposed control group. Those people who live 30 to 35 miles from high-tension wires could be misclassified as unexposed although they may truly have a similar degree of exposure as those within 30 miles. In fact, families living 60 miles from the wires may be equally affected by the electrical field if the wires have four times the amount of current.

Cointervention occurs when one group or the other receives different medical care based partly or totally upon their group assignment. This occurs more often in randomized trials, but could be present in an observational study when the group exposed to one particular treatment also receives different therapy than the unexposed group. This can easily occur in studies with historical controls, since patients in the past may not have had access to the same advances in medical care as the patients who are currently being treated. The end results of the historical comparison would be different if both groups had received the same level of medical care.

Patient attrition

Patient attrition occurs when patients drop out of a study or are lost to follow-up, leading to a loss of valuable information. Patients who drop out may do so because a treatment or placebo is ineffective or there are too many unwanted side effects. Therefore, it is imperative for researchers to account for all patients enrolled in the study. In practice a drop-out rate less than 20% is an acceptable level of attrition. However, even a lower rate of attrition may bias the study if the reason patients were lost from the study is directly related to one of the study variables. If there is a differential rate of attrition between the intervention and comparison groups, an even lower rate of attrition may be very important.

How the authors dealt with outcome measurements of subjects who dropped out, were lost to follow-up, or for whom the outcome is unknown is extremely important. These study participants cannot be ignored and left out of final data calculations; this will certainly introduce bias into the final results. In this instance, the data can be analyzed using a **best case/worst case** strategy, assuming that missing patients all had a poor outcome in one analysis and a good outcome in the other. The researcher can then compare the results obtained from each group and see if the loss of patients could have made a big difference.

For subjects who switch groups or don't complete therapy and for whom the outcome is known, an **intention-to-treat** strategy should be used. The final outcome of those patients who changed groups or dropped out of the study is analyzed with the group to which they were originally assigned. We will discuss the issues of attrition and intention to treat further in the chapter on the randomized clinical trial (Chapter 15).

External validity and surrogate markers

External validity refers to all problems in applying the study results to a larger or different population. External validity can be called into question when the subjects of a study are from only one small subgroup of the general population. Age, gender, ethnic or racial groups, socioeconomic groups, and cultural groups are examples of variables that can affect external validity. Simply having a clearly identified group of patients in a study does not automatically mean there will be lack of external validity. There ought to be an a-priori reason that the results could be different in other groups. For example, we know that women respond differently than men to various drugs. Therefore, a study of a particular drug performed only on men could lack external validity when it comes to recommending the drug to women. Overall, each study must be looked at separately and the reader must determine whether external validity exists.

Poor external validity can lead to inappropriate extrapolation or generalization of the results of a study to groups to which they do not apply. In a study of patients with myocardial infarction (MI), those who had frequent premature ventricular contractions (PVCs) had increased mortality in the hospital. This led to the recommendation that antiarrhythmic drugs to suppress the PVCs should be given to all patients with MI. Later studies found an increased number of deaths among patients on long-term antiarrhythmic drug therapy. Subsequent recommendations were that these drugs only be used to treat immediately life-threatening PVCs. The original study patients all had acute ischemia (lack of oxygen going to the heart muscle) while the long-term patients did not, making extrapolation to that population inappropriate.

The outcome chosen to be measured should be one that matters to the patient. Ideally it is a measure of faster resolution of the problem such as reduction of pain or death rate due to the illness. In these cases, all patients would agree that the particular outcome is important. However, there are studies that look at other outcomes. These may be important in the overall increase in medical knowledge, but not immediately important to an individual patient. In fact, these results, called **surrogate endpoints,** may not translate into improved health at all.

Suppose that a researcher wanted to see if there was any relationship between the timing of students' taking of Step I of the USMLE and their final score. The researcher would look at all of the scores and correlate them with the date the test is taken. The researcher finds that there is a strong association between board scores and date, with the higher scores occurring among students taking the boards at earlier dates. The study would conclude that medical students should be taking the boards as early as possible in the cycle. What the researcher might be missing is that the timing of taking the exam and the score are both dependent on another factor, class rank. Therefore the variable of timing of the USMLE is a surrogate marker for overall class rank.

Final concerns

There are a few more miscellaneous concerns for validity when evaluating outcome measurements. Are the measured outcomes those that are important to patients? Were all of the important outcomes included and reported upon or were only certain main outcomes of the research project included? If certain outcomes were measured to the exclusion of others, suspect foul play. A study may find a significant improvement in one outcome, for instance disease-free survival, while the outcome of importance for patients is overall survival, which shows no improvement. The problems associated with subgroup analysis and composite endpoints will be discussed in the chapter on Type I errors (Chapter 11).

There is a definite **publication bias** toward the publication of studies that show a positive result. Studies that show no effect or a negative result are more difficult to get published or may never be submitted for publication. Authors are aware of the decreased publication of negative studies, and as a result, it takes longer for negative studies to be written.

Chance can also lead to errors in the study conclusions. The action of chance error causes distortion of the study results in a random way. Researchers can account for this problem with the appropriate use of statistical tests, which will be addressed in the next several chapters.

Studies supported by or run by drug companies or other proprietary interests are inherently biased. Since these companies want their products to do well in clinical trials, the methods used to bias these studies can be quite subtle. Drug-company sponsorship should be a red flag to look more carefully for sources of bias in the study. In general, all potential conflicts of interest should be clearly stated in any medical study article. Many journals now have mandatory

Table 8.1. Looking for sources of bias: a checklist

Check the methods section for the following

(1) The methods for making all the measurements were fully described with a clearly defined protocol for making these measurements.

(2) The observers were trained to make the measurements and this training was adequately described and standardized.

(3) All measurements were made unobtrusively, the subjects were blinded to the measurement being made, and the observers (either the ones providing care or the ones making the measurements or interpreting the results) were blinded.

(4) Paired measurements were made (test–retest reliability) or averaged and intra-observer or inter-observer reliability of repeated measurements was measured.

(5) The measurements were checked against a known "gold standard" (the measurement accepted as being the truth) and checked for their validity either through citations from the literature or by a demonstration project in the current study. Readers may have to decide for themselves if a measurement has face validity. You will know more about this as you learn more background material about the subject.

(6) The reasons for inclusion and exclusion must be spelled out and appropriate.

(7) Patients who drop out or cross over must be clearly identified and the results appropriately adjusted for this behavior.

(8) The most appropriate outcome measure should be selected. Be suspicious of composite or surrogate outcome measures.

requirements that this be included and prominently displayed. However, as the examples below illustrate, there are still some problems with this policy.

In one case, Boots Pharmaceuticals, the maker of Synthroid, a brand of levothyroxine, a thyroid hormone commonly taken to replace low thyroid levels, sponsored a study of their thyroid hormone against generic thyroid replacement medication. The study was done at Harvard and when the researchers found that the two drugs were equivalent, they submitted their findings to *JAMA*. The company notified both Harvard and *JAMA* that they would sue them in court if the study were printed. Harvard and *JAMA* both stepped down and pulled the article. That news was leaked to the *Wall Street Journal*, which published an account of the study. Finally, Boots relented and allowed the study to be published in *JAMA*.

In the second case, a researcher at the Hospital for Sick Children in Toronto was the principal investigator in a study of a new drug to prevent the side effect of iron accumulation in children who needed to receive multiple transfusions. The drug appeared to be associated with severe side effects. When the researcher attempted to make this information known to authorities at the university, the company threatened legal action and the researcher was removed from the project. When other scientists at the university stood up to support the researcher, the researcher was fired. When the situation became public and the government stepped in, the researcher was rehired by the university, but in a lower position. The issues of conflict of interest in clinical research will be discussed in more detail in Chapter 16.

This chapter was an introduction to common sources of bias. Students must evaluate each study on its own merits. If readers think bias exists, one must be able to demonstrate how that bias could have affected the study results. For more information, there is an excellent article by Dr. David Sackett on sources of bias.[1] The accompanying checklist (Table 8.1) will help the novice reader identify potential sources of bias.

[1] D. L. Sackett. Bias in analytic research. *J. Chronic Dis.* 1979; 32: 51–63.

9

Review of basic statistics

There are three kinds of lies: lies, damned lies, and statistics.

Benjamin Disraeli, Earl of Beaconsfield (1804–1881)

Learning objectives

In this chapter you will learn:
- evaluation of graphing techniques
- measures of central tendency and dispersion
- populations and samples
- the normal distribution
- use and abuse of percentages
- simple and conditional probabilities
- basic epidemiological definitions

Clinical decisions ought to be based on valid scientific research from the medical literature. Useful studies consist of both epidemiological and clinical research. The competent interpreter of these studies must understand basic epidemiological and statistical concepts. Critical appraisal of the literature and good medical decision making require an understanding of the basic tools of probability.

What are statistics and why are they useful in medicine?

Nature is a random process. It is virtually impossible to describe the operations of a given biological system with a single, simple formula. Since we cannot measure all the parameters of every biological system we are interested in, we make approximations and deduce how often they are true. Because of the innate variation in biological organisms it is hard to tell real differences in a system from random variation or noise. Statistics seek to describe this randomness by telling us how much noise there is in the measurements we make of a system. By filtering out this noise, statistics allow us to approach a correct value of the underlying facts of interest.

Descriptive and inferential statistics

Descriptive statistics are concerned with the presentation, summarization, and utilization of data. These include techniques for graphically displaying the results of a study and mathematical indices that summarize the data with a few key numbers. These key numbers are **measures of central tendency** such as the **mean, median,** and **mode** and **measures of dispersion** such as **standard deviation, standard error of the mean, range, percentile,** and **quartile.**

In medicine, researchers usually study a small number of patients with a given disease, a **sample**. What researchers are actually interested in finding out is how the entire population of patients with that disease will respond. Researchers often compare two samples for different characteristics such as use of certain therapies or exposure to a risk factor to determine if these changes will be present in the population. **Inferential statistics** are used to determine whether or not any differences between the research samples are due to chance or if there is a true difference present. Also inferential statistics are used to determine if the data gathered can be generalized from the sample to a larger group of subjects or the entire population.

Visual display of data

The purpose of a graph is to display the data visually in a form that allows the observer to draw conclusions about the data. Although graphs seem straightforward, they can be deceptive. The reader is responsible for evaluating the accuracy and truthfulness of graphic representations of the data. There are several common features that should be present in a proper graph. Lack of these items can lead to deception.

First, there must be a well-defined zero point. Lack of zero point (Fig. 9.1) is always improper. A lack of a well-defined zero point makes small differences look bigger by emphasizing only the upper portion of the scale. It is proper to start at zero, break the line up with two diagonal hash marks just above the zero point, and then continue from a higher value (as in Fig. 9.2). This still exaggerates the changes in the graph, but now the reader is warned and will consider the results accordingly.

The axes of the graph should be relatively equally proportioned. **Lack of proportionality**, a much more subtle technique than lack of a well-defined zero, is also improper. It serves to emphasize the drawn-out axis relative to the other less drawn-out axis. This visually exaggerates smaller changes in the axis that is drawn to the larger scale (Fig. 9.3). Therefore, both axes should have their variables drawn to roughly the same scale (Fig. 9.4).

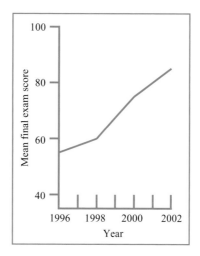

Fig. 9.1 Improper graph due to the lack of a defined zero point. This makes the change in mean final exam scores appear to be much greater (relatively) than they truly are.

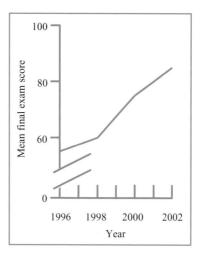

Fig. 9.2 Proper version of the graph in Figure 9.1 created by putting in a defined zero point. Although the change in mean final exam scores still appears to be relatively greater than they truly are, the reader is notified that this distortion is occurring.

Another deceptive graphing technique can be seen in some pharmaceutical advertisements. This consists of the use of three-dimensional shapes to demonstrate the difference between two groups, usually the effect of a drug on a patient outcome. One example uses cones of different heights to demonstrate the difference between the endpoint of therapy for the drug produced by the company and its closest competitor. The height of each cone is the percentage of patients responding in each group. Visually, the cones represent a larger volume than simple bars or even triangles, making the drug being advertised look like it caused a much larger effect. For more information on deceptive graphing techniques, please refer to E.R. Tufte's classic book on graphing.[1]

[1] E. R. Tufte. *The Visual Display of Quantitative Information.* Cheshire, CT: Graphics Press, 1983.

Fig. 9.3 Improper graph due to the lack of proportionality of the x and y axes. This makes it appear as if the change in mean final exam scores occurred over a much shorter time period than in reality.

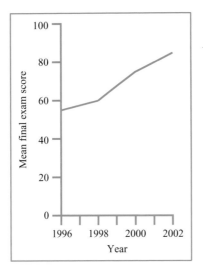

Fig. 9.4 Proper graph with proportioned x and y axes, giving a true representation of the rise in exam scores gradually over time.

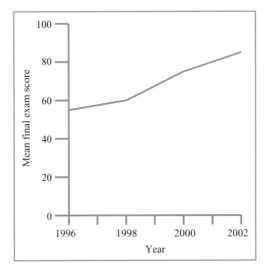

Types of graph

Stem-and-leaf plots

Stem-and-leaf plots are shortcuts used as preliminary plots for graphs called simple histograms. The stem is made up of the digits on the left side of each value (tens, hundreds, or higher) and the leaves are the digits on the right side (units, or lower) of each number. Let's take, for example, the following grades on a hypothetical statistics exam:

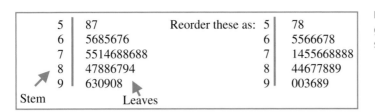

Fig. 9.5 Stem-and-leaf plot of grades in a hypothetical statistics exam.

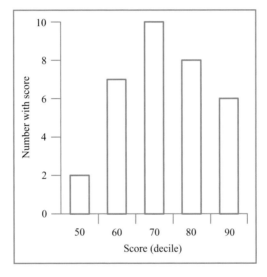

Fig. 9.6 Bar graph of the data in Fig. 9.5.

96 93 84 75 75 71 65 74 58 87 66 90 76 68 65 78 78 66 76 88 99 88 78
90 86 98 67 66 87 57 89 84 78

In this example, the first digit forms the stem and the second digit, the leaves. In creating the stem-and-leaf plot, first list the tens digits, and then next to them all the units digits which have that 'tens' digit in common. Our example becomes the stem-and-leaf plot in Fig. 9.5.

This can be rotated 90° counterclockwise and redrawn as a bar graph or histogram. The x-axis shows the categories, the tens digits in our example, and the y-axis shows the number of observations in each category. The y-axis can also show the percentages of the total that each observation occurs in each category. This shows the relationship between the independent variable, in this case the exam scores, and the dependent variable, in this instance the number of students with a score in each 10% increment of grades.

Fig. 9.7 Histogram of the data in
Fig. 9.5.

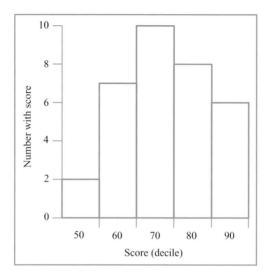

Bar graphs, histograms, and frequency polygons

The most common types of graphs used in the medical articles are bar graphs, histograms, and frequency polygons. The **bar graph** (Fig. 9.6) that would represent the data in our previous stem-and-leaf plot is drawn by replacing the numbers with bars. A **histogram** is a bar graph in which the bars touch each other (Fig. 9.7). As a rule, the author should attempt to make the contrast between bars on a histogram as clear as possible. A **frequency polygon** shows how often each observation occurs (Fig. 9.8 is a frequency polygon of the data in Fig. 9.5). A cumulative frequency polygon (Fig. 9.9) shows how the number of accumulated events is distributed. Here the y-axis is usually the percentage of the total events.

Box-and-whisker plots

Box-and-whisker plots (Fig. 9.10) are common ways to represent the range of values for a single variable. The central line in the box is the median, the middle value of the data as will be described below. The box edges are the 25th and 75th percentile values and the lines on either side represent the limits of 95% of the data. The stars represent extreme outliers.

Measures of central tendency and dispersion

There are two numerical measures that describe a data set, the central tendency and the dispersion. There are three measures of central tendency, describing the center of a set of variables: the mean, median, and mode.

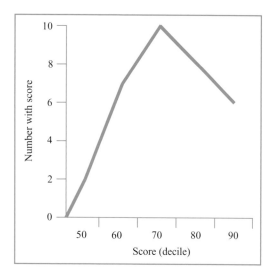

Fig. 9.8 Frequency polygon of the data in Fig. 9.5.

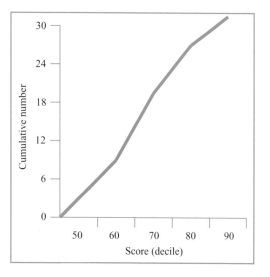

Fig. 9.9 Cumulative frequency polygon of the data in Fig. 9.5.

The **mean** (μ or $\bar{x}$) is the arithmetical center, commonly called the arithmetic average. It is the sum of all measurements divided by the number of measurements. Mathematically, $\mu = (\Sigma x_i)/n$. In this equation, x_i is the numerical value of the i th data point and n is the total number of data points. The mean is strongly effected by **outliers**. These are extreme numbers on either the high or low end of the distribution that will produce a high degree of skew. There will not be a truly representative central value if the data are highly skewed and the mean can misstate the data. It makes more sense to

Fig. 9.10 Box-and-whisker plot
of scores on the statistics test by
student height.

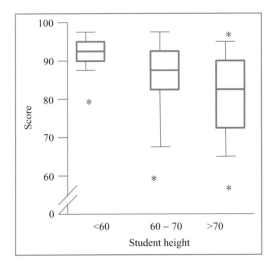

use the median if this is the case. The mean should not be used for ordinal data and is meaningless in that setting unless the ordinal data has been shown to behave like continuous data in a symmetrical distribution. This is a common error and may invalidate the results of the experiment or portray them in a misleading manner.

The **median** (M) is the middle value of a set of data points. There are the same number of data points above and below M. For an even number of data points, M, is the average of the two middle values. The median is less affected by outliers and by data that are highly skewed. It should be used when dealing with ordinal variables or when the data are highly skewed. There are special statistical tests for dealing with these types of data.

The **mode** is the most common value or the one value with the largest number of data points. It is used for describing nominal and ordinal data and is rarely used in clinical studies.

There are several ways to describe the degree of dispersion of the data. The common ones are the range, percentiles, variance, and standard deviation. The standard error of the mean is a measure that describes the dispersion of a group of samples.

The **range** is simply the highest value to the lowest value. It gives an overview of the data spread around a central value. It should be given whenever there is either a large spread of data values with many outliers or when the range is asymmetrical about the value of central tendency. It also should be given with ordinal data.

Quartiles divide the data into fourths, and **percentiles** into hundredths. The lowest quarter of values lie below the lower quartile or 25th percentile, the lower half below the 50th percentile, and the lowest three-quarters below the upper quartile or 75th percentile. The **interquartile range** is the range of values from the 25th to the 75th percentile values.

The **variance** (σ^2 or s^2) is a statistical measure of variation. It is the average of the squares of the difference between each value and the mean or the sum of the squares of the difference between each value and the mean divided by n (the number of data points in the sample). It is often divided by $n - 1$, and either method is correct. This assumes a normal distribution of the variables (see below). Mathematically, $s^2 = (\Sigma (x_i - \mu)^2)/(n - 1)$. The **standard deviation** (SD, s, or σ) is simply the square root of the variance.

The **standard error of the mean** (SEM) is the standard deviation of the means of multiple samples that are all drawn from the same population. If the population size is greater than 30 and the distribution is normal, the SEM is estimated by the equation $\mathbf{SEM = SD/\sqrt{n}}$, (where n is sample size).

Populations and samples

A **population** is the set of all possible members of the group being studied. The members of the population have various attributes in common and the more characteristics they have in common, the more homogeneous and therefore restrictive the population. An example of a fairly restricitive population would be all white males between 40 and 65 years of age. With a restrictive population, the **generalizability** of the population is often a problem. The less the members of the sample have in common, the more generalizable the results of data gathered for that population. For example, a population that included all males is more generalizable than one that only includes white males between 40 and 65 years of age. The population size is symbolized by capital N.

A **sample** is a subset of the population chosen for a specific reason. An example could be all white males available to the researcher on a given day for a study. Reasons to use a sample rather than the entire population include **convenience**, **time**, **cost**, and **logistics**. The sample may or may not be representative of the entire population, an issue which has been discussed in the chapter on sources of bias (Chapter 8). The sample size is symbolized by lower-case n.

Histograms or frequency polygons show how many subjects in a sample or population (the y-axis) have a certain characteristic value (the x-axis). When plotted in this manner, we call the graph a distribution of values for the given sample. Distributions can be symmetrical or skewed. By definition, a **symmetrical** distribution is one for which the mean, median, and mode are identical. Many curves or distributions of variables are asymmetrical. **Skew** describes the degree to which the curve is asymmetrical. Figures 9.11 and 9.12 show symmetrical and skewed distributions. They are said to be skewed to the right (positive

Fig. 9.11 Symmetrical curve. Mean, median, and mode are the same.

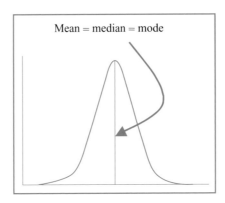

Fig. 9.12 Skewed curve (to the right). Mode<median<mean.

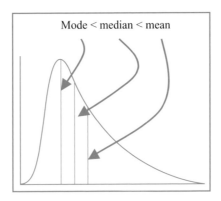

Fig. 9.13 Curve with skew to the right (positive skew).

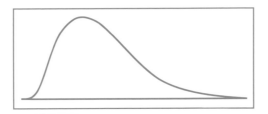

skew, Fig. 9.13) when the outlier values are to the right side or positive side of the bulk of the data. Those skewed left or with negative skew (Fig. 9.14) have the extreme values to the left of, or negative relative to, the majority of the data points. Skew should be discussed when presenting and evaluating data and the range of the data given in addition to the standard measures of central tendency and dispersion. One clue to the presence of skewed data is if twice the standard deviation is larger than the mean. The mathematical measures used to describe data are different for skewed distributions than for symmetrical ones.

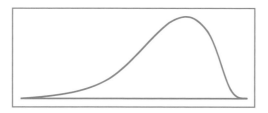

Fig. 9.14 Curve with skew to the left (negative skew).

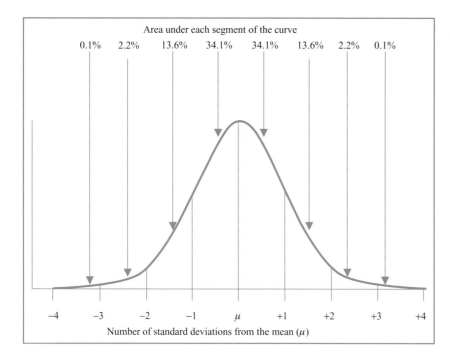

Fig. 9.15 The normal distribution.

The normal distribution

The Gaussian or normal distribution (Fig. 9.15) is also called the bell-shaped curve. It is named after Carl Frederick Gauss, a German mathematician. However, he did not discover the bell-shaped curve. Abraham de Moivre, a French mathematician, discovered it about 50 years before Gauss published his thesis. It is a special case of a symmetrical distribution, and it describes the frequency of occurrence of many naturally occurring phenomena. For the purposes of most statistical tests, we assume normality in the distribution of a variable. It is better defined by giving its properties:

(1) The mean, median, and mode are equal so that we can say that the curve is **symmetric** around the mean and not skewed or has a skew = 0.

Table 9.1. Properties of the normal distribution

(1) One standard deviation ($\pm$ 1 SD) on either side of the mean encompasses 68.2% of the population
(2) Two standard deviations ($\pm$ 2 SD) is an additional 27.2% (95.4% of total)
(3) Three ($\pm$ 3 SD) is an additional 4.4% (99.8% of total)
(4) Four ($\pm$ 4 SD) is an additional 0.2% (99.99% of total)
(5) Five ($\pm$ 5 SD) includes (essentially) everyone (99.9999% of total)

(2) The tails of the curve approach the x-axis asymptotically, that is they get closer and closer to the x-axis as you move away from the mean and they never quite reach it no matter how far you go.

There are specific numerical equivalents to the standard deviations of the normal distribution, as shown in Table 9.1. For all practical purposes **68%** of the population are within one standard deviation of the mean ($\pm$ 1 SD), **95%** are within two standard deviations of the mean ($\pm$ 2 SD), and **99%** are within three standard deviations of the mean ($\pm$ 3 SD). The 95% interval ($\pm$ 2 SD) is a range commonly referred to as the normal range or the Gaussian definition of the normal range. The normal distribution is the basis of most statistical tests and concepts we will use in critical interpretation of the statistics used in the medical literature.

Percentages

Percentages are commonly used in reporting results in the medical literature. Percentage improvement or percentage of patients who achieve one of two dichotomous endpoints are the preferred method of reporting the results. These are commonly called **event rates**. A percentage is a ratio or fraction, the numerator divided by the denominator, multiplied by 100 to create a whole number. Obviously, inaccuracies in either the numerator or denominator will result in inaccuracy of the percentage.

Percentages can be misleading in two important ways. **Percent of a percent** will usually show a very large result, even when there is only a small absolute change in the variables. Consider two drugs, we'll call them t-PA and SK, which have different mortality rates. In a particular study, the mortality rate for patients given t-PA was 7%, which is referred to as the experimental event rate (EER) while the mortality for SK was 8%, which is the control event rate (CER). The absolute difference, called the absolute risk reduction, is calculated as ARR = |EER – CER| and is 1% in this example. The relative improvement in mortality, referred to as the relative risk reduction, is calculated by RRR = |EER – CER|/CER) is (1/8 × 100% = 12.5%, a much larger and more impressive number than the 1% ARR.

Using the latter without prominently acknowledging the former is misleading and is a commonly used technique in pharmaceutical advertisements.

The second misleading technique is called the **percentages of small numbers,** and can be misleading in a more subtle way. In this case, the percentage is most likely to be simply inaccurate. Twenty percent of ten subjects seems like a large number, yet represents only two subjects. For example, the fact that those two subjects had an adverse reaction to a drug could have occurred simply by chance and the percentage could be much lower ($< 1\%$) or higher ($> 50\%$) when the same intervention is studied in a larger sample of the population. To display these results properly when there are only a small number of subjects in a study, the percentage may be given as long as the overall numbers are also given with equal prominence. The best way to deal with this is through the use of confidence intervals, which will be discussed in the next chapter.

Probability

Probability tells you the likelihood that a certain event will or will not occur relative to all possible related events of interest. Mathematically it is expressed as the number of times the event of interest occurs divided by the number of times all possible related events occur. This can be written as $P(x) = n_x/N$ where $P(x)$ is the probability of an event x occurring in a total of N possible outcome events. In this equation, n_x is the number of times x occurs. The letter P (or p) symbolizes probability. For flipping a coin once, the probability of a head is $P(\text{head})$. This is calculated as $P(\text{head}) = 1/2,$ **or** the outcome of interest (one head)/the total number of possible outcomes of the coin toss (one head plus one tail).

Two events are said to be **independent**, not to be confused with the independent variable of an experiment, when the occurrence of one of the events does not depend on the occurrence of the other event. In other words, the two events occur by independent mechanisms. The toss of a coin is a perfect example. Each toss is an independent event. The previous toss has no influence on the next one. Since the probability of a head on one toss is 1/2, if the same coin is tossed again, the probability of flipping a head does not change. It is still 1/2. The probability will continue to be 1/2 no matter how many heads or tails are thrown, unless of course, the coin is rigged.

Similarly, events are said to be **dependent**, not to be confused with the dependent variable of an experiment, if the probability of one event affects the outcome of the other. An example would be the probability of first drawing a red ball and then a yellow ball from a jar of colored balls, without replacing the one you drew out first. This means that the probabilities of selecting one or another colored ball will change each time one is selected and removed from the jar.

Events are said to be **mutually exclusive** if the occurrence of one absolutely precludes the occurrence of the other. For example, gender in humans is a mutually exclusive property. If someone is a biological male they cannot also be a biological female. Another example is a coin flip. Heads or tails obtained on the flip of a coin are mutually exclusive events as a coin will only land on the head or tail.

Conditional probability allows us to calculate complex probabilities, such as the probability that one event occurs given that another event has occurred. If the two events are a and b, the notation for this is $P(a \mid b)$. This is read as "the probability of event a if event b occurs." The vertical line means "conditional upon." This construct can be used to calculate otherwise complex probabilities in a very simple manner.

If two events are mutually exclusive, the probability that either event occurs can be easily calculated. The probability that **event a or event b** occurs is simply the sum of the two probabilities. $P(a \text{ or } b) = P(a) + P(b)$. The probability of a head or a tail occurring when a coin is flipped is $P(\text{head}) + P(\text{tail})$, which is $1/2 + 1/2 = 1$, or a certain event. Similarly, the probability that **event a and event b** occurs is the product of the two probabilities. $P(a \text{ and } b) = P(a) \times P(b)$. The probability of getting two heads on two flips of a coin is $P(\text{head on 1st flip}) \times P(\text{head on 2nd flip})$ which is $1/2 \times 1/2 = 1/4$.

Determining the probability that at least one of several mutually exclusive events will occur is a bit more complex, but the above rules allow us to make this a simple calculation: **$P(\text{at least one event will occur}) = 1 - P(\text{none of the events will occur})$**. We can calculate $P(\text{none of the events occurring}) = P(\text{not } a) \times P(\text{not } b) \times P(\text{not } c) \times \cdots$ For example, if we want to know the probability of getting at least one head in three flips of a coin, we could calculate the probability of getting one head, two heads, and three heads and add them up, then subtract the probabilities of events that overlap, in this case getting two heads and one tail can be done three ways with three coins. Using the above rule, the probability of at least one head is $1 - P(\text{no heads})$. The probability of no heads is the probability of three tails $(1/2)^3 = 1/2 \times 1/2 \times 1/2 = 1/8$, thus making the probability of at least one head $1 - 1/8 = 7/8$. This is an important concept in the evaluation of the statistical significance of the results of studies and the interpretation of simple lab tests.

Many lab tests use the Gaussian distribution to define the normal values. This considers ± 2 SD as the cutoff point for normal vs. abnormal results. This means that 95% of the population will have a normal result and 5% will have an abnormal result. Physicians routinely do a number of tests at once, such as a Complete Metabolic Profile, SMA-C, or SMA-20. What is the significance of one abnormal result out of the 20 tests ordered in these panels? We want to know the probability that a normal person will have at least one abnormal lab test in a panel of 20 tests by chance alone. The probability that each test will be normal is 95%. Therefore, the probability that all the tests are normal is $(0.95)^{20} = 0.36$. Then, the

Table 9.2. Commonly used probabilities in epidemiology

Prevalence	Probability of the presence of disease: number of existing cases of a disease/total population
Incidence	Probability of the occurrence of new disease: number of new cases of a disease/total population
Attack rate	A specialized form of incidence relating to a particular epidemic, expressed as a percentage: the number of new cases of a disease/number of persons exposed in the outbreak under surveillance
Crude mortality rate	Number of deaths for a given time period and place/mid-period population during the same time period and at the same place
Age-specific mortality rate	Number of deaths in a particular age group/total population of the same age group in the same period of time, using the mid-period population
Infant mortality rate	Deaths in infants under 1 year of age/total number of live births
Neonatal mortality rate	Deaths in infants under 28 days of age/total number of live births
Perinatal mortality rate	(Stillbirths + deaths in infants under 7 days of age)/(total number of live births + total number of stillbirths)
Maternal mortality rate	All pregnancy related deaths/total number of live births.

probability that at least one test is abnormal becomes $1 - 0.36 = 0.64$. This means that there is a 64% chance that a normal person will have at least one abnormal test result that occurred purely by chance alone, when in reality that person is normal.

Basic epidemiology

Epidemiology is literally the study of epidemics, but is commonly used to describe the study of disease in populations. Many of the studies that medical students will learn how to evaluate are epidemiological studies. On a very simplistic level, epidemiology describes the probability of certain events occurring in a population (Table 9.2). These probabilities are described in terms of rates. This could be a rate of exposure to a toxin, disease, disability, death, or any other important outcome. In medicine, rates are usually expressed as number of cases per unit of population. The unit of population most commonly used is 100 000, although other numbers can be used. The rates can also be expressed as percentages.

The **prevalence** of disease is the percentage of the population that has existing cases of the disease at a given time. It is the probability that a given person in this population has the disease of interest. It is calculated as the number of cases of a disease divided by the total population at risk for the disease. The number of new cases and the resolution of existing cases affect prevalence. Prevalence increases as the number of new cases increases and as the mortality rate decreases.

The **incidence** of a disease is the number of new cases of the disease for a given unit of population in a given unit of time. It is the probability of the occurrence of a new patient with that disease. It is the number of new cases in a given time period divided by the total population. Incidence is only affected by the occurrence of new cases of disease. The occurrence of new cases can be influenced by factors such as mass exposure to a new infectious agent or a change in the diet of the society.

The **mortality rate** is the incidence or probability of death in a certain time period. It is the number of people who die within a certain time divided by the entire population at risk of death during that time.

An excellent resource for learning more statistics is a CD-ROM called *ActivStats*,[2] a review of basic statistics and probability. There is also an electronic textbook called StatSoft,[3] which includes some good summaries of basic statistical information.

[2] P. Velleman. *ActivStats 3.0*. Ithaca, NY: Data Description, 2006.
[3] StatSoft. www.statsoftinc.com/textbook/stathome.html.

10

Hypothesis testing

Medicine is the science of uncertainty and the art of probability.

Sir William Osler (1849–1919)

Learning objectives

In this chapter you will learn:
- steps in hypothesis testing
- potential errors of hypothesis testing
- how to calculate and describe the usage of control event rates (CER), experimental event rates (EER), relative rate reduction (RRR), and absolute rate reduction (ARR)
- the concepts underlying statistical testing

Interpretation of the results of clinical trials requires an understanding of the statistical processes used to analyze data. Intelligent readers of the medical literature must be able to interpret these results and determine for themselves if they are important enough to use for their patients.

Introduction

Hypothesis testing is the foundation of the scientific method. Roger Bacon suggested the beginnings of this process in the thirteenth century. Sir Francis Bacon further defined it in the fifteenth century, and it was first regularly used in scientific research in the eighteenth and nineteenth centuries. It is a process by which new scientific information is added to previously discovered facts and processes. Previously held beliefs can be tested to determine their validity, and expected outcomes of a proposed new intervention can be tested against a previously used intervention. If the result of the experiment shows that the newly thought-up hypothesis is true, then researchers can design a new experiment to further

Table 10.1. Steps in hypothesis testing

(1) Gather background information
(2) State hypothesis
(3) Formulate null hypothesis (H_0)
(4) Design a study
(5) Decide on a significance level (α)
(6) Collect data on a sample
(7) Calculate the sample statistic (P)
(8) Reject or accept the null hypothesis (by comparing P to α)
(9) Begin all over again, step 1

increase our knowledge. If the hypothesis being tested is false, it is "back to the drawing board" to come up with a new hypothesis (Table 10.1).

The hypothesis

A **hypothesis** is a statement about how the study will relate the predictors, cause or independent variable, and outcomes, effect or dependent variable. For example, a study is done to see if taking aspirin reduces the rate of death among patients with myocardial infarction (heart attack). The hypothesis is that there is a relationship between daily intake of aspirin and a reduction in the risk of death caused by myocardial infarction. Another way to state this hypothesis is that there is a reduced death rate among myocardial infarction patients who are taking aspirin. This is a statement of what is called the **alternative hypothesis** (H_a or H_1). The alternative hypothesis states that a difference does exist between two groups or there is an association between the predictor and outcome variables. The alternative hypothesis cannot be tested directly by using statistical methods.

The **null hypothesis** (H_0) states that no difference exists between groups or there is no association between predictor and outcome variables. In our example, the null hypothesis states that there is no difference in death rate due to myocardial infarction between those patients who took aspirin daily and those who did not. The null hypothesis is the basis for formal testing of statistical significance. By starting with the proposition that there is no association, statistical tests estimate the probability that an observed association occurred due to chance alone. The customary scientific approach is to accept or reject the null hypothesis. Rejecting the null hypothesis is a vote in favor of the alternative hypothesis, which is then accepted by default.

The only knowledge that can be derived from statistical testing is the probability that the null hypothesis was falsely rejected. Therefore the validity of the alternative hypothesis is accepted by exclusion if the test of statistical significance rejects the null hypothesis. For statisticians, the reference point for significance of the results is the probability that the null hypothesis is rejected when in fact the null hypothesis is true and there really is no difference between groups. This appears to be a lot of double talk, but is actually the way statisticians talk. The goal is for this to occur less than 5% of the time ($P < 0.05$) which is the basis to the usual definition of statistical significance, $P < 0.05$. The letter P stands for the probability of obtaining the observed difference or effect size between groups by chance if in reality the null hypothesis is true and there is no difference between the groups. In other words, the probability of falsely rejecting the null hypothesis.

Where did this 5% notion come from and what does it mean statistically? Sir Ronald Fisher, a twentieth-century British mathematician and founder of modern statistics one day said it, and since he was the expert it stuck. He reasoned that "if the probability of *such an event (falsely rejecting the null hypothesis)* were sufficiently small – say, 1 chance in 20, then one might regard the result as significant." Prior to this, a level of $P = 0.0047$ (or one chance in 212) had been accepted as the level of significance.

His reasoning was actually pretty sound, as the following experiment shows. How much would you bet on the toss of a coin? You pay $1.00, or £1.00 in Sir Ronnie's experiment, if tails come up and you get paid the same amount if it's heads. How many tails in a row would you tolerate before beginning to suspect that the coin is rigged? Sir Ronald reasoned that in most cases the answer would be about four or five tosses. The probability of four tails in a row is $(1/2)^4$ or 1 in 16, and for five tails in a row $(1/2)^5$ or 1 in 32. One in 20 (5%) is about halfway between.[1] Is it coincidental that 95% of the population corresponds almost exactly to ± 2 SD of the normal distribution? It is sobering to realize that in experimental physics, the usual P value is 0.0001 as physicists want to be really sure where a particular subatomic particle is or what its mass or momentum are before telling the press. There is always talk in biomedical research circles, usually by pharmaceutical or biotech companies, that the level of significance of 0.05 is too low and should be increased to 0.1. This means that we would accept one chance in ten that the difference found was not true and only occurred by chance! This would be a poor decision, and the reasoning why will be evident by the end of this book.

Errors in hypothesis testing

The results of a clinical study are tested by application of a statistical test to the experimental results. The researcher asks the question "what is the probability that the difference between groups that I found was obtained purely by chance,

---

[1] From G. R. Norman & D. L. Streiner. *Biostatistics: The Bare Essentials.* St Louis: Mosby, 1994.

	Is the study actually valid?	
	Actually is a positive result (absolute truth)– H_0 actually false	Actually is a negative result (absolute truth)– H_0 actually true
Experiment found positive results – H_0 found to be false	Correct conclusion (Power = $1 - \beta$)	Type I error α
Experiment found negative results – H_0 found to be true	Type II error β	Correct conclusion

and that there is actually no difference between the two groups?" Statistical tests are able to calculate this probability.

In general there are four possible outcomes of a study. These are shown in Fig. 10.1. They compare the result found in the study with the actual state of things. The universal truth cannot always be determined, and this is what's referred to as **clinical uncertainty**. Researchers can only determine how closely they are approaching this universal truth by using statistical tests.

A **Type I error** occurs when the null hypothesis is rejected even though it is really true. In other words, concluding that there is a difference or association when in actuality there is not. This is also called a **false positive** study result. There are many ways in which a Type I error can occur in a study, and the reader must be aware of these since the writer will rarely point them out. Often the researcher will spin the results to make them appear more important and significant than the study actually supports. Manipulation of variables using techniques such as data dredging, snooping or mining, one-tailed testing, subgroup analysis, especially if done post hoc, and composite-outcome endpoints may result in the occurrence of this type of error.

A **Type II error** occurs when the null hypothesis is not rejected even though it is really false. In other words, the researcher concludes that there is not a difference when in reality there is. This is also called a **false negative** study result. An example would be concluding there is no relationship between hyperlipidemia and coronary artery disease when there truly is a relationship. **Power** represents the ability of the study to detect a difference when it exists. By convention the power of a study should be greater than 80% to be considered adequate. Think of an analogy to the microscope. As the power of the microscope increases, smaller differences between cells can be detected.

A Type II error can only be made in negative clinical trials or those trials that report no statistically significant difference between groups or no association between cause and effect. Therefore, when reading negative clinical trials, one needs to assess the chance that a Type II error occurred. This is important because a negative result may not be due to the lack of an effect but simply because of low power or the inability to detect the effect. From an interpretation perspective, the question one asks is "for a given Type II error level and an effect difference that I consider clinically important, did the researcher use a large enough sample size"? Both of these concepts will be discussed in more detail in the next two chapters.

Type III and IV errors are not usually found in biostatistical or epidemiological textbooks and yet are extremely common. **Type III** errors are those that compare the intervention to the wrong comparator, such as a drug that is not usually used for the problem or the incorrect dose of a drug. This is fairly common in the literature and includes studies of new drugs against placebo instead of older drugs. Studies of drugs for acute treatment of migraine headaches may be done against drugs that are useful for that indication, but in doses that are inadequate for the management of the pain. The reader must have a working knowledge of the standard therapy and determine if the new intervention is being tried against the best current therapy. Studies of new antibiotics are often done against an older antibiotic that is no longer used as standard therapy.

Type IV errors are those in which the wrong study was done. For example, a new antiviral drug for influenza is tested against placebo. The drug should at least have been tested against an old antiviral drug previously shown to be effective, and not against placebo, which is a Type III error. But, since the current standard is prevention in the form of influenza vaccine, the correct study should in fact have been comparing the new drug against the strategy of prevention with vaccine. This is a much more complex study, but would really answer the question posed about the drugs. Any study of a new treatment should be compared to the effect of both currently available standard therapies and prevention programs.

Effect size

The actual results of the measurements showing a difference between groups are given in the results section of a scientific paper. There are many different ways to express the results of a study. The **effect size,** commonly called δ, is the magnitude of the outcome, association, or difference between groups that one observes. This result can be given either as an absolute or as a relative number. It often can be expressed as either an absolute difference or the percentage with the outcome in each group or the event rate.

The expression of the results will be different for different types of data. The effect size for outcomes that are dichotomous can be expressed as percentages that achieved the result of interest in each of the groups. When continuous outcomes are evaluated, the mean and standard deviations of two or more groups can be compared. If the distribution of values is skewed, the range should also be given. A statistical test will then calculate the P value for the difference between the two mean values, and will show the probability that the difference found occurred by chance alone. If the measure is an ordinal number, the median is the measure that should be compared. In that case, special statistical methods can be used to determine the P value for the difference found.

The **clinically significant** effect size is the difference that is estimated to be important in clinical practice. It is statistically easier to detect a large effect like one representing a 90% change than a small effect like one representing a 2% change. Therefore, it should be easier to detect a difference which is likely to be clinically important. However, if the sample size is very large, even a small effect size may be detected. This effect size may not be clinically important even though it is **statistically significant**. This concept will be addressed in more detail later.

Event rates

In any study, researchers are interested in how many events of interest happen within each of two treatment groups. The outcome of interest must be a dichotomous variable for this set of calculations. The most common varilables are survival, admission to the hospital, patients who had relief of pain, or patients who were cured of infection. Usually a positive outcome such as survival or cure is used. However, a negative outcome such as death can also be used. The reader ought to be able to clearly determine the outcome being measured and the differences between the groups are usually expressed as percentages. The **control group** consists of those subjects treated with placebo, comparison, or the current standard therapy. The **experimental group** consists of those subjects treated with the experimental therapy. For studies of risk, the control group is those not exposed to the risk factor, while the experimental group is those exposed to the risk factor being studied.

The rate of success or failure can be calculated for each group. The **control event rate** (**CER**) is the percentage of control patients who have the outcome of interest. Similarly, the **experimental event rate** (**EER**) is the percentage of experimental patients who have the outcome of interest. The absolute difference between the two is the **absolute rate reduction** (**ARR**). Similarly, the **relative rate reduction** (**RRR**) is the percentage of the difference between the groups. This is the difference between the two outcome rates as a percentage of one of the event rates, usually by convention, the CER. This is, in fact, a percentage of a percentage and the reader must be careful when interpreting this result. The RRR always overestimates the effect of therapy when compared with the ARR (Fig. 10.2).

	Events of interest	Other events	Totals
Control or placebo group	A	B	CE = Control group events
Experimental group	C	D	EE = Experimental group events

Formulas

CER = control patients with outcome of interest / total control patients = A/CE

EER = experimental patients with outcome of interest / total experimental patients = C/EE

ARR = |CER – EER| RRR = |CER – EER|/CER

Fig. 10.2 Event rates.

Confidence = $\sqrt{n}$ × (signal / noise)

Where the signal is the event rate, the noise is the standard deviation, and n is the sample size

SEM = $\sigma/\sqrt{n}$

where n is the sample size and σ is the standard deviation

Fig. 10.3 Confidence and standard error of the mean (SEM).

Signal-to-noise ratio

Nearly all commonly used statistical tests are based on the concept of the signal-to-noise ratio. The **signal** is the relationship the researcher is interested in and the **noise** represents random error. Statistical tests determine how much of the difference between two groups is likely due to random noise and how much is likely due to systematic or real differences in the results of interest. The statistical measure of noise for continuous variables is the standard deviation or standard error of the mean (Fig. 10.3).

The confidence of the statistical results of a study can be expressed as proportional to the signal times the square root of the sample size (n) divided by the noise. Confidence is analogous to the power of a study. The signal is the effect size and the noise is the standard deviation of the effect size. Confidence in a particular result increases when the strength of the signal or effect size increases. It also increases as the noise level or standard deviation decreases. Finally, it increases as the sample size increases, but only in proportion to the square root of the sample size. To double the confidence, you must quadruple the sample size. Remember this relationship when evaluating study results.

Standard deviation tells the reader how close individual scores cluster around their mean value. A related number, the standard error of the mean (SEM) tells the reader how close the mean scores from repeated samples will be to the true

Fig. 10.4 The 95% confidence
intervals (95% CI).

$$95\% \ CI = \mu \pm Z_{95\%} \ (\sigma/\sqrt{n})$$

Where $Z_{95\%} = 1.96$ (the number of standard deviations which defines 95% of the data),
$\sigma/\sqrt{n} = SEM$, and $\mu = mean$

Therefore, $95\% \ CI = \mu \pm 1.96(SEM)$

population mean. This is the mathematical basis for many statistical tests. There are some limitations on the use of SEM. It should not be used to describe the dispersion of data in a sample. The standard deviation does this and using SEM is dishonest since it under-represents differences between groups. The SEM is a measure of the variability of the sample means if the study were repeated. For all practical purposes, the SEM is the standard deviation of the means of all the possible samples taken from the population. The 95% confidence interval may be calculated from the SEM and the clearest way to report variation in a study would be simply to show the 95% confidence intervals. A more detailed explanation of standard deviation and SEM can be found in an excellent article by David Streiner.[2]

Confidence intervals

Confidence intervals (CI) are another way to represent the level of significance and are the preferred way to do this. The actual definition is that 95% of such intervals calculated from the same experiment repeated multiple times contain the true value of the variable for that population. For all practical purposes in plain English, the 95% CI means that 95% of the time we expect the true mean to be between the upper and lower limits of the confidence interval. This means that if we were to repeat the experiment 20 times, in 19 of those repeated experiments the value of the effect size would lie within the stated CI range. This gives more information than a simple P value, since one can see a range of potentially likely values. If the data assume a normal distribution and we are measuring independent events, the SEM can be used to calculate 95% confidence intervals (Fig. 10.4).

Statistical tests

The **central limit theorem** is the theoretical basis for most statistical tests. It states that if we select equally sized samples of a variable from a population with

[2] D. L. Streiner. Maintaining standards: differences between the standard deviation and standard error, and when to use each. *Can. J. Psychiatry* 1996; 41: 498–502.

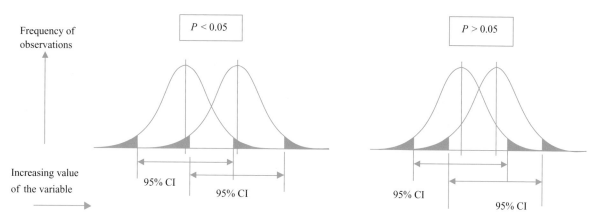

Fig. 10.5 The relationship between the overlap of 95% of possible variable values and the level of statistical significance.

a non-normal distribution the distribution of the means of these samples will be a normal distribution. This is true as long as the samples are large enough. For most statistical tests, the sample size considered large enough is 30. For smaller sample sizes, other more complex statistical approximations can be used.

Statistical tests calculate the probability that a difference between two groups obtained in a study occurred by chance. It is easier to visualize how statistical tests work if we assume that the distribution of each of two sample variables is two normal distributions graphed on the same axis. Very simplistically and for visual effectiveness, we can represent two sample means with their 95% confidence intervals as bell-shaped curves. There are two tails at the ends of the curves, each representing half of the remaining 5% of the confidence interval. If there is only some overlap of the areas on the tails or if the two curves are totally separate with no overlap, the results are statistically significant. If there is more overlap such that the value central tendency of one distribution is inside the 95% confidence interval of the other, the results are not statistically significant (Fig. 10.5). While this is a good way to visualize the process, it cannot be translated into simple overlap of the two 95% confidence intervals, as statistical significance depends on multiple other factors.

Statistical tests are based upon the principle that there is an expected outcome (E) that can be compared to the observed outcome (O). Determining the value of E is problematic since we don't actually know what value to expect in most cases. One estimate of the expected value is that found in the control group. Actually, there are complex calculations for determining the expected value that are part of the statistical test. Statistical tests calculate the probability that O is different from E or that the absolute difference between O and E is greater than zero and occurred by chance alone. This is done using a variety of formulas, is the meat of statistics, and is what statisticians get paid for. They also get paid to help researchers decide what to measure and how to ensure that the measure of interest is what is actually being measured. To quote Sir Ronnie Fisher again: "To call in the statistician after the experiment is done may be no more than asking him to perform a postmortem examination: he may be able to say what the experiment died of."[3]

One does not need to be a trained statistician to know which statistical test to use, but it helps. What is the average physician to do? The list in Appendix 3 is one place to start. It is an abbreviated list of the specific statistical tests that the reader should look for in evaluating the statistics of a study. As one becomes more familiar with the literature, one will be able to identify the correct statistical tests more often. If the test used in the article is not on this list, the reader ought to be a bit suspicious that perhaps the authors found a statistician who could save the study and generate statistically significant results, but only by using an obscure test.

The placebo effect

There is an urban myth that the placebo effect occurs at an average rate of about 35% in any study. The apparent placebo effect is actually more complex and made up of several other effects. These other effects, which can be confused with the true placebo effect, are the natural course of the illness, regression to the mean, other timed effects, and unidentified parallel interventions. The true placebo effect is the total perceived placebo effect minus these other effects.

The natural course of the disease may result in some patients getting better regardless of the treatment given while others get worse. In some cases, it will appear that patients got better because of the treatment, when really the patients got better because of the disease process. This was demonstrated in a previous example when patients with bronchitis appeared to get better with antibiotic treatment, when in reality, the natural course of bronchitis is clinical improvement. This concept is true with almost all illnesses including serious infections and advanced cancers.

Regression to the mean is the natural tendency for a variable to change with time and return toward the population mean. If endpoints are re-measured they are likely to be closer to the mean than an initial extreme value. This is a commonly seen phenomenon with blood pressure values. Many people initially found to have an elevated blood pressure will have a reduction in their blood pressure over time. This is partly due to their relaxing after the initial pressure reading and partly to regression to the mean.

Other timed effects that may affect the outcome measurements include the learning curve. A person gets better at a task each time it is performed. Similarly, a patient becomes more relaxed as the clinical encounter progresses. This explains the effect known as white coat hypertension, the phenomenon by which

---

[3] Indian Statistical Congress, Sankhya, 1938. Sir Ronald Fisher, 1890–1962.

a person's blood pressure will be higher when the doctor takes it and lower when taken later by a machine, a non-physician, or repeatedly by their own physician. Some of this effect is due to the stress engendered by the presence of the doctor; as a patient becomes more used to having the doctor take their blood pressure, the blood pressure decreases.

Unidentified parallel interventions may occur on the part of the physician, health-care giver, investigator, or patient. This includes things such as unconscious or conscious changes in lifestyle instituted as a result of the patient's medical problem. For example, patients who are diagnosed with elevated cholesterol may increase their exercise while they also began taking a new drug to help lower their cholesterol. This can result in a greater-than-expected rate of improvement in outcomes both in those assigned to the drug and in the control or placebo group.

The reader's goal is to differentiate the true treatment effect from the perceived treatment effect. The true treatment effect is the difference between the perceived treatment effect and the various types of placebo effect as described above. Studies should be able to differentiate the true treatment effect from the perceived effect by the appropriate use of a control group. The control group is given the placebo or a standard therapy that is equivalent to the placebo since the standard therapy would be given regardless of the patients' participation in the study.

A recent meta-analysis combined the results of multiple studies that had placebo and no-treatment arms. They compared the results obtained by all the patients in these two groups and found that the overall effect size for these two groups was the same. The only exception was in studies for pain where an overall positive effect favored the placebo group by the amount of 6.5 mm on a 100-mm pain scale.[4] As demonstrated by previous pain studies, this difference is not clinically significant.

---

[4] A. Hróbjartsson & P. C. Gøtzsche. Is the placebo powerless? An analysis of clinical trials comparing placebo with no treatment *N. Engl. J. Med.* 2001; 344: 1594–1602.

11

Type I errors and number needed to treat

If this be error, and upon me prov'd,
I never writ, nor no man ever lov'd.

William Shakespeare (1564–1616): Sonnet 116

Learning objectives

In this chapter you will learn:

- how to recognize Type I errors in a study
- the concept of data dredging or data snooping
- the meaning of number needed to treat to benefit (NNTB) and number needed to treat to harm (NNTH)
- how to differentiate statistical from clinical significance
- other sources of Type I errors

Interpreting the results of a clinical trial requires an understanding of the statistical processes that are used to analyze these results. Studies that suffer from a Type I error may show statistical significance when the groups are not actually different. Intelligent readers of the medical literature must be able to interpret these results and determine for themselves if these results are important enough to use for their patients.

Type I error

This occurs when the null hypothesis is rejected even though it is really true. In other words, studies that have a Type I error conclude that there is a positive effect size or difference between groups when in reality there is not. This is a **false positive** study result. Alpha (α), known as the **level of significance**, is defined as the maximum probability of making a Type I error that the researcher is willing to accept. Alpha is the probability of rejecting the null hypothesis when it is really

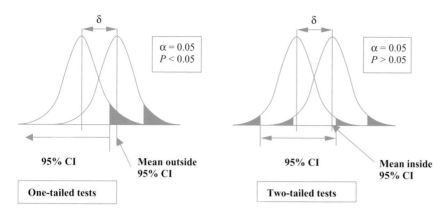

Fig. 11.1 One- and two-tailed tests for the same effect size δ.

true and is predetermined before conducting a statistical test. The probability of obtaining the actual difference or effect size by chance if the null hypothesis is true is P. This is calculated by performing a statistical test.

The researcher minimizes the risk of a Type I error by setting the level of significance (α) very low. By convention, the alpha level is usually set at 0.05 or 0.01. In other words, with $\alpha = 0.05$ the researcher expects to make a Type I error in one of 20 trials. The researcher then calculates P using a statistical test. He or she compares P to α. If $\alpha = 0.05$, P must be less than 0.05 ($P < 0.05$) to show statistical significance. There are two situations for which this must be modified: two-tailed testing and multiple variables.

One-tailed vs. two-tailed tests

If researchers have an a-priori reason to believe that one group is clearly going to be different from the other and they know the direction of that difference, they can use a one-tailed statistical test. It is important to note that the researcher must hypothesize either an increase or a decrease in the effect, not just a difference. This means that the normal distribution of one result is only likely to overlap the normal distribution of the other result on one side or in one direction. This is demonstrated in Fig. 11.1.

One-tailed tests specify the direction that researchers think the result will be. When asking the question "is drug A better than drug B?" the alternative hypothesis, H_a is that drug A is better than drug B. The null hypothesis, H_0 is that either there is no difference or drug A is worse than drug B. This states that we are only interested in drug A if it is better and we have good a-priori reason to think that it really is better. It removes from direct experimentation the possibility that drug A may actually be worse that drug B.

It is best to do a two-tailed test in almost all circumstances. The use of a one-tailed test can only be justified if previous research demonstrated that drug A actually appears to be better and certainly is no worse than drug B. When doing a two-tailed test, there is no a-priori assumption about the direction of the result. A **two-tailed test** asks the question "is there any difference between groups?" In this case, the alternative hypothesis H_a is that drug A is different from drug B. This can mean that drug A is either better or worse, but not equivalent to drug B. The null hypothesis H_0 states that there is no difference between the two drugs or that they are equivalent.

For $\alpha = 0.05$, P must only be < 0.10 for statistical significance with the one-tailed test. It must be < 0.05 for the two-tailed test. This means that we will accept a Type I error one in 10 trials with a one-tailed test rather than one in 20 with a two-tailed test. Conceptually this means that for a total probability of a randomly occurring error of 0.05, each tail of the normal distribution contributes 0.025 of alpha. For a one-tailed test, each tail contributes 0.05 of alpha. This requirement for $\alpha = 0.05$ is less stringent if a one-tailed test is used.

Multiple outcomes

The probability of making a Type I error is α for each outcome being measured. If two variables are measured, the probability of a Type I error or a false positive result is α for each variable. The probability that at least one of these two variables is a false positive is one minus the probability that neither of them is a false positive. The probability that neither is a false positive is the probability that the first variable is not a false positive $(1 - \alpha)$ and that the second variable is not a false positive $(1 - \alpha)$. This makes the probability that neither variable is a false positive $(1 - \alpha) \times (1 - \alpha)$, or $(1 - \alpha)^2$. The probability that at least one of the two is falsely positive then becomes $1 - (1 - \alpha)^2$. Therefore, the probability that one positive and incorrect outcome will occur only by chance if n variables are tested is $1 - (1 - \alpha)^n$.

This probability becomes sizable as n gets very large. **Data dredging, mining, or snooping** is a technique by which the researcher looks at multiple variables in the hope that at least one will show statistical significance. This result is then emphasized as the most important positive result in the study. This is a common example of a Type I error. Suspect this when there are many variables being tested, but only a few of them show statistical significance. This can be substantial in studies of DNA sequences looking for genetic markers of disease. Typically the researcher will look at hundreds or thousands of DNA sequences and see if any are related to phenotypic signs of disease. A few of these may be positively associated by chance alone if α of 0.05 is used as the standard for statistical significance.

For example, if a researcher does a study that looks at 20 clinical signs of a given disease, it is possible that any one of them will be statistically significantly associated with the disease. For one variable, the probability that this association occurred by chance only is 0.05. Therefore the probability that no association occurred by chance is $1 - 0.05 = 0.95$. The probability that at least one of the 20 variables tested will be positively associated with the disease by chance alone is 1 minus the probability of no association. Since this is 0.95 for each variable, the probability that at least one occurred by chance becomes $1 - 0.95^{20}$ or $1 - 0.36 = 0.64$. Therefore, there is a 64% likelihood of coming up with one association that is falsely positive and occurred only by chance. If there are two values that show an association, one cannot know if both occurred by chance alone or if one result is truly statistically significant. Then the question becomes which result is the significant value and which result is a false positive.

One way to get around this problem is by applying the **Bonferroni correction**. First we must create a new level of α, which will be α/n. This is the previous α divided by n, the number of variables being compared, not the sample size. Therefore, P must be $< \alpha/n$ for the result to be statistically significant. The Bonferroni correction is used when the variables being tested are independent of each other and there are only 10 or fewer variables being measured. This correction is not a true assumption in most cases and other means of estimating α' must be used.

Data dredging is a proper device if the study is a **derivation set**. The variables that came up statistically significant will then be measured in another study using only those variables and a new sample called the **validation set** to see if this relationship still holds. One clue to data dredging is the absence of an explicit hypothesis. This allows the researcher to find a statistically significant relationship that exists only by chance and claim it as the reason for the study. This technique is only legitimate if the variable that comes up statistically significant in the derivation set can then become the explicit hypothesis of a validation set. This is the correct way that studies of DNA sequences as markers of disease ought to be done.

Confidence intervals

Confidence intervals (CI) are used more frequently now to represent the level of significance (Table 11.1). As mentioned earlier, the true definition of the 95% CI is that 95% of such intervals calculated by repeating the same experiment contain the true value of the variable for that population. For all practical purposes the 95% CI is a range of values within which we would expect the true value to lie 95% of the time, or with 95% certainty. If one repeats the experiment 20 times, 19 of those times the true value will be within the stated CI range. This gives

Table 11.1. Rules of thumb for 95% confidence intervals

(1) If the point value for one (experimental) group is within the 95% CI for the other (control) group, there is likely to be no statistical significance for the difference between values.

(2) If the point value for one (experimental) group is outside the 95% CI for the other (control) group, there is likely to be statistical significance for the difference between values.

(3) If the 95% CI for a difference includes 0, the difference found is not statistically significant.

(4) If the 95% CI for a ratio includes 1, the ratio is not statistically significant.

more information than a simple $P < 0.05$ value since one can see a statistically plausible range of values.

The limits of the 95% CI display the precision of the results. If the CI is very wide, the results are not very precise. This means that there is a great deal of random variation in the result and a very large or small value could be the true effect size. Similarly if the CI is very narrow, the results are very precise and we are more certain of the true result.

If the 95% confidence interval around the difference between two groups in studies of the therapy includes the zero point, $P > 0.05$. The zero point is the point at which there is no difference between the two groups or the null hypothesis is true. If one limit of the CI is just near, and the interval does not cross the zero point, the result may only be slightly statistically significant. The addition of a few more subjects could make the result more statistically significant. However, the true effect may be very small and not clinically important.

Statistical significance vs. clinical significance

A study of a population with a very large sample size can show statistical significance at the $\alpha = 0.05$ level when the actual clinical difference between the two groups is very small. For example, if a study measuring the level of pain perception using a visual analog scale showed a statistically significant difference in pain scores of 6.5 points on a scale 0–100, one might think this was important. But, another study found that patients could not actually discriminate a difference on this scale of less than 13 points. Therefore, although statistically significant, a difference of 6.5 points would not be clinically important.

Clinicians must decide for themselves whether a result has reasonable clinical significance. They must then help their patients decide how much benefit will accrue from the therapy and how much risk they are willing to accept as a result

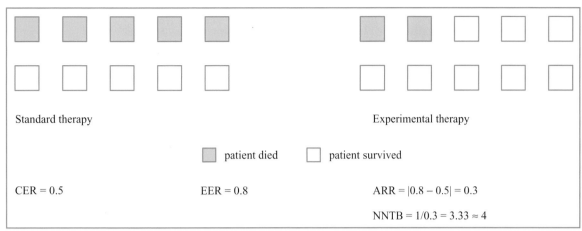

Standard therapy   Experimental therapy

□ patient died   □ patient survived

CER = 0.5   EER = 0.8   ARR = |0.8 − 0.5| = 0.3

NNTB = 1/0.3 = 3.33 ≈ 4

Fig. 11.2 Number needed to treat to benefit. For every 10 patients treated with the experimental treatment, there are three additional survivors. The number needed to treat is $10/3 = 3.33 \approx$ (rounded up to) 4. Therefore we must treat four patients to get one additional survivor.

of potential side effects or failure of the treatment. If a difference in effect size of the magnitude found in the study will not change the clinical situation of a given patient, then that is not an important result. Clinicians must look at the overall impact of small effect size on patient care. This may include issues of ultimate survival, potential side effects and toxicities, quality of life, adverse outcomes, and costs to the patient and society. We will cover formal decision analysis in Chapter 30 and cost-effectiveness analysis in Chapter 31.

Number needed to treat

A useful numerical measure of clinical significance is the **number needed to treat to benefit** (**NNTB**). The NNTB is the number of patients that must be treated with the proposed therapy in order to have one additional successful result. To calculate NNTB one must first calculate the absolute risk reduction (ARR). This requires that the study outcomes are dichotomous and one can calculate the experimental (EER) and control (CER) event rates. The ARR is the absolute difference of the event rates of the two groups being compared (|EER − CER|). The NNTB is one divided by the ARR. By convention, NNTB is given as 1/ARR rounded up to the nearest integer. Figure 11.2 is a pictorial description of NNTB.

It is ideal to see small NNTBs in studies of treatment as this means that the new and experimental treatment is a lot better than the standard, control, or placebo treatment. One can compare the NNTB to the risk of untreated disease and the risks of side effects of treatment. The related concept, the **number needed to treat to harm** (NNTH), is the number of patients that one would need to expose to a risk factor before an additional patient is harmed by side effects of the treatment. The concepts of NNTB and NNTH help physicians balance the benefit and risk of therapy. The NNTH is usually calculated from studies of risk, and will be discussed in the chapter on risk assessment (Chapter 13).

For studies of prevention, NNTB tends to be much larger than for studies of therapy. This difference is fine if the intervention is relatively cheap and not dangerous. For example, one aspirin taken daily can prevent death after a heart attack. The NNTB to prevent one death in the first 5 weeks after a heart attack is 40. Since aspirin is very cheap and has relatively few side effects, this is a reasonable number. The following two examples will demonstrate the use of NNTB.

(1) A study of treatment for migraine headache tested a new drug sumatriptan against placebo. In the sumatriptan group, 1067 out of 1854 patients had mild or no pain at 2 hours. In the placebo group, 256 out of 1036 patients had mild or no pain at 2 hours. First the event rates are calculated, then the ARR and RRR, and finally the NNTB:

EER $= 1067/1854 = 58\% = 0.58$ and CER $= 256/1036 = 25\% = 0.25$.

ARR $= 0.58 - 0.25 = 0.33$. In this case we ought to say absolute rate increase (ARI) since this is the absolute increase in well-being due to the drug. This means that 33% more patients taking sumatriptan for headache will have clinical improvement compared to patients taking placebo.

RRR $= 0.33/0.25 = 1.33$. This is the relative risk reduction or in this case relative rate increase (RRI) and means that patients treated with sumatriptan are one-and-a-third times more likely to show improvement in their headache compared with patients treated with placebo therapy. The RRR always makes the improvement look better than the ARR.

NNTB $= 1/0.33 = 3$. You must treat three patients with sumatriptan to reduce pain of migraine headaches in one additional patient. This looks like a very reasonable number for NNTB. However, bear in mind that clinicians would never recommend placebo, and it is likely that the NNTB would not be nearly this low if sumatriptan were compared against other migraine medications. This is an example of a false comparison, very common in the medical literature, especially among studies sponsored by pharmaceutical companies.

(2) Streptokinase (SK) and tissue plasminogen activator (t-PA) are two drugs that can dissolve blood clots in the coronary arteries and can treat myocardial infarction (MI). A recent study called GUSTO compared the two in the treatment of MI. In the most positive study comparing the use of these in treating MI, the SK group had a mortality of 7% (CER) and the t-PA group had a mortality of 6% (EER). This difference was statistically significant ($P < 0.05$).

ARR $= |6\% - 7\%|$ or 1%. This means that there is a 1% absolute improvement in survival when t-PA is used rather than SK.

RRR $= (|6 - 7|)/6$ or 16%. This means that there is a relative increase in survival of 16% when t-PA is used rather than SK. This is the figure that was used in advertisements for the drug that were sent out to cardiologists, family-medicine, emergency-medicine, and critical-care physicians.

NNTB $= 1/1\% = 1/0.01 = 100$. This means that you must treat 100 patients with the experimental therapy to save one additional life. This may not be reasonable especially if there is a large cost difference or significantly more side effects. In this case, SK costs $200 per dose while t-PA costs $2000 per dose. There was also an increase in the number of symptomatic intracranial bleeds with t-PA. The ARR for symptomatic intracranial bleeds was about 0.3%, giving an NNTH of about 300. That means for every 300 patients who get t-PA rather than streptokinase, one additional patient will have a symptomatic intracranial bleed.

The **number needed to screen to benefit** (NNSB) is a related concept that looks at how many people need to be screened for a disease in order to prevent one additional death. For example, to prevent one additional death from breast cancer one must screen 1200 women beginning at age 50. Since the potential outcome of not detecting breast cancer is very bad and the screening test is not invasive with very rare side effects, it is a reasonable screening test. We will discuss screening tests in Chapter 28.

The **number needed to expose to harm** (NNEH) is the number of patients that must be exposed to a risk factor in order for one additional person to have the outcome of interest. This can be a negative outcome such as lung cancer from exposure to secondhand smoke or a positive one such as reduction in dental caries from exposure to fluoride in the water. The NNEH to secondhand smoke to cause one additional case of lung cancer in a non-smoking spouse after 14 years of exposure is 1300. This NNEH is very high, meaning that very few of the people who are at risk will develop the outcome. However, the baseline exposure rate is high, with 25% of the population being smokers and the cost of intervention is very low, thus making reduction of secondhand smoke very desirable.

For all values of NNTB and other similar numbers, confidence intervals should be given in studies that calculate these statistics. The formulas for these are very complex and are given in Appendix 4. There are several convenient NNTB calculators on the Web. Two recommended sites are those of the University of British Columbia[1] and the Centre for Evidence-Based Medicine at Oxford University.

Other sources of Type I error

There are three other common sources of Type I error that are seen in research studies and may be difficult to spot. Authors with a particular bias will do many things to make their preferred treatment seem better than the comparison

[1] www.spph.ubc.ca/sites/healthcare/files/calc/clinsig.html

treatment. Authors may do this because of a conflict of interest, or simply because they are zealous in defense of their original hypothesis.

An increasingly common device for reporting results uses **composite endpoints**. A composite endpoint is the combination of two or more endpoints or outcome events into one combined event. These are most commonly seen when a single important endpoint such as a difference in death rates shows results that are small and not statistically significant. The researcher then looks at other endpoints such as reduction in recurrence of adverse clinical events. The combination of both decreased death rates and reduced adverse events may be decreased enough to make the study results statistically significant. A recent study looked at the anticoagulant low-molecular-weight heparin (LMWH) for the prevention of death in certain types of cardiac events such as unstable angina and non-Q-wave myocardial infarctions. The final results were that death, heart attack, urgent surgery, or angioplasty revascularization occurred in fewer of the LMWH group than in the standard heparin group. However, there was no difference between groups for death. It was only when all the outcomes were put together that the difference achieved statistical significance. In addition, the LMWH group had more intracranial bleeds and the NNTB for the composite endpoint was almost equal to the NNTH for the bleeds.

Sometimes a study will show a non-significant difference between the intervention and comparison treatment for the overall sample group being studied. In some cases, the authors will then look at subgroups of the study population to find one that demonstrates a statistically significant association. This **post-hoc subgroup analysis** is not an appropriate way to look for significance and is a form of data dredging. The more subgroups that are examined, the more likely it is that a statistically significant outcome will be found – and that it will have occurred by chance. This can determine a hypothesis for the next study of the same intervention. In that subsequent study, only that subgroup will be the selected study population and improvement looked for in that group only.

A recent study of stroke found that patients treated with thrombolytic therapy within 3 hours did better than those treated later than 3 hours. The authors concluded that this was the optimal time to begin treatment and the manufacturer began heavily marketing these very expensive and possibly dangerous drugs. Subsequent studies of patients within this time frame have not found the same degree of reduction in neurological deficit found in the original study. It turns out that the determination of the 3-hour mark was a post-hoc subgroup analysis performed after the data were obtained. The authors looked for some statistically significant time period in which the drug was effective, and came to rest on 3 hours. To obtain the true answer to this 3-hour mark question, a randomized controlled clinical trial explicitly looking at this time window should be done to determine if the results are reproducible.

Finally, there can be a serious problem if a clinical trial is stopped early because of apparently excellent results early in the study. The researchers may feel that it is unethical to continue the trial when the results are so dramatic that they have achieved statistical significance even before the required number of patients have been enrolled. This is becoming more common, having more than doubled in the past 20 years. One problem is that there may be an apparently large treatment effect size initially, when in reality only a few outcome events have occurred in a small study population. The reader can tell if this is likely to have happened by looking at the 95% confidence intervals and seeing that they are very wide, and often barely statistically significant. When a trial is stopped early, there is also a danger that the trial won't discover adverse effects of therapy and the trial will not determine if the side effects are more or less likely to occur than the beneficial events. One proposed solution to this problem is that there be prespecified stopping rules. These might include a minimum number of patients to be enrolled and also a more stringent statistical threshold for stopping the study. It has been suggested that an α level of 0.001 be set as the statistically significant level that must be met if the study is stopped early. Even this may not prevent overly optimistic results from being published, and all research must be reviewed in the context of other studies of the same problem. If these other studies are congruent with the results of the study stopped early, it is very likely that the results are valid. However, if the results seem too good to be true, be careful, they probably are.

12

Negative studies and Type II errors

If I had thought about it, I wouldn't have done the experiment. The literature was full of examples that said you can't do this.

Spencer Silver on the work that led to the unique adhesives for 3M Post-It ® Notepads

Learning objectives

In this chapter you will learn:
- how to recognize Type II errors in a study
- how to interpret negative clinical trials using 95% confidence intervals
- how to use a nomogram to determine the appropriate sample size and interpret a Type II error

Interpretation of the results of negative clinical trials requires an understanding of the statistical processes that can account for these results. Intelligent readers of the medical literature must be able to interpret these results and determine for themselves if they are important enough to ignore in clinical practice.

The problem with evaluating negative studies

Negative studies are those that conclude that there is no statistically significant association between the cause and effect variables or no difference between the two groups being compared. This may occur because there really is no association or difference between groups, a **true negative** result, or it can occur because the study was unable to determine that the association or difference was statistically significant. If there really is a difference or association, the latter finding would be a **false negative** result and this is a critical problem in medical research.

In a college psychology class, an interesting experiment was done. There were two sections of students in the lab portion of the class and each section did the same experiment. On separate days, each student was given a cup of coffee; one day they got real Java and the next day decaf. After drinking the coffee, they were given a simple test of math problems that had to be completed in a specified time and each of the students' scores was then calculated. For both groups, the scores under the influence of caffeine were higher. However, when a statistical test was applied to the results, they were not statistically significant, meaning that the results could have occurred by chance greater than 5% of the time. Does caffeine improve scores on a simple math test? Are the results really no different or was the study falsely negative?

Type II error

This type of error occurs when the null hypothesis H_0, is accepted and no difference is found between the groups even though the groups truly are different. In other words, the researcher concludes that there isn't a difference, when in fact there is a difference. An example would be concluding there is no relationship between familial hyperlipidemia and the occurrence of coronary artery disease when there truly is a relationship. Another would be concluding that caffeine intake does not increase the math scores of college psychology students when in fact it does. This is called a β or **Type II error**.

The researcher should define beta (β) as the maximum probability of making a Type II error or failing to reject the null hypothesis when it is actually false. This is a convoluted way of saying that it finds the alternative hypothesis to be false, when it ain't! Beta is the probability of the occurrence of this wrong conclusion that an investigator must be willing to accept. The researcher does not set β directly. It can be calculated from the expected study results before a study is done. Practically, the value of β is estimated from the conditions of the experiment.

Power is the ability to detect a statistically significant difference when it actually exists. Power is one minus the probability that a type II error is made and is equal to $1 - \beta$. The researcher can reduce β, and thereby increase the power, by selecting a sufficiently large sample size (n). Other changes that can be made to lower the probability of making a Type II or β error include increasing the difference one wants to detect, using a one-tailed rather than a two-tailed test, and increasing the level of α from 0.05 to 0.1 or even higher.

Determining power

In statistical terminology, power means that the study will reject the null hypothesis when it really is false. By convention one sets up the experiment so that β

is no greater than 0.20. Equivalently, power should be more than 0.80 to be considered adequate for most studies. Remember, that a microscope with greater power will be able to detect smaller differences between cells.

Power depends on several factors. These include the type of variable, statistical test, degree of variability, effect size, and the sample size. The type of variable can be dichotomous, ordinal, or continuous, and for a high power, continuous variables are best. For the statistical test, a one-tailed test has more power than a two-tailed test. The degree of variability is based on the standard deviation, and in general, the smaller the standard deviation, the greater the power. The bigger the better is the basic principle when using the effect size and the sample size to increase a study's power. These concepts are directly related to the concept of confidence discussed in Chapter 10. The confidence formula (confidence = (signal/noise) $\times \sqrt{n}$) can be written as confidence = (effect size/standard deviation) $\times \sqrt{n}$. According to this formula, as effect size or sample size increases, confidence increases, thus the power increases. As the standard deviation increases, confidence decreases and the power decreases.

Effect of sample size on power

Sample size (n) has the most obvious effect on the power of a study with power increasing in proportion to the square root of the sample size. If the sample size is very large, an experiment is more likely to show statistical significance even if there is a small effect size. This is a purely mathematical issue. The smaller the sample size, the harder it is to find statistical significance even if one is looking for a large effect size. Remember the two groups of college psychology students at the start of this chapter. It turns out, when the scores for the two groups were combined, the results were statistically significant. Figure 12.1 demonstrates the effect of increasing sample size to obtain a statistically significant result.

For example, one does a study to find out if ibuprofen is good for relieving the pain of osteoarthritis. The results were that patients taking ibuprofen had 50% less pain than those taking placebo. However, in this case. there were only five patients in each group and the result, although very large in terms of effect size, was not statistically significant. If one then repeats the study and gets exactly the same results with 25 patients in each group, then the result turns out to be statistically significant. This change in statistical significance occurred because of an increase in power.

In the extreme, studies of tens of thousands of patients will often find very tiny effect sizes, such as 1% difference or less, to be statistically significant. This is the most important reason to use the number needed to treat instead of only $P < 0.05$ as the best indicator of the clinical significance of a study result. In

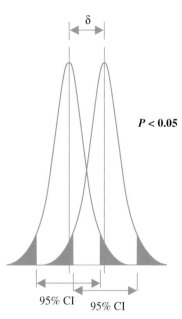

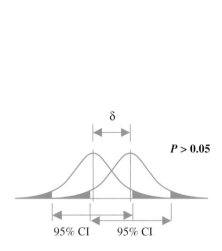

Fig. 12.1 Effect of changing sample size. Two variables with different sample sizes and the same effect size (δ). The area under the curves is proportional to the sample size (n). The samples on the left with a small sample size are not statistically significantly different ($p > 0.05$). The ones on the right with a larger sample size have an effect size that is statistically significant ($p < 0.05$).

cases like this, although the results are statistically significant, the patient will most likely have minimal, if any, benefit from the treatment. In terms of confidence intervals, a larger sample size will lead to narrower 95% confidence intervals.

Effect of effect size on power

Before an experiment is done, effect size is estimated as the difference between groups that will be clinically important. The sample size needed to detect the predetermined effect size can then be calculated. Overall, it is easier to detect a large effect such as a 90% change rather than a small one like a 2% change (Fig. 12.2). However, as discussed above, if the sample size is large enough, even a very small effect size may be statistically significant but not clinically important. Another technique to be aware of is that the conditions of the experiment can be manipulated to show a large effect size, but this is usually at the cost of making a Type III or IV error.

Effect of level of significance on power

The magnitude of the level of significance, α, tells the reader how willing the researchers are to have a result that occurred only by chance. If α is large, the study will have more power to find a statistically significant difference between

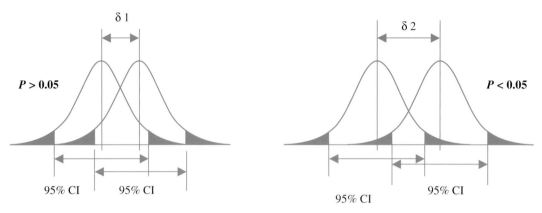

Fig. 12.2 Effect of changing effect size. Two variables with different effect sizes and the same sample size. The results of the group on the left with a small effect size are not statistically significantly different ($p > 0.05$). The ones on the right with a larger effect size have a result that is statistically significant ($p < 0.05$).

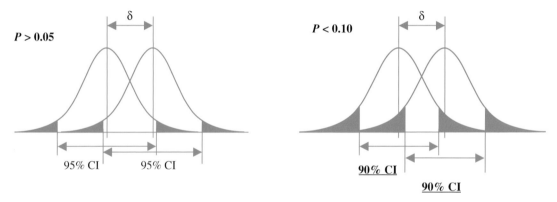

Fig. 12.3 Effect of changing alpha. Two variables with different levels of α. The samples on the left with a small α ($= 0.05$) are not statistically significantly different ($p > 0.05$). The ones on the right with a larger α ($= 0.1$) have an effect size that is statistically significant ($p < 0.10$).

groups. If α is very small, researchers are willing to accept only a tiny likelihood that the effect size found occurred by chance alone. In general, as the level of α increases, we are willing to have a greater likelihood that the effect size occurred by chance alone (Fig. 12.3). We are more likely to find the difference to be statistically significant if the level of α is larger rather than smaller. In medicine, we generally set α at 0.05, while in physics α may be set at 0.0001 or lower. Those in medicine today who believe that 0.05 is too stringent and we should go to an α level of 0.1 might not be comfortable knowing that the treatment they were

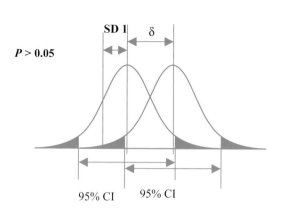

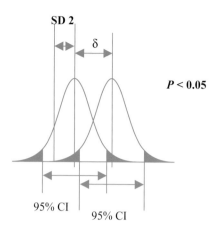

Fig. 12.4 Effect of changing precision (standard deviation). Two variables with the same sample size and effect size. In the case on the left there is a large standard deviation, while on the right there is a small standard deviation. The situation on the right will be statistically significant ($p < 0.05$) while the one on the left will not ($p > 0.05$).

receiving was better than something cheaper, less toxic, or more commonly used by a chance factor of 10%.

Effect of standard deviation on power

The smaller the standard deviation of the data-sets, the better the power of the study. If two samples each have small standard deviations, a statistical test is more likely to find them different than if they have large standard deviations. Think of the standard deviation as defining the width of a normal distribution around the mean value found in the study. When the two normal distributions are compared, the one with the smallest spread will have the most likelihood of being found statistically significant (Fig. 12.4).

Negative studies

A Type II error can only be made in a negative clinical trial. These are trials reporting no statistically significant difference or association. Therefore, when reading negative clinical trials, one needs to assess the chance that a Type II error occurred. This is important because a negative result may not be due to the lack of an important effect, but simply because of the inability to detect that effect statistically. This is called a study with low power. From an interpretation perspective, the question one asks is, "For a given β level and a difference that I consider clinically important, did the researcher use a large enough sample size?"

Since the possibility of a Type II error is a non-trivial problem, one must perform his or her own interpretation of a negative clinical trial. The three common ways of doing this are through the interpretation of the confidence intervals, by using sample size nomograms, and with published power tables. We will discuss the first two methods since they can be done most simply without specialized references.

Evaluating negative studies using confidence intervals

Confidence intervals (CI) can be used to represent the level of significance. There are several rules of thumb that must be remembered before using CIs to determine the potential of a Type II error. First, if the point estimate value of one variable is within the 95% CI range of the other variable, there is no statistical significance to the difference between the two groups. Second, if the 95% CI for a difference includes 0, the difference found is not statistically significant. Last, if the 95% CI for a ratio includes 1, the ratio found is not statistically significant.

Unlike P values, which are only a single number, 95% CIs allow the reader to actually see a range of possible values that includes the true value with 95% certainty. For the difference between two groups, it gives the range of the most likely difference between the two groups under consideration. For a given effect size, one can look at the relationship between the limits of the CI and the **null point**, the point at which there is no difference or association. A 95% CI that is skewed in one direction and where one end of the interval is very near the null point can have occurred as a result of low power. In that case, a larger sample size might show a statistically significant effect.

For example, in a study of the effect of two drugs on pain, the change in the visual analog score (VAS) was found to be 25mm with a 95% CI from –5mm to 55mm. This suggests that a larger study could find a difference that was statistically significant, although maybe not as large as 25mm. If one added a few more patients, the CI would be narrower and would most likely not include the null point, 0 in this case. If there were no other evidence available, it might be reasonable to use the better drug until either a more powerful study or a well-done meta-analysis showed a clear-cut superiority of one treatment over the other, or showed equivalence of the two drugs. On the other hand, if the 95% CI were –15mm to 60mm, it would be unlikely that adding even a large number of additional patients would change the results. There is approximately the same degree of the 95% CI on either side of the null point, suggesting that the true values are most likely to be near the null point and less likely to be near either extreme. In this case, consider the study to be negative, at least until another and much larger study comes along.

The 95% CI can also be used to evaluate positive studies. If the absolute risk reduction (ARR) for an intervention is 0.05 with a 95% CI of 0.01 to 0.08, the intervention achieves statistical significance, but barely achieves clinical

Begin with the sample size that was used in the study

Use the nomogram to determine the effect size (δ) that could be found with this sample

Potential δ < clinically important δ
Ignore results (lacks power)

Potential δ > clinically important δ
Accept results

Fig. 12.5 Sequence of events for analyzing negative studies using sample size.

significance. In this case, if the intervention is extremely expensive or dangerous, its use should be strongly debated based upon such a small effect size.

Evaluating negative studies using a nomogram

There are two ways to analyze the results of a negative study using published nomograms from an article by Young and others.[1] These begin either with the sample size or with the effect size. Either method will show, for a study with sufficient power, what sample size was necessary or what effect size could be found to produce statistical significance.

In the first method, use the nomogram to determine the effect size that the sample size of the study had the power to find. Begin with the sample size and work backward to find the effect size. If the effect size that could potentially have been found with this sample size was larger than the effect size that a clinician or patient would consider clinically important, accept the study as negative. In other words, in this study, the clinically important difference could have been found and was not. On the other hand, if the clinically important effect size could not have been found with the sample size that was enrolled, the study was too small. Ignore the study and consider the result a Type II error. Wait for confirmatory studies before using the information (Fig. 12.5).

The second way of analyzing a negative study is to determine the sample size needed to get a clinically important effect size. Use the nomograms starting from the effect size that one considers clinically important and determine the sample size that would be needed to find this effect size. This clinically important effect size will most likely be larger than the actual difference found in the study. If the actual sample size is greater than the sample size required to find a clinically important difference, accept the results as negative. The study had the power

[1] M. J. Young, E. A. Bresnitz & B. L. Strom. Sample size nomograms for interpreting negative clinical studies. *Ann. Intern. Med.* 1983; 99: 248–251.

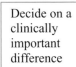

| Decide on a clinically important difference | | Use the nomogram to determine the sample size (*n*) needed to find this difference | | Actual n < required n Ignore results (lacks power) |
| | | | | Actual n > required n Accept results |

Fig. 12.6 Schematic of sequence of events for analyzing negative studies using effect size.

to find a clinically important effect size and did not. If the actual study sample size is less than the required sample size to find a clinically important difference, ignore the results with the caveats listed below. The study didn't have the power to find a difference that is clinically important (Fig. 12.6).

There are some caveats which must be considered in using this method to evaluate negative studies. If the needed sample size is huge, it is unlikely that a group that large can ever be studied, so accept the results as a negative study. If the needed sample size is within about one order of magnitude greater than the actual sample size, wait for the bigger study to come along before using the information. This process is illustrated in Fig. 12.7 (dichotomos variables) and Fig. 12.8 (continuous variables). The CD-ROM has some sample problems that will help you understand this process.

Using a nomogram for dichotomous variables

Dichotomous variables are those for which there are only two possible values (e.g., cured or not cured).
(1) Identify one group as the control group and the other as the experimental group, which should be evident from the study design.
(2) Decide what relative rate reduction (RRR) would be clinically important.
(3) RRR = (CER – EER)/CER, where CER = control event rate and EER = experimental event rate.
(4) Locate this % change on the horizontal axis.
(5) Extend a vertical line to intersect with the diagonal line representing the percentage response rate of the control group (CER).
(6) Extend a horizontal line from the intersection point to the vertical axis and read the required sample size (*n*) for each group.

Using a nomogram for continuous variables

Continuous variables are those for which multiple possible values can exist and which have proportional intervals.

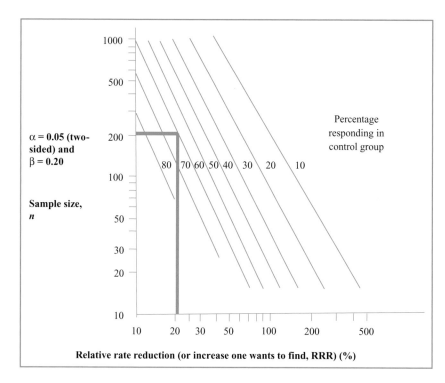

Fig. 12.7 Nomogram for dichotomous variables. If a study found a 20% relative risk reduction and there was a 60% response rate in the control group (vertical line), you would find this effect size statistically significant only if there was a sample size of more than 200 in each group (horizontal line). If the actual study had only 100 patients in each group and found a 20% relative risk reduction, which was not statistically significant, you should wait until a slightly larger study (200 per group) is done. After M. J. Young, E. A. Bresnitz & B. L. Strom. Sample size nomograms for interpreting negative clinical studies. *Ann. Intern. Med.* 1983; 99: 248–251 (used with permission.)

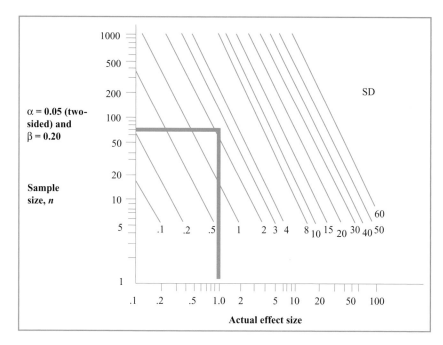

Fig. 12.8 Nomogram for continuous variables. If a study found a difference of 1 unit and the control group had a standard deviation of 2 (vertical line), you would find this effect size statistically significant only if there was a sample size of more than 70 per group (horizontal line). If the actual study found an effect size of only 0.5, and you thought that was clinically but not statistically significant, you would need to wait for a larger study (about 250 in each group) to be done before accepting that this was a negative study. After M. J. Young, E. A. Bresnitz & B. L. Strom. Sample size nomograms for interpreting negative clinical studies. *Ann. Intern. Med.* 1983; 99: 248–251 (used with permission.)

(1) Decide what difference (absolute effect size) is clinically important.
(2) Locate this difference on the horizontal axis.
(3) Extend a vertical line to the diagonal line representing the standard deviation of the data being measured. You can use the SD for either group.
(4) Extend a horizontal line to the vertical axis and read the required sample size (*n*) for each group.

Non-inferiority studies and equivalence studies

Sometimes a goal of a research study can be to determine that the experimental treatment is no worse than the standard treatment or placebo. In that case, an approach has been suggested that only seeks to show non-inferiority of the experimental therapy to the comparison. In these studies, the alternative hypothesis is that the experimental therapy is inferior to the standard therapy. This comes from a null hypothesis that states that the experimental treatment is equal to or better than the placebo or control treatment. In order for this study to be done, there must have been previous research studies showing that when compared to standard therapy or placebo, there is either no difference or the results were not statistically significant. It is also possible that there was a difference but the studies were of very poor quality, possibly lacking correct randomization and blinding so that the majority of physicians would not accept the results.

It is important for the reader to recognize that what the authors are essentially saying is that they are willing to do a one-tailed test for showing that the treatment is equal to or better than the control or placebo group. This leads to a value of P for statistical significance on one tail that should be less than 0.05 rather than the traditional 0.025. The standard two-tailed statistical tests should not be done as they are more likely to lead to a failure to find statistical significance, which in this case would be most likely a Type II error. In other words, they will most likely find that there is no difference in the groups when in fact there is a difference. Non-inferiority studies are most often seen in drug studies used by manufacturers to demonstrate that a new drug is at least as good as the standard drugs that are available. Of course, common sense would dictate that if a new drug is more expensive than a standard one and if it does not have a track record of safety, there ought to be no reason to use the new drug simply because it is not inferior.

13

Risk assessment

We saw the risk we took in doing good,
But dared not spare to do the best we could.

Robert Frost (1874–1963): The Exposed Nest

Learning objectives

In this chapter you will learn:

- the basic concept and measures of risk
- the meanings, calculations, uses, and limitations of:
  - absolute risk
  - relative risk
  - odds ratios
  - attributable risk and number needed to harm
  - attributable risk percent
- the use of confidence intervals in risk
- how to interpret the concept of "zero risk"

Risk is present in all human activities. What is the risk of getting breast cancer if a woman lives on Long Island and is exposed to organochlorines? What is the risk of getting lung cancer because there is a smoke residue on a co-worker's sweater? What is the risk of getting paralyzed as a result of spinal surgery? How about the risk of getting diarrhea from amoxicillin? Some of these risks are real and others are, at best, minimally increased risks of modern life. Risks may be those associated with a disease, with therapy, or with common environmental factors. Physicians must be able to interpret levels of risk for better care of their patients.

Measures of risk

First one must understand that risk is the probability that an event, disease, or outcome will occur in a particular population. The **absolute risk** of an event, disease, or outcome in exposed subjects is defined as the ratio of patients who are exposed to the risk factor and develop the outcome of interest to all those patients exposed to the risk. For example, if we study 1000 people who drink more than two cups of coffee a day and 60 of them develop pancreatic cancer, the risk of developing pancreatic cancer among people drinking more than two cups of coffee a day is 60/1000 or 6%. This can also be written as a conditional probability, *P* **outcome | risk = probability of the outcome if exposed to the risk factor**. The same calculation can be done for people who are not exposed to the risk and who nevertheless get the outcome of interest. Their absolute risk is the ratio of those not exposed to the risk factor and who have the outcome of interest to all those not exposed to the risk factor.

Risk calculations can help us in many clinical situations. They can help associate an etiology such as smoking to an outcome such as lung cancer. Risk calculations can estimate the probability of developing an outcome such as the increased risk of endometrial cancer because of exposure to estrogen therapy. They can demonstrate the effectiveness of an intervention on an outcome such as showing a decreased mortality from measles in children who have been vaccinated against the disease. Finally, they can target interventions that are most likely to be of benefit. For example, they can measure the effect of aspirin as opposed to stronger blood thinners like heparin or low-molecular-weight heparin on mortality from heart attacks.

The data used to estimate risk come from research studies. The best estimates of risk come from randomized clinical trials (RCTs) or well done cohort studies. These studies can separate groups by the exposure and then measure the risk of the outcome. They can also be set up so that the exposure precedes the outcome, thus showing a cause and effect relationship. The measure of risk calculated from these studies is called the relative risk, which will be defined shortly. Relative risk can also be measured from a cross-sectional study, but the cause and effect cannot be shown from that study design. Less reliable estimates of risk may still be useful and can come from case–control studies, which start with the assumption that there are equal numbers of subjects with and without the outcome of interest. The estimates of risk from these studies approximate the relative risk calculated from cohort studies using a calculation known as an odds ratio, which will also be defined shortly.

There are several measures associated with any clinical or epidemiological study of risk. The study design determines which way the data are gathered and this determines the type of risk measures that can be calculated from a given

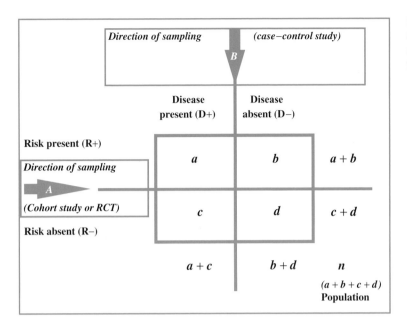

Fig. 13.1 A pictorial way to look at studies of risk. Note the difference in sampling direction for different types of studies.

study. Patients are initially identified either by exposure to the risk factor as in cohort studies or RCTs, by their outcome as in case–control studies, or by both as in cross-sectional studies. These are summarized in Fig. 13.1.

Absolute risk

Absolute risk is the probability of the outcome of interest in those exposed or not exposed to the risk factor. It compares those with the outcome of interest and the risk factor (*a*) to all subjects in the population exposed to the risk factor (*a* + *b*). In probabilistic terms, it is the probability of the outcome if exposed to the risk factor, also written as *P* **outcome | risk** = *P* (**O**+ | **R**+). One can also do this for patients with the outcome of interest who are not exposed to the risk factor (*c*) and compare them to all of those who are not exposed to the risk factor [*c*/(*c* + *d*)]. Probabilistically it is written as *P* **outcome | no risk** = *P* (**O**+ | **R**−). Absolute risk only gives information about the risk of one group, either those exposed to the risk factor or those not exposed to the risk factor. It can only be calculated from cross-sectional studies, cohort studies, or randomized clinical trials, because in these study designs, you can calculate the incidence of a particular outcome for those exposed or not exposed to the risk factor. One must know the relative proportions of the factors in the total population in order to calculate this number, as demonstrated in the rows of the 2 × 2 table in Fig. 13.1.

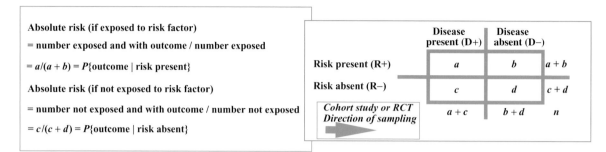

Fig. 13.2 Absolute risk.

The absolute risk is the probability that someone with the risk factor has the outcome of interest. In the 2×2 diagram (Fig. 13.2), patients labeled a are those with the risk factor who have the outcome and those labeled $a + b$ are all patients with the risk factor. The ratio $a/(a + b)$ is the probability that one will have the outcome if exposed to the risk factor. This is a statement of conditional probability. The same can be done for the row of patients who were not exposed to the risk factor. The absolute risk for them can be written as $c/(c + d)$. These absolute risks are the same as the incidence of disease in the cohort being studied.

Relative risk

Relative risk (RR) is the ratio of the two absolute risks. This is the absolute risk of the outcome in subjects exposed to the risk factor divided by the absolute risk of the outcome in subjects not exposed to the risk factor. It shows whether that risk factor increases or decreases the outcome of interest. In other words, it is the ratio of the probability of the outcome if exposed to the probability of the outcome if not exposed. Relative risk can only be calculated from cross-sectional studies, cohort studies or randomized clinical trials. The larger or smaller the relative risk, the stronger the association between the risk factor and the outcome.

If the RR is greater than 1, the risk factor is associated with an increase in the rate of the outcome. If the RR is less than 1, the risk factor is associated with a reduction in the rate of the outcome. If it is 1, there is no change in risk from the baseline risk level and it is said that the risk factor has no effect on the outcome. The higher the relative risk, the stronger the association that is discovered. A relative risk greater than 4 is usually considered very strong. Values below this could have been obtained because of systematic flaws in the study. This is especially true for observational studies like cross-sectional and cohort studies where there may be many confounding variables that could be responsible for the results. In

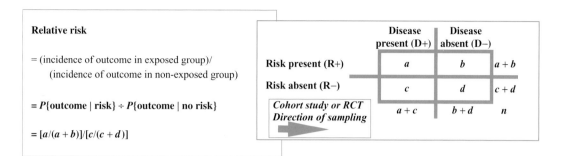

Relative risk

= (incidence of outcome in exposed group)/
(incidence of outcome in non-exposed group)

= P{outcome | risk} ÷ P{outcome | no risk}

= [a/(a + b)]/[c/(c + d)]

	Disease present (D+)	Disease absent (D−)	
Risk present (R+)	a	b	a + b
Risk absent (R−)	c	d	c + d
Cohort study or RCT Direction of sampling	a + c	b + d	n

Fig. 13.3 Relative risk.

studies showing a reduction in risk, look for RR to be less than 0.25 for it to be considered a strong result.

A high relative risk does not prove that the risk factor is responsible for outcome: it merely quantifies the strength of association of the two. It is always possible that a third unrecognized factor, a **surrogate** or **confounding variable,** is the cause of the association because it equally affects both the risk factor and the outcome. The calculation of relative risk is pictured in Fig. 13.3.

Data collected for relative-risk calculations come from cross-sectional studies, cohort studies, non-concurrent cohort studies, and randomized clinical trials. These studies are used because they are the only ones capable of calculating incidence. Importantly, cohort studies should demonstrate complete follow-up of all study subjects, as a large drop-out rate may lead to invalid results. The researchers should allow for an adequate length of follow-up in order to ensure that all possible outcome events have occurred. This could be years or even decades for cancer while it is usually weeks or days for certain infectious diseases. This follow-up cannot be done in cross-sectional studies, which can only show the strength of association but not that the cause preceded the effect.

Odds ratio

An **odds ratio** is the calculation used to estimate the relative risk or the association of risk and outcome for case–control studies. In case–control studies, subjects are selected based upon the presence or absence of the outcome of interest. This study design is used when the outcome is relatively rare in the population and calculating relative risk would require a cohort study with a huge number of subjects in order to find enough patients with the outcome. In case–control studies, the number of subjects selected with and without the outcome of interest are independent of the true ratio of these in the population. Therefore the incidence, the rate of occurrence of new cases of each outcome associated with and without

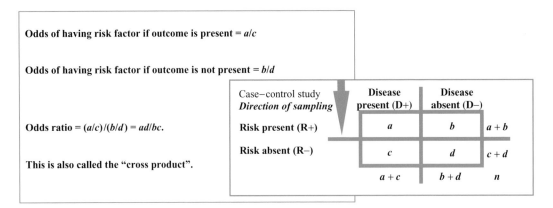

Fig. 13.4 Odds ratio.

the risk factor, cannot be calculated. Relative risk cannot be calculated from this study design.

Odds are a different way of saying the same thing as probabilities. Odds tell someone the number of times an event will happen divided by the number of times it won't happen. Although they are different ways of expressing the same number, odds and probability are mathematically related. In case–control studies, one measures the individual odds of exposure in subjects with the outcome as the ratio of subjects with and without the risk factor among all subjects with that outcome. The same odds can be calculated for exposure to the risk factor among those without the outcome.

The odds ratio compares the odds of having the risk factor present in the subjects with and without the outcome under study. This is the odds of having the risk factor if a person has the outcome divided by the odds of having the risk factor if a person does not have the outcome. Overall, it is an estimate of the relative risk for case–control studies (Fig. 13.4).

Using the odds ratio to estimate the relative risk

The odds ratio best estimates the relative risk when the disease is very rare. The rationale for this is not intuitively obvious. Cohort-study patients are evaluated on the basis of exposure and then outcome is determined. Therefore, one can calculate the absolute risk or the incidence of disease if the patient is or is not exposed to the risk factor and subsequently the relative risk can be calculated.

Case–control study patients are evaluated on the basis of outcome and exposure is then determined. The true ratio of patients with and without the outcome in the general population cannot be known from the study, but is an arbitrary ratio set by the researcher. One can only look at the ratio of the odds of risk in the diseased and non-diseased groups, hence the odds ratio. In the case–control

In the cohort study, the **relative risk (RR)** is **[$a/(a+b)$]/[$c/(c+d$)].** If the disease or

outcome is very rare, $a <<< b$ and $c <<< d$, making $(a+b) \rightarrow b$ and $(c+d) \rightarrow d$ and RR $\approx (a/b)/(c/d) = ad/bc$

RR approximates **odds ratio** = $(a/c)/(b/d) = ad/bc$

	Disease present (D+)	Disease absent (D−)	
Risk present (R+)	a	b	$a + b$
Risk absent (R−)	c	d	$c + d$
	$a + c$	$b + d$	n

Fig. 13.5 Odds ratio as estimate of relative risk. From S. B. Hulley & S. R. Cummings. *Designing Clinical Research*. Baltimore, MD, Williams & Wilkins, 1988.

study, we are looking at the disease as if it were present in a preset ratio, usually half of the population or an equal number of cases and controls. In reality, this preset ratio is not true and there are actually many fewer patients with known disease than people without known disease in the population. This fact allows the odds ratio to approximate the relative risk. We can prove this mathematically using two hypothetical studies of the same risk and outcomes (Fig. 13.5).

We assume that the true incidence of disease is represented by the results of the cohort study. In the case–control study, groups with and without outcome are equal. The ratios a/b and c/d approximate the incidence with and without exposure to the risk factor when the number of cases of the outcome of interest (a and c) is much smaller than the number of cases of no outcome (b and d). Then the value of the ratio $a/(a + b)$ approaches a/b and that of $c/(c + d)$ approaches c/d.

A word of caution is needed here. In order for the above to be absolutely true, the sample must be representative of the population, the outcome of disease must be much rarer than non-disease, and the systematic and random sampling error must be small. When the incidence of disease is high, the odds ratios and relative risk values diverge dramatically. This becomes greater as the value of RR and OR increases above 1 or decreases below 1. The differences are minimal when the RR or OR is equal to 1 regardless of the actual incidence of the outcome.

Attributable risk and the number needed to treat to harm (NNTH)

Attributable risk estimates how much of the risk of an outcome in exposed subjects is attributable to the risk factor. There are two numbers that are called attributable risk. The first is known as the absolute attributable risk (AAR), which is the same as either the absolute risk reduction (ARR) or the absolute risk increase (ARI). This is the difference in absolute risks with and without the risk factor. The second is the attributable risk percent or relative attributable risk. It is calculated by dividing the absolute risk increase or decrease by the absolute risk

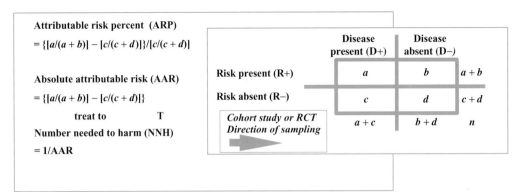

Fig. 13.6 Attributable risk and the number needed to harm.

for those not exposed to the risk factor. It can also be reported relative to those exposed to the risk factor. It tells you how much of the change in risk is due to the risk factor either absolutely or relative to the risk in the control group. For example, 95% of cases of lung cancer can be attributed to smoking. This percentage is risk of cases of lung cancer relative to people who don't smoke. The attributable risk of lung cancer in non smokers would be 5% and is the absolute attributable risk divided by the absolute risk in smokers. Attributable risk can only be calculated from cross-sectional studies, cohort studies or randomized clinical trials that can provide good measurement of the incidence of the outcome. This construct tries to quantify the contribution of other unidentifiable risk factors to the differences in outcomes between exposed and non-exposed groups.

Attributable risk quantitates the contribution of the risk factor in producing the outcome in those exposed to the risk factor. It is helpful in calculating the cost–benefit ratio of eliminating the risk factor from the population. Absolute attributable risk, also known as the absolute risk increase, is analogous to absolute risk reduction between the control and experimental event rates that was mentioned in the previous chapters. It allows for the calculation of the **number needed to treat to harm** (NNTH = 1/AAR or 1/ARI). This was previously called the number needed to harm (NNH). It tells us how many people need to be exposed before one additional person will be harmed or one additional harmful outcome will occur (Fig. 13.6).

Putting risk into perspective

A large increase in relative risk may represent a clinically unimportant increase in personal risk. This is especially true if the outcome is relatively rare in the population. For instance, several years ago there was a concern that the influenza vaccine could cause a serious and potentially fatal neurologic syndrome called Guillain–Barré syndrome (GBS). This syndrome consists of progressive weakness of the muscles of the body in an ascending pattern. It is usually reversible, but may require a period of time on a ventilator getting artificial respiration. There were 74 cases of this related to the influenza vaccine in 1993–1994. The odds ratio for that season was 1.5, meaning a 50% increase in the number of cases. Since the base incidence of this disease is approximately two in one million, even a 10-fold increase in risk would have little impact on the general population. This risk needed to be balanced against the number of lives saved by the influenza vaccine. That number is thousands of times greater than the small increased risk of GBS with the vaccine. Although the news of this possible reaction was alarming to many patients, it had very little clinical significance.

Similarly, a small increase in relative risk may represent a clinically important increase in personal risk if the outcome is common in the population. For example, if an outcome has an incidence of 12 in 100, increasing the risk even by 1.5, the same 50% increase as seen in the previous example, will have a significant impact on the general population. In this case, the examination of all possible outcome data is necessary to determine if eliminating the risk is associated with appropriate gains. For example, it is known that the use of conjugated estrogens in postmenopausal women can reduce the rate of osteoporosis but these estrogens are associated with an increased risk of endometrial carcinoma. Would the decreased morbidity and mortality due to osteoporosis balance the increase in morbidity and mortality due to endometrial cancer among women using conjugated estrogens? Good clinicians must be able to interpret these risks for patients and help them make an informed decision.

Confidence intervals give an idea of the relative precision of a study result. They represent the standard error of the relative risk or odds ratio. They should always be reported whenever relative risk or odds ratios are reported! Small, or as the statisticians say tight, confidence intervals suggest that the sampling error due to random events is small, leading to a very precise result. A large confidence interval is also called loose and suggests that there is a lot of random error leading to a very imprecise result. For example if the RR is 2 and the CI is 1.01 to 6, there is indeed an association, but it may be very strong (6) or very weak (1.01). Remember, if the confidence interval for a relative risk or odds ratio includes the number 1, there is no statistical association between risk factor and outcome. Statistically this is equivalent to a study result with $P > 0.05$.

The confidence interval allows someone to look at the spread of the results, and interpret the strengths and weaknesses of the results. Loose confidence intervals should suggest a need for more research. Usually they represent small samples and the addition of one or two new events could dramatically change the numbers. Very tight intervals that are close to one suggest a high degree of precision in the result, but also a low strength of association which may not be clinically important.

Reporting relative risk and odds ratios

Over the past 15 years, more and more epidemiologic cohort and case–control studies have been reporting their results in terms of relative risk and odds ratios. The intelligent consumer of the medical literature will be able to determine whether these resulting measures of risk were used correctly. Sometimes these measures are not used correctly, as illustrated below.

A recent example of this was a report in the *New England Journal of Medicine* about the effect of race and gender on physician referral for cardiac catheterization.[1,2] The original study reported that physicians, when given standardized scenarios, were more likely to refer white men, white women, and black men than black women for evaluation of coronary artery disease (CAD). The newspapers reported that blacks and women were 40% less likely to be referred for cardiac catheterization than whites and men. The actual study showed that 90.6% of the white men, white women, and black men were referred while 78.8% of the black women were referred. The authors incorrectly calculated the odds ratios for these numbers and came up with an odds ratio of 0.4. The actual odds associated with a 90.6% probability are 9.6 to 1 while those associated with a 78.8% probability are 3.7 to 1. When the data were recalculated for men and women or whites and blacks, the results showed that men were referred more often (90.6%) than women (84.7%) and whites (90.6%) more often than blacks (84.7%). The odds here were men (9.6), women (5.5), whites (9.6) and blacks (5.5), making the odds ratio for both of these comparisons equal to 0.6.

However, there were two problems with these numbers. First, the outcome was not rare in the diseased group. All of the groups were equal in size and the outcome was not rare in the general population. This distorts the odds ratio as an approximation of the relative risk. Second, the study was a clinical trial with the risk factors of race and gender being the independent variable and the referral for catheterization, the dependent variable. Therefore, the relative risk and not the odds ratio should have been calculated. Had this been done, the relative risk for white vs. black and men vs. women was 0.93 with the 95% CI from 0.89 to 0.99. Not only is the risk much smaller than reported in the news, but it approaches the null point suggesting lack of clinical significance or the possibility of a type I error. Ultimately, the original report using odds ratios led to a distortion in reporting of the study by the media.

[1] K. A. Schulman, J. A. Berlin, W. Harless, J. F. Kerner, S. Sistrunk, B. J. Gersch, R. Dubé, C. K. Taleghani, J. E. Burke, S. Williams, J. M. Eisenberg & J. J. Escarce. The effect of race and sex on physicians' recommendations for cardiac catheterization. *N. Engl. J. Med.* 1999; 340: 618–626.
[2] L. M. Schwartz, S. Woloshin & H. G. Welch. Misunderstandings about the effects of race and sex on physicians' referrals for cardiac catheterization. *N. Engl. J. Med.* 1999; 341: 279–283.

A user's guide to the trials of harm or risk

The following standardized set of methodological criteria can be used for the critical assessment of a trial studying risk, also called harm. It is based upon the Users' Guides to the Medical Literature published by *JAMA* and used with permission.[3] The University of Alberta (www.med.ualberta.ca/ebm) has online worksheets for evaluating articles of therapy that use this guide and are available as free use documents.

(1) Was the study valid?

   (a) Except for the exposure under study, were the compared groups similar to each other? Was this an RCT, a cross-sectional, cohort, or case–control study? Were other known prognostic factors similar or adjusted for?

   (b) Were the outcomes and exposures measured in the same way in the compared groups? Was there recall or interviewer bias? Was the exposure opportunity similar?

   (c) Was follow-up sufficiently long and complete? What were the reasons for incomplete follow-up?

   (d) Were risk factors similar in those lost and not lost to follow-up?

   (e) Is the temporal relationship correct? Did the exposure precede the outcome?

   (f) Is there a dose–response relationship? Did the risk of the outcome increase with the quantity or duration of the exposure?

(2) What are the results?

   (a) How strong is the association between exposure and outcome? What are the RR's or OR's? Was the correct measure of risk used for the study? RR used for cross-sectional, cohort, or RCTs and OR for case–control studies.

   (b) How precise is the estimate of risk? Were there wide or narrow confidence intervals?

   (c) If the study results were negative, did the study have a sufficiently large sample size?

(3) Will the results help me in patient care?

   (a) Can the results be applied to my patients? Were patients similar for demographics, severity, co-morbidity, and other prognostic factors?

   (b) Are treatments and exposures similar?

   (c) What is the magnitude of the risk? What is the absolute increase and its reciprocal, NNTH?

   (d) Should I attempt to stop the exposure? How strong is the evidence? What is the magnitude of the risk? Are there any adverse effects of reducing exposure?

---

[3] G. H. Guyatt & D. Rennie (eds.). *Users' Guides to the Medical Literature: a Manual for Evidence-Based Practice.* Chicago: AMA, 2002. See also Bibliography.

What does a zero numerator mean? Is there ever zero risk?

What if you read a study that found no instances of a particular outcome? A zero numerator does not mean that there is no risk. One can still infer an estimate of the potential size of the risk. There is an excellent article by Hanley and Lippman-Hand that shows how to handle this eventuality.[4] Their example is used here.

Suppose a given study shows no adverse events in 14 consecutive patients. What is the largest number of adverse events we can reasonably expect? What we are doing here is calculating the upper limit of the 95% CI for this sample. The rule of three can be used to determine this risk. The maximum number of events that can be expected to occur when none have been observed is $3/n$. For this study finding no adverse events in a study of 14 patients, the upper limit of the 95% CI is $3/14 = 21.4\%$. One could expect to see as many as one adverse event in every 5 patients and still have come up with no events in the 14 patients in the initial study.

Assume that the study of 14 patients resulted in no adverse outcomes. What if in reality there is an adverse outcome rate of 1:1000? The probability of no adverse events in one patient is 1 minus the probability of at least one adverse event in one patient. Another way of writing this is p(no adverse event in one patient) $= 1 - p$(at least one adverse event in one patient). This makes the probability of no adverse events $= 1 - 0.001 = 0.999$. Therefore p(no adverse events in n patients) is 0.999^n. For 14 patients this is 0.986, or there is a 98.6% chance that in 14 patients we would find no adverse outcome events.

Now suppose that the actual rate of adverse outcomes is 1:100. p(no adverse outcomes in one patient) $= 1 - 0.01 = 0.99$. p(no adverse events in 14 patients) $= 0.99^{14}$. This means that there is a 86.9% chance that we would find no adverse outcome in these 14 patients. We can continue to reduce the actual adverse event rate to 1:10, and using the same process we get p(no adverse events in 14 patients) $= (0.90)^{14}$. Now 22.9% is the chance we would find no adverse outcome events in these 14 patients.

Similarly, for an actual rate of 1:5 p(no adverse event in 14 patients) $= 0.8^{14}$ or 3.5%, and for an actual rate of 1:6 you get you will get a potential event rate of 7.7%. Therefore the 95% CI lies between event rates of 1:5 and 1:6. The rate estimated by our rule of three for adverse events is $3/n = 1/4.7 = 21.4\%$. When actually calculated the true number is $1/5.5 = 18.2\%$.

Mathematically one must solve the equation $(1 - \text{maximum risk})^n = 0.05$ to find the upper limit of 95% CI. Solving the equation for the maximum risk, $1 - \text{maximum risk} = \sqrt[n]{0.05}$, and maximum risk $= 1 - \sqrt[n]{0.05}$. For $n > 30$, $\sqrt[n]{0.05}$ is close to $(n-3)/n$, making the maximum risk $= 1 - [(n-3)/n] = 3/n$. The actual numbers are shown in Table 13.1. One can use a similar process to approximate

[4] J. A. Hanley & A. Lippman-Hand. If nothing goes wrong, is everything all right? Interpreting zero numerators. *JAMA* 1983; 249: 1743–1745.

Table 13.1. Actual vs. estimated rates of adverse events if there is a zero numerator

Rate found in study	Exact 95% CI	Rule $3/n$
0/10	26%	30%
0/20	14%	15%
0/30	10%	10%
0/100	0.3%	0.3%

Table 13.2. Approximate maximum event rate for small numerators

Number of events in the numerator	Estimate of maximum number of events
0	3/n
1	4/n
2	5/n
3	7/n
4	9/n

the upper limit of the 95% CI if there are 1, 2, 3, or 4 events in the numerator. Table 13.2 is the estimate of the maximum number of events one might expect if the actual number of events found is from 0 to 4.

For example, studies of head-injured patients to date have shown that none of the 2700 low-risk patients, those with laceration only or bump without loss of consciousness, headache, vomiting, or change in neurological status, had any intracranial bleeding or swelling. Therefore, the largest risk of intracranial injury in these low-risk patients would be $3/2700 = 1/900 = 0.11\%$. This is the upper limit of the 95% confidence interval.

To find the upper limit of the 99% CI, use rule of $4.6/n$, which can be derived in a similar manner. Table 13.3 gives the 95% CIs for extreme results with a variety of sample sizes.

General observations on the nature of risk

Most people don't know how to make reasonable judgments about the nature of risk, even in terms of risks that they know they are exposed to. This was articulated in 1662 by the Port Royal monks in their treatise about the nature of risk. If people did have this kind of judgment, very few people would be smoking. There

Table 13.3. 95% confidence limits on extreme results

	And the % is 0, the true	And the % is 100, the true
If the denominator is	% could be as *high* as	% could be as *low* as
10	26%	74%
20	14%	86%
30	10%	90%
40	7%	93%
50	6%	94%
60	5%	95%
70	4%	96%
80	4%	96%
90	3%	97%
100	3%	97%
150	2%	98%
300	1%	99%

are several important biases that come into play when talking about risk. The physician should be aware of this when discussing risks with their patient.

People are more likely to risk a poor outcome if due to voluntary action rather than imposed action. They are likely to smoke and accept the associated risks because they think it is their choice rather than an addiction. Similarly, they will accept risks that they feel they have control over rather than risks controlled by others. Because of this, people are much more likely to be very upset when they find out that their medication causes a very uncommon, but previously known, side effect.

One only has to read the newspapers to know that there are more stories on the front page about catastrophic accidents like plane crashes or fatal automobile accidents than minor automobile accidents. This is also true of medical situations. Patients are more willing to accept the risk of death from cancer or sudden cardiac death than death due to unforeseen complications of routine surgery. If there is a clear benefit to avoiding a particular risk, for example that one shouldn't drink poison, patients are more likely to accept a bad outcome if they engage in that risky behavior. A major exception to this rule is cigarette smoking, because of the social nature of smoking and the addictive nature of nicotine.

People are democratic about their perception of risk. They are more willing to accept risk that is distributed to all people rather than risk that is biased to some people. Natural risks are more acceptable than man-made risks. There is a perception that man-made objects ought not to fail, while if there is a natural disaster it is God's will. Risk that is generated by someone in a position of trust such as a doctor is less acceptable than that generated by someone not in that position like one's neighbor. We are more accepting of risks that are likely to affect adults than of those primarily affecting children, risks that are more familiar over those that are more exotic, and random events like being struck by lightning rather than catastrophes such as a storm without adequate warning.

14

Adjustment and multivariate analysis

Stocks have reached what looks like a permanently high plateau.

Irving Fisher, Professor of Economics, Yale University, 1929

Learning objectives

In this chapter you will learn:

- the essential features of multivariate analysis
- the different types of multivariate analysis
- the limitations of multivariate analysis
- the concept of propensity scoring
- the Yule–Simpson paradox

Studies of risk often look at situations where there are multiple risk factors associated with a single outcome, which makes it hard to determine whether a single statistically significant result is a chance occurrence or a true association between cause and effect. Since most studies of risk are observational rather than interventional studies, confounding variables are a significant problem. There are several ways of analyzing the effect of these confounding variables. Multivariate analysis and propensity scores are methods of evaluating data to determine the strength of any one of multiple associations uncovered in a study. They are attempts to reduce the influence of confounding variables on the study results.

What is multivariate analysis?

Multivariate analysis answers the question "What is the importance of one risk factor for the risk of a disease, when controlling for all other risk factors that could contribute to that disease?" Ideally, we want to quantitate the added risk for each individual risk factor. For example, in a study of lipid levels and the risk for coronary-artery disease, it was found that after adjusting for advancing age, smoking, elevated systolic blood pressure, and other factors, there was a 19% decrease in coronary heart disease risk for each 8% decrease in total cholesterol level.

In studies of diseases with multiple etiologies, the dependent variable can be affected by multiple independent variables. In the example described above, coronary heart disease is the dependent variable. Smoking, advancing age, elevated systolic blood pressure, other factors, and cholesterol levels are the independent variables. The process of multivariate analysis looks at the changes in magnitude of risk associated with each independent variable when all the other contributing independent variables are held fixed.

In studies using multivariate analysis, the dependent variable is most often an outcome variable. Some of the most commonly used outcome variables are incidence of new disease, death, time to death, and disease-free survival. In studies involving small populations or uncommon outcomes, there may not be enough outcome endpoints for analysis. In these cases, composite variables are often used to get enough outcome endpoints to enable a valid statistical analysis to be done. The independent variables are the risk factors that are suspected of influencing the outcome.

How multivariate analysis works: determining risk

Multivariate analysis looks at the changes in magnitude of the risk of a dependent variable associated with each suspected risk factor when the other suspected risk factors are held fixed. A schematic example of how this works can be seen in Fig. 14.1.[1]

If more variables are to be adjusted for, further division into even smaller groups must be done. This is shown in Fig. 14.2. One will notice that as more and more variables are added, the number of patients in each cell of every 2×2 table gets smaller and smaller. This will result in the confidence intervals of each odds ratio or relative risk getting larger and larger.

What can multivariate analysis do?

Some studies will look at multiple risk factors to determine which are most important in making a diagnosis or predicting the outcome of a disease. The output of these studies is often the result of a multivariate analysis. Although this can suggest which variables are most important, those important variables should be

---

[1] Demonstrated to me by Karen Rossnagel from the Institute of Social Medicine, Epidemiology and Health Economics of the Charité University Medical Center in Berlin, Germany.

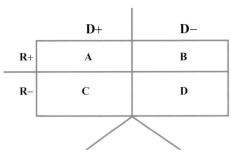

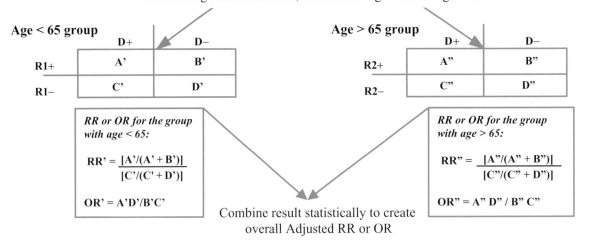

Fig. 14.1 The method of adjusting for a single variable in a multivariate analysis.

specifically evaluated in more detail in another study. The important variables are referred to as the **derivation set** and if the statistical significance found initially is still present after the multivariate analysis, it is less likely to be due to a Type I error. The researchers still need to do a follow-up or **validation study** to verify that the association did not occur purely by chance. Multivariate analysis can also be used for data dredging to confirm statistically significant results already found as a result of simple analysis of multiple variables. Finally, multivariate analysis can combine variables and measure the magnitude of effect of different combinations of variables on the outcome.

There are four basic types of multivariate analysis depending on the type of outcome variable. **Multiple linear regression** analysis is used when the outcome variable is continuous. **Multiple logistic regression analysis** is used when the outcome variable is a binary event like alive vs dead, or disease-free vs recurrent disease. **Discriminant function analysis** is used when the outcome variable is categorical such as better, worse, or about the same. **Proportional hazards regression analysis (Cox regression)** is used when the outcome variable is the

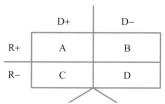

Separate into two groups by the presence or absence of the first potential confounding risk factor (age < 65 or > 65)

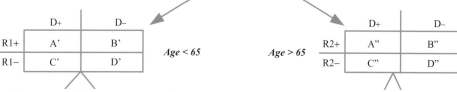

Separate each group further into two groups by the presence or absence of the second potential confounding risk factor (systolic blood pressure > 150mm Hg or <150mm Hg)

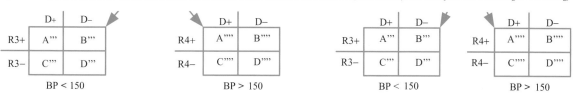

Fig. 14.2 Two confounding variables tested to see if the relationship between risk and outcome would still be true.

time to the occurrence of a binary event. An example of this is the time to death or time to tumor recurrence among treated cancer patients.

Assumptions and limitations

There are several types of problems associated with the interpretation of the results of multivariate analysis. These include overfitting, underfitting, linerarity, interaction, concomitance, coding, and outliers. All of these can produce error during the process of adjustment and should be considered by the author of the study.

Overfitting occurs when too many independent variables allow the researcher to find a relationship when in fact none exists. Overfitting leads to a Type I error. For example, in a cohort of 1000 patients there are 20 deaths due to cancer. If there are 15 baseline characteristics considered as independent variables, it is likely that one or two will cause a result which has statistical significance by chance alone. As a rule of thumb, there should be at least 10, and some statisticians say at least 20, outcome events per independent variable of importance for statistical tests to be valid. In the example here, with only 20 outcome events, adjustment for one or at most two independent variables is all that should be done. Overfitting of variables is characterized by large confidence intervals for each outcome measure.

Fig. 14.3 Non-linear curves and
the effect of crossing curves.

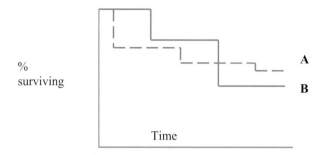

Underfitting occurs when there are too few outcome events to find a difference that actually exists. Underfitting causes a Type II error. For example,
a study of cigarette smokers followed 200 patients of whom two got lung
cancer over 10 years. This may not have been long enough time to follow the cohort and the number of cancer cases is too small to find a relationship between smoking and lung cancer. Too few cases of the outcome
of interest may make it impossible to find any statistical relationship with
any of the independent variables. Like overfitting, underfitting of variables
is also characterized by large confidence intervals. To minimize the effects
of underfitting, the sample size should be large enough for there to be at
least 10 and preferably 20 outcome events for each independent variable
chosen.

Linearity assumes that a linear relationship exists between the independent
and dependent variables, and this is not always true. Linearity means that
a change in the independent variable always produces the same proportional change in the dependent variable. If this is not true, one cannot use
linear regression analysis. In the Cox method of proportional hazards, the
increased risk due to an independent variable is assumed to be constantly
proportional over time. This means that when the risks of two treatments are
plotted over time, the curves will not cross. If there is a crossover (Fig. 14.3),
the early survival advantage of treatment B may not be noted since the initial improvement in survival in that group may be cancelled out by the later
reduction in survival.

Interaction between independent variables must be evaluated. For example,
smoking and oral contraceptive (OC) use are both risk factors for pulmonary
embolism in young women. When considering the risk of both of these
factors, it turns out that they interact. The risk of pulmonary embolism is
greater in smokers using OCs than with either risk factor alone. In cases like
this, the study should include enough patients with simultaneous presence
of both risk factors so that the adjustment process can determine the degree
of interaction between the independent variables.

Concomitance refers to a close relationship between variables. Unless there is no relationship between two apparently closely related independent variables being evaluated, only one should be used. If one measures both ventricular ejection fraction and ventricular contractility and correlates them to cardiovascular mortality, it is possible that one will get redundant results. In most cases, both independent variables will predict the dependent variable, but it is possible that only one variable would be predictive, when in fact they both ought to give the same result. This is an example of **concomitance**. Researchers should use the variable that is most important clinically as the primary independent variable. In this example, ventricular ejection fraction is easier to measure clinically and therefore more useful in a study.

Coding of the independent variables can affect the final result in unpredictable ways. For example, if the age is used as an independent variable and is recorded in 1-year intervals, 10-year intervals or as a dichotomous value such as less than or greater than 65, the results of a study will likely be different. There should always be a clear explanation about how the independent variables were coded for the analysis and why that method of coding was chosen. One can suspect that the authors selected the coding scheme that led to the best possible results and should be skeptical when reading studies in which this information is not explicitly given. Some authors might participate in post-hoc coding as a method of data dredging.

Outliers are influential observations that occur when one data point or a group of points clearly lie outside the majority of data. These should be explained during the discussion of the results and an analysis that includes and excludes these points should be presented. Outliers can be caused by error in the way the data are measured or by extreme biological variation in the sample. A technique called stratified analysis can be used to evaluate outliers.

In evaluation of any study using multivariate analysis, the standard processes in critical appraisal should be followed. There should be an explicit hypothesis, the data collection should be done in an objective, non-biased and thorough manner, and the software package used should be specified. An excellent overview on multivariate analysis is by J. Concato and others.[2]

Finally, it may not be possible to completely identify all of the confounders present in a study, especially when studying multifactorial chronic illnesses. Any study that uses multivariate analysis should be followed up with a study that looks specifically at those factors that are most important.

---

[2] J. Concato, A. R. Feinstein & T. R. Holford. The risk of determining risk with multivariable models. *Ann. Intern. Med.* 1993; 118: 201–210.

Propensity scores

Propensity scores are another mathematical method for adjusting results of a study to attempt to decrease the effect of confounders. They were developed specifically to counteract selection bias that can occur in an observational study. Patients may be selected based upon characteristics that are not explicitly described in the methods of the study. They have become a popular tool for adjustment over the past few years. Standard adjustment is done after the final results of the study are complete. Propensity scores are used before any calculations are done and typically use a scoring system to create different levels of likelihood or propensity for placing a particular patient into one or the other group. Patients with a high propensity score are those most likely to get the therapy being tested when compared to those with a low propensity score. The propensity score can then be used to stratify the results and determine whether one group will actually have a different result than the other groups. Usually the groups being compared are the ones with the highest or lowest propensity scores.

Patients who are likely to benefit the most from the chosen therapies will have the highest propensity scores. If a study is done using a large sample including patients who are less likely to benefit from the therapy, the study results may not be clinically or statistically important. But if the data are reanalyzed using only those groups with high propensity scores, it may be possible to show that there is improvement and justify the use of the drug at least in the group most likely to respond positively. The main problem with propensity scores is that the external validity of the result is limited. Ideally, the treatment should only be used for groups that have the same propensity scores as the group in the study. Those with much lower propensity scores should not have the drug used for them unless a study shows that they would also benefit from the drug.

Another use of propensity scores is to determine the effect of patients who drop out of a research study. The patients' propensity to attain the outcome of interest can be calculated using this score. Be aware, if there are too many coexisting confounding variables, it is unlikely that these approximations are reasonable and valid. One downfall of propensity scores is that they are often used as a means of obtaining statistically significant results, which are then generalized to all patients who might meet the initial study inclusion criteria. Propensity scores should be critically evaluated using the same rules applied to multivariate analysis as described in the start of this chapter.

Yule–Simpson paradox

This statistical anomaly was discovered independently by Yule in 1903 and rediscovered by Simpson in the 1950s. It states that it is possible for one of two groups to be superior overall and for the other group to be superior in multiple sub-groups. For example, one hospital has a lower overall mortality rate while a second competing hospital has a higher overall mortality rate but lower mortality in the various subgroups such as high risk and low risk patients. This is a purely mathematical phenomenon that occurs when there are large discrepancies in the sizes of these two subgroups between the two hospitals. Table 14.1 below demonstrates how this might occur.

Ideally, adjustment of the data should compensate for the potential for the Yule–Simpson paradox. However, this is not always possible and it is certainly reasonable to assume that particular factors may be more important than others and that these may not be adjusted for in the data. Readers should be careful to determine that all important factors have been included in the adjustments and still consider the possibility of the Yule–Simpson paradox if the results are fairly close together or if discrepant results occur for subgroups.

Table 14.1. Yule–Simpson paradox: mortality of patients with pneumonia in two hospitals[a]

Characteristic	High risk patients	Low risk patients	Total mortality
Hospital A	$30/100 = 30\%$	$1/10 = 10\%$	$31/110 = 28\%$
Hospital B	$6/10 = 60\%$	$20/100 = 20\%$	$26/110 = 24\%$

[a] Hospital A has lower mortality for each of the subgroups while Hospital B has lower total mortality.

15

Randomized clinical trials

One pill makes you larger,
and one pill makes you small.
And the ones your mother gives you,
don't do anything at all.

Grace Slick, The Jefferson Airplane: White Rabbit, from Surrealistic Pillow, 1967

Learning objectives

In this chapter you will learn:

- the unique features of randomized clinical trials (RCTs)
- how to undertake critical interpretation of RCTs

The randomized clinical trial (RCT) is the ultimate paradigm of clinical research. Many consider the RCT to be the most important medical development of the twentieth century, as their results are used to dictate clinical practice. Although these trials are often put on a pedestal, it is important to realize that as with all experiments, there may be flaws in the design, implementation, and interpretation of these trials. The competent reader of the medical literature should be able to evaluate the results of a clinical trial in the context of the potential biases introduced into the research experiment, and determine if it contains any fatal flaws.

Introduction

The clinical trial is a relatively recent development in medical research. Prior to the 1950s, most research was based upon case series or uncontrolled observations. James Lind, a surgeon in the British Navy, can claim credit for performing the first recorded clinical trial. In 1747, aboard the ship *Salisbury*, he took 12 sailors with scurvy and divided them into six groups of two each. He made sure they were similar in every way except for the treatment they received for scurvy.

Dr. Lind found that the two sailors who were given oranges and lemons got better while the other ten did not. After that trial, the process of the clinical trial went relatively unused until it was revived with studies of the efficacy of streptomycin for the treatment of tuberculosis done in 1948. The randomized clinical trial or randomized controlled trial has remained the premier source of new knowledge in medicine since then.

A **randomized clinical trial** is an experiment. In an RCT, subjects are randomly assigned to one of two or more therapies and then treated in an identical manner for all other potential variables. Subjects in an RCT are just as likely or unlikely to get the therapy of interest as they are to get the comparator therapy. Ideally the researchers are blinded to the group in which the subjects are allocated. The randomization code is not broken until the study is finally completed. There are variations on this theme using blinded safety committees to determine if the study should be stopped. Sometimes it is warranted to release the results of the study, which is stopped early because it showed a huge benefit and continuing the study would not be ethical.

Physician decision making and RCTs

There are several ways that physicians make decisions on the best treatment for their patients. **Induction** is the retrospective analysis of uncontrolled clinical experience or extension of the expected mechanism of disease as taught in pathophysiology. It is doing that which "seems to work," "worked before," or "ought to work." **"Abdication"** or seduction is someone doing something because others tell them that it is the right thing to do. These may be teachers, consultants, colleagues, advertisements, pharmaceutical representatives, authors of medical textbooks, and others. One accepts their analysis of the medical information on faith and this dictates what one actually does for his or her patient.

Deduction is the prospective analysis and application of the results of critical appraisal of formal randomized clinical trials. This method of decision making will successfully withstand formal attempts to demonstrate the worthlessness of a proven therapy. Therapy proven by well-done RCTs is what physicians should be doing for their patients, and it is what medical students should integrate into clinical practice for the rest of their professional lives. One note of caution belongs here. It is not possible to have an RCT for every question about medicine. Some diseases are so rare or therapies so dangerous that it is unlikely that a formal large RCT will ever be done to answer that clinical query. For these types of questions, observational studies or less rigorous forms of evidence may need to be applied to patients.

Table 15.1. Schema for randomized clinical trials

Ultimate objective	Specific treatment	Target disorder
cure	drug therapy	disease
reduce mortality	surgery	illness
prevent recurrence	other therapies	predicament
limit deterioration	nutrition	
prevention	psychological support	
relieve distress		
deliver reassurance		
allow the patient to die comfortably		

There are three global issues to identify when evaluating an RCT (Table 15.1). These are (1) the ultimate objective of treatment, (2) the nature of the specific treatment, and (3) the treatment target. The ultimate objective of treatment must be defined before the commencement of the trial. While we want therapy to cure and eliminate all traces of disease, more often than not other outcomes will be sought. Therapy can reduce mortality or prevent a treatable death, prevent recurrence, limit structural or functional deterioration, prevent later complications, relieve the current distress of disease including pain in the terminal phase of illness, or deliver reassurance by confidently estimating the prognosis. These are all very different goals and any study should specify which ones are being sought.

After deciding on the specific outcome one wishes to achieve, one must then decide which element of sickness the therapy will most affect. This is not always the disease or the pathophysiologic derangement itself. It may be the illness experience of the patient or how that pathophysiologic derangement affects the patient through the production of certain signs and symptoms. Finally, it could also be how the illness directly or indirectly affects the patient through disruption of the social, psychological, and economic function of their lives.

Characteristics of RCTs

The majority of RCTs are drug studies or studies of therapy. Often, researchers or drug companies are trying to prove that a new drug is better than drugs that are currently in use for a particular problem. Other researched treatments can be surgical operations, physical or occupational therapy, procedures, or other modalities to modify illness. We will use the example of drug trials for most of this discussion. However, any other medical question can be substituted for the subject of an RCT. The basic rules to apply to critically evaluate RCTs are covered in the following pages.

Hypothesis

The study should contain a hypothesis regarding the use of the drug in the general medical population or the specific population tested. There are two basic types of drug study hypotheses. First, the drug can be tested against placebo, or second, the drug can be tested against another regularly used active drug for the same indication. "Does the drug work better than nothing?" looks at how well the drug performs against a placebo or inert treatment. The placebo effect has been shown to be relatively consistent over many studies and has been approximated to account for up to 35% of the treatment effect. A compelling reason to compare the drug against a placebo would be in situations where there is a question of the efficacy of standard therapies. The use of Complementary and Alternative Medicines (CAM) is an example of testing against placebo and can often be justified since the CAM therapy is expected to be less active than standard medical therapy. Testing against placebo would also be justified if the currently used active drug has never been rigorously tested against active therapy. Otherwise, the drug being tested should always be compared against an active drug that is in current use for the same indication and is given in the correct dose for the indication being tested.

The other possibility is to ask "Does the drug work against another drug which has been shown to be effective in the treatment of this disease in the past?" Beware of comparisons of drugs being tested against drugs not commonly used in clinical practice, with inadequate dosage, or uncommon routes of administration. These caveats also apply to studies of medical devices, surgical procedures, or other types of therapy. Blinding is difficult in studies of modalities such as procedures and medical devices, and should be done by a non-participating outside evaluation team. Another way to study these modalities is by 'expert based' randomization. In this method, various practitioners are selected as the basis of randomization and patients enrolled in the study are randomized to the practitioner rather than the modality.

When ranking evidence, the well-done RCT with a large sample size is the highest level of evidence for populations. A subgroup of RCTs called the n-of-1 trial is stronger evidence in the individual patient and will be discussed later. An RCT can reduce the uncertainty surrounding conflicting evidence obtained from lesser quality studies as illustrated in the following example. Over the past 20 years, there were multiple studies that demonstrated decreased mortality if magnesium was given to patients with acute myocardial infarction (AMI). Most of these studies were fairly small and showed no statistically significant improvement in survival. However, when they were combined in a single systematic review, also called a meta-analysis, there was definite statistical and clinical improvement. Since then, a single large randomized trial called ISIS-4, enrolled thousands of patients with AMI and showed no beneficial effect attributable to giving magnesium. It is therefore very unlikely that magnesium therapy would benefit AMI patients.

RCTs are the strongest research design capable of proving cause-and-effect relationships. The cause is often the treatment, preventive medicine, or diagnostic test being studied, and the effect is the outcome of the disease being treated, disease prevention by early diagnosis or disease diagnosis by a test. The study design alone does not guarantee a quality study and a poorly designed RCT can give false results. Thus, just like all other studies, critical evaluation of the components is necessary before accepting the results.

The hypothesis is usually found at the end of the introduction. Each study should contain at least one clearly stated, unambiguous hypothesis. One type of hypothesis to be aware of is a single hypothesis attempting to prove multiple cause-and-effect relationships. This cannot be analyzed with a single statistical test and will lead to data dredging. Multiple hypotheses can be analyzed with multivariate analysis and the risks noted in Chapter 14 should be considered when analyzing these studies. The investigation should be a direct test of the hypothesis, although occasionally it is easier and cheaper to test a substitute hypothesis. For example, drug A is studied to determine its effect in reducing cardiovascular mortality, but what is measured is its effect on exercise-stress-test performances. In this case, the exercise-stress-test performance is a surrogate outcome and is not necessarily related to the outcome in which most patients are interested, mortality.

Inclusion and exclusion criteria

Inclusion and exclusion criteria for subjects should be clearly spelled out so that anyone reading the study can replicate the selection of patients. These criteria ought to be sufficiently broad to allow generalization of the study results from the study sample to a large segment of the population. This concept is also called **external validity** and was discussed in Chapter 8. The source of patients recruited into the study should minimize sampling or referral bias. For instance, patients selected from specialty health-care clinics often are more severely ill or have more complications than most patients. They are not typical of all patients with a particular disease so the results of the RCT may not be generalizable to all patients with the disorder. A full list of the reasons for patients' exclusion, the number of patients excluded for each reason, and the methods used to determine exclusion criteria must be defined in the study. Additionally, these reasons should have face validity. Commonly accepted exclusions are patients with rapidly fatal diseases that are unrelated to the disease being studied, those with absolute or relative contraindications to the therapy, and those likely to be lost to follow-up. Beware if there are too many subjects excluded without sound reasons, as this may be a sign of bias.

Randomization

Randomization is the key to the success of the RCT. The main purpose of randomization is to create study groups that are equivalent in every way except for the intervention being studied. Proper randomization means subjects have an equal chance of inclusion into any of the study groups. By making them as equal as possible, the researcher seeks to limit potential confounding variables. If these factors are equally distributed in both groups, bias due to them is minimized.

Some randomization schemes have the potential for bias. The date of admission to hospital, location of bed in hospital (Berkerson's bias), day of birth, and common physical characteristics such as eye color, all may actually be confounding variables and result in unequal qualities of the groups being studied. The first table in most research papers is a comparison of baseline variables of the study and control groups. This documents the adequacy of the randomization process. In addition, statistical tests should be done to show the absence of statistically significant differences between groups. Remember that the more characteristics looked at, the higher the likelihood that one of them will show differences between groups, just by chance alone. The characteristics listed in this first table should be the most important ones or those most likely to confound the results of the study.

Allocation of patients to the randomization scheme should be concealed. This means that the process of randomization itself is completely blinded. If a researcher knew to which study group the next patient was going to be assigned, it would be possible to switch their group assignment. This can have profound effects on the study results, acting as a form of selection bias. Patients who appeared to be sicker could be assigned to the study group preferred by the researcher, resulting in better or worse results for that group. Current practice requires that the researcher states whether allocation was concealed. If this is not stated, it should be assumed that it was not done and the effect of that bias assessed.

There are two new randomization schemes that merit consideration as methods of solving more and more complex questions of efficacy. The first is to allow all patients requiring a particular therapy to choose whether they will be randomized or be able to freely choose their own therapy. The researchers can then compare the group that chose randomization with the group that chose to self-select their therapy. This has an advantage if the outcome of the therapy being studied has strong components of quality of life measures. It answers the question of whether the patient's choice of being in a randomized trial has any effect on the outcome when compared with the possibility of having either of the therapies being studied as a choice. Another method of randomization is using expertise as the point of randomization. In this method, the patients are not randomized, but the therapy is randomized by the provider, with one provider or group of providers using one therapy and another, the comparison therapy. This is a useful method for studying surgical techniques or complementary and alternative medicine therapies.

Blinding

Blinding prevents confounding variables from affecting the results of a study. If all subjects, treating clinicians, and observers are blinded to the treatment being given during the course of the research, any subjective effects that could lead to biased results are minimized. Blinding prevents observer bias, contamination, and cointervention bias in either group. Lack of blinding can lead to finding an effect where none exists, or vice versa. No matter how honest, researchers may subconsciously tend to find what they want to find. Ideally, tests for adequacy of blinding should be done in any RCT. The simplist test is to ask participants if they knew which therapy they were getting. If there is no difference in the responses between the two groups, the blinding was successful and there is not likely to be any bias in the results due to lack of blinding.

   Some types of studies make blinding challenging, athough they can be done. Studies of different surgical methods or operations can be done with blinding by using sham operations. This has been successfully performed and in some cases found that standard therapeutic surgical procedures were not particularly beneficial. A recent series of studies showed that when compared to sham arthroscopic surgery for osteoarthritis, actual arthroscopic surgery had no benefit on outcomes such as pain and disability. Similar use of sham with acupuncture showed an equal degree of benefit from real acupuncture and sham acupuncture, with both giving better results than patients treated with no acupuncture. A recent review of studies of acupuncture for low back pain found that there was a dramatic effect of blinding on the outcomes of the studies. The non-blinded studies found acupuncture to be relatively useful for the short-term treatment of low back pain with a very low NNTB. However, when blinded studies were analyzed, no such effect was found and the results, presented in Table 15.2, were not statistically significant.[1]

---

[1] E. Ernst & A. R. White. Acupuncture for back pain: a meta-analysis of randomized controlled trials. *Arch. Intern. Med.* 1998; 158: 2235–2241.

Table 15.2. Effects of acupuncture on short-term outcomes in back pain

Type of study	Number of trials	Improved with acupuncture (%)	Improved with control (%)	Relative Benefit (95 % CI)	NNT (95% CI)
Blinded	4	73/127 (57)	61/123 (50)	1.2 (0.9 to 1.5)	13 (5 to no benefit)
Non-blinded	5	78/117 (67)	33/87 (38)	1.8 (1.3 to 2.4)	3.5 (2.4 to 6.5)

Description of methods

The methods section should be so detailed that the study could be duplicated by someone uninvolved with the study. The intervention must be well described, including dose, frequency, route, precautions, and monitoring. The intervention also must be reasonable in terms of current practice since if the intervention being tested is being compared to a non-standard therapy, the results will not be generalizable. The availability, practicality, cost, invasiveness, and ease of use of the intervention will also determine the generalizability of the study. In addition, if the intervention requires special monitoring it may be too expensive and difficult to carry out and therefore, impractical in most ordinary situations.

Instruments and measurements should be evaluated using the techniques discussed in Chapter 7. Appropriate outcome measures should be clearly stated, and their measurements should be reproducible and free of bias. Observers should be blinded and should record objective outcomes. If there are subjective outcomes measured in the study, use caution. Subjective outcomes don't automatically invalidate the study and observer blinding can minimize bias from subjective outcomes. Measurements should be made in a manner that ensures consistency and maximizes objectivity in the way the results are recorded. For statistical reasons, beware of composite outcomes, subgroup analysis, and post-hoc cutoff points, which can all lead to Type I errors.

The study should be clear about the method, frequency, and duration of patient follow-up. All patients who began the study should be accounted for at the end of the study. This is important because patients may leave the study for important reasons such as death, treatment complications, treatment ineffectiveness, or compliance issues, all of which will have implications on the application of the study to a physician's patient population. A study attrition rate of > 20% is a rough guide to the number that may invalidate the final results. However, even a smaller percentage of patient drop-outs may affect the results of a study if not taken into consideration. The results should be analyzed with an intention-to-treat analysis or using a best case/worst case analysis.

Analysis of results

The preferred method of analysis of all subjects when there has been a significant drop-out or crossover rate is to use an intention-to-treat methodology. In this method, all patient outcomes are counted with the group to which the patient was originally assigned even if the patient dropped out or switched groups. This approximates real life where some patients drop out or are non-compliant for various reasons. Patients who dropped out or switched therapies must still be accounted for at the end of the trial since if their fates are unknown, it is impossible to accurately determine their outcomes. Some studies will attempt to use statistical models to estimate the outcomes that those patients should have had if they had completed the study, but the accuracy of this depends on the ability of the model to mimic reality.

A good example of intention-to-treat analysis was in a study of survival after treatment with surgery or radiation for prostate cancer. The group randomized to radical prostatectomy surgery or complete removal of the prostate gland, did much better than the group randomized to either radiation therapy or watchful waiting with no treatment. Some patients who were initially randomized to the surgery arm of the trial were switched to the radiation or watchful waiting arm of the trial when, during the surgery, it was discovered that they had advanced and inoperable disease. These patients should have been kept in their original surgery group even though their cancerous prostates were not removed. When the study was re-analyzed using an intention-to-treat analysis, the survival in all three groups was identical. Removing those patients biased the original study results since patients with similarly advanced cancer spread were not removed from the other two groups.

Another biased technique involves removing patients from the study. Removing patients after randomization for reasons associated with the outcome is patently biased and grounds to invalidate the study. Leaving them in the analysis as an intention-to-treat is honest and will not inflate the results. However, if the outcomes of patients who left the study are not known, a best case/worst case scenario should be applied and clearly described so that the reader can determine the range of effects applicable to the therapy.

In the best case/worst case analysis, the results are re-analyzed considering that all patients who dropped out or crossed over had the best outcome possible or worst outcome possible. This should be done by adding the drop-outs of the intervention group to the successful patients in the intervention group and at the same time subtracting the drop-outs of the comparison group from the successful patients in that group. The opposite process, subtracting drop out patients from the intervention group and adding them to the comparison group, should then be done. This will give a range of possible values of the final effect size. If this range is very large, we say that the results are **sensitive** to small changes that could result from drop-outs or crossovers. If the range is very small, we call the results **robust**, as they are not likely to change drastically because of drop-outs or crossovers.

Compliance with the intervention should be measured and noted. Lack of compliance may influence outcomes since the reason for non-compliance may be directly related to the intervention. High compliance rates in studies may not be duplicated in clinical practice. Other clinically important outcomes that should be measured include adverse effects, direct and indirect costs, invasiveness, and monitoring of an intervention. A blinded and independent observer should measure these outcomes, since if the outcome is not objectively measured, it may limit the usefulness of the therapy. Remember, no adverse effects among n patients could signify as many as $3/n$ adverse events in actual practice.

Results should be interpreted using the techniques discussed in the sections on statistical significance (Chapters 9–12). Look for both statistical and clinical significance. Look at confidence intervals and assess the precision of the results. Remember, narrow CIs are indicative of precise results while wide CIs are imprecise. Determine if any positive results could be due to Type I errors. For negative studies determine the relative likelihood of a Type II error.

Discussion and conclusions

The discussion and conclusions should be based upon the study data and limited to settings and subjects with characteristics similar to the study setting and subjects. Good studies will also list weaknesses of the current research and offer directions for future research in the discussion section. Also, the author should compare the current study to other studies done on the same intervention or with the same disease.

In summary, no study is perfect, all studies have flaws, but not all flaws are fatal. After evaluating a study using the standardized format presented in this chapter, the reader must decide if the merits of a study outweigh the flaws before accepting the conclusions as valid.

Further problems

A study published in *JAMA* in February 1995 reviewed several systematic reviews of clinical trials, and found that if the trials were not blinded or the results were incompletely reported there was a trend of showing better results.[2] This highlights the need for the reader to be careful in evaluating these types of trials.

[2] K. F. Schulz, I. Chalmers, R. J. Hayes & D. G. Altman. Empirical evidence of bias. Dimensions of methodological quality associated with estimates of treatment effects in controlled trials. *JAMA* 1995; 273: 408–412.

Fig. 15.1 Effect of blinding and sample size on results in trials of acupuncture for low back pain. From E. Ernst & A. R. White. *Arch. Intern. Med.* 1998; 158: 2235–2241.

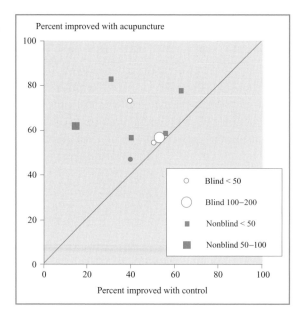

Always look for complete randomization, total double blinding, and reporting of all potentially important outcomes. An example of this phenomenon can be seen in the systematic review of studies of acupuncture for back pain that was described earlier.

L'Abbé plots are a graphic technique for presenting the results of many individual clinical trials.[3] The plot provides a simple visual representation of all the studies of a particular clinical question. It is a way of looking for the presence of bias in the studies done on a single question. The plot shows the proportion of patients in each study who improved taking the control therapy against the proportion who improved taking the active treatment. Each study is represented by one point and the size of the circle around that point is proportional to the sample size of the study. The studies closest to the diagonal show the least effect of therapy, and farther from the diagonal show a greater effect. In addition to getting an idea of the strength of the difference between the two groups, one can also look for the effects of blinding, sample size, or any other factor on the study results. Figure 15.1 shows the results of studies of the effectiveness of acupuncture on short-term improvements in back pain. The studies are divided by blinded vs. non-blinded and by size of sample. One can clearly see that the results of the blinded trials were less spectacular than the unblinded ones.

[3] K. A. L'Abbé, A. S. Detsky & K. O'Rourke. Meta-analysis in clinical research. *Ann. Intern. Med.* 1987; 107: 224–233.

The n-of-1 trial

An n-of-1 trial is done like any other experiment, but with only one patient as a subject. Some have called this the highest level of evidence available. However, it is only useful in the one patient to whom it is applied. It is a useful technique to determine optimal therapy in a single patient when there appears to be no significant advantage of one therapy over another based on reported clinical trials. In order to justify the trial, the effectiveness of therapy must really be in doubt, the treatment should be continued long-term if it is effective, and the patient must be highly motivated to allow the researcher to do an experiment on them. It is helpful if there is a rapid onset of action of the treatment in question and rapid cessation when treatment is discontinued. There should be easily measurable and clinically relevant outcome measures and sensible criteria for stopping the trial.

Additionally, the patient should give informed consent before beginning the trial. The researcher must have a willing pharmacist and pharmacy that can dispense identical, unlabeled active and placebo or comparison medications. Endpoints must be measurable with as much objectivity as possible. Also, the patient should be asked if they knew which of the two treatments they were taking and a statistician should be available to help evaluate the results.[4]

A user's guide to the randomized clinical trial of therapy or prevention

The following is a standardized set of methodological criteria for the critical assessment of a randomized clinical trial article looking for the best therapy which can be used in practice. It is based, with permission, upon the Users' Guides to the Medical Literature published by *JAMA*.[5] The University of Alberta (www.med.ualberta.ca.ebm) has online worksheets for evaluating articles of therapy that use this guide.

(1) Was the study valid?
    (a) Was the assignment of patients to treatments really randomized?
        (i) Was similarity between groups documented?
        (ii) Was prognostic stratification used in allocation?
        (iii) Was there allocation concealment?
        (iv) Were both groups of patients similar at the start of the study?
    (b) Were all patients who entered the study accounted for at its conclusion?

---

[4] For more information on the n-of-1 RCT, consult D. L. Sackett, R. B. Haynes, P. Tugwell & G. H. Guyatt. *Clinical Epidemiology: a Basic Science for Clinical Medicine.* 2nd edn. Boston: Little Brown, 1991, pp. 225–238.

[5] G. H. Guyatt & D. Rennie (eds.). *Users' Guides to the Medical Literature: A Manual for Evidence-Based Practice.* Chicago: AMA, 2002. See also Bibliography.

      (i) Was there complete follow-up of all patients?

      (ii) Were drop-outs, withdrawals, non-compliers, and those who crossed over handled appropriately in the analysis?

  (c) Were the patients, their clinicians, and the study personnel including recorders or measurers of outcomes blind to the assigned treatment?

  (d) Were the baseline factors the same in both groups at the start of the trial?

  (e) Aside from the intervention being tested, were the two groups of patients treated in an identical manner?

      (i) Was there any contamination?

      (ii) Were there any cointerventions?

      (iii) Was the compliance the same in both groups?

(2) What are the results?

  (a) How large was the effect size and were both statistical and clinical significance considered? How large is the treatment effect?

      (i) If statistically significant, was the difference clinically important?

      (ii) If not statistically significant, was the study big enough to show a clinically important difference if it should occur?

      (iii) Was appropriate adjustment made for confounding variables?

  (b) How precise are the results? What is the size of the 95% confidence intervals?

(3) Will the results help me care for my patient?

  (a) Were the study patients recognizably similar to my own?

      (i) Are reproducibly defined exclusion criteria stated?

      (ii) Was the setting primary or tertiary care?

  (b) Were all clinically relevant outcomes reported or at least considered?

      (i) Was mortality as well as morbidity reported?

      (ii) Were deaths from all causes reported?

      (iii) Were quality-of-life assessments conducted?

      (iv) Was outcome assessment blind?

  (c) Is the therapeutic maneuver feasible in my practice?

      (i) Is it available, affordable, and sensible?

      (ii) Was the maneuver administered in an adequately blinded manner?

      (iii) Was compliance measured?

  (d) Are the benefits worth the costs?

      (i) Can I identify all the benefits and costs, including non-economic ones?

      (ii) Were all potential harms considered?

The CONSORT statement

Beginning in 1993, the Consolidated Standards of Reporting Trials Group, known as the CONSORT group began their attempt to standardize and improve the

Table 15.3. Template for the CONSORT format of an RCT showing the flow of participants through each stage of the study

1. Assessed for eligibility (n = . . .)
2. Enrollment: Excluded (n = . . .) Not meeting inclusion criteria (n = . . .), Refused to participate (n = . . .), Other reasons (n = . . .)
3. Randomized (n = . . .)
4. Allocation: Allocated to intervention (n = . . .), Received allocated intervention (n = . . .), Did not receive allocated intervention (n = . . .) (give reasons)
5. Follow-up: Lost to follow up (n = . . .) (give reasons), Discontinued intervention (n = . . .) (give reasons)
6. Analysis: Analyzed (n = . . .), Excluded from analysis (n = . . .) (give reasons)

reporting of the process of randomized clinical trials. This was as a result of laxity of reporting of the results of these trials. Currently most medical journals require that the CONSORT requirements be followed in order for an RCT to be published. Look for the CONSORT flow diagram at the start of any RCT and be suspicious that there are serious problems if there is no flow diagram for the study. The CONSORT flow diagram is outlined in Table 15.3.

Ethical issues

Finally, there are always ethical issues that must be considered in the evaluation of any study. Informed consent must be obtained from all subjects. This is a problem in some resuscitation studies, where other forms of consent such as substituted or implied consent may be used. Look for Institutional Review Board (IRB) approval of all studies. If it is not present, it may be an unethical study. It is the responsibility of the journal to publish only ethical studies. Therefore most journals will not publish studies without IRB approval. Decisions about whether or not to use the results of unethical studies are very difficult and beyond the scope of this book. As always, in the end, readers must make their own ethical judgment about the research.

All the major medical journals now require authors to list potential conflicts of interest with their submissions. These are important to let the reader know that there may be a greater potential for bias in these studies. However, there are always potential reasons to suspect bias based upon other issues that may not be so apparent. These include the author's need to "publish or perish," desire to gain fame, and belief in the correctness of a particular hypothesis. A recent study on the use of bone-marrow transplantation in the treatment of stage 3 breast cancers showed a positive effect of this therapy. However, some time after publication, it was discovered that the author had fabricated some of his results, making the therapy look better than it actually was.

All RCTs should be described, before initiation of the research, in a registry of clinical trials. This can be seen on the ClinicalTrials.gov website, a project of the National Institutes of Health in the United States. This is a registry of clinical trials conducted around the world. The site gives information about the purpose of the clinical trial, who may participate, locations, and phone numbers for more details. These details should be adequate for anyone else to duplicate the trial. The purpose of the registry is to get the details of the trial published on-line prior to initiation of the trial itself. This way, the researchers cannot spin the results to look better by reporting different outcomes than were originally specified or by using different methods than originally planned. Most journals will no longer publish trials that are not registered in this or a similar international registry.

The question of placebo controls is one ethical issue which is constantly being discussed. Since there are therapies for almost all diseases, is it ever ethical to have a placebo control group? This is still a contentious area with strong opinions on both sides. One test for the suitability of placebo use is clinical equipoise. This occurs when the clinician is unsure about the suitability of a therapy and there is no other therapy that works reasonably well to treat the condition. Here placebo therapy can be used. Both the researcher and the patient must be similarly inclined to choose either the experimental or a standard therapy. If this is not true, placebo ought not to be used.

16

Scientific integrity and the responsible conduct of research

John E. Kaplan, Ph.D.

Integrity without knowledge is weak and useless, and knowledge without integrity is dangerous and dreadful.

Samuel Johnson (1709–1784)

Learning objectives

In this chapter you will learn:

- what is meant by responsible conduct of research
- how to be a responsible consumer of research
- how to define research misconduct and how to deal with it
- how conflicts of interest may compromise research, and how they are managed
- why and how human participants in research studies are protected
- what constitutes responsible reporting of research findings
- how peer review works

The responsible conduct of research

The conduct and ethics of biomedical researchers began to receive increased attention after World War II. This occurred in part as a response to the atrocities of Nazi medicine and in part because of the increasing rate of technological advances in medicine. This interest intensified in the United States in response to the publicity surrounding improper research practices, particularly the Tuskegee syphilis studies, studies of the effects of LSD on unsuspecting subjects, and studies of radiation exposure. While these issues triggered important reforms, the focus was largely restricted to protection of human experimental subjects.

The conduct of scientists again became an area of intense interest in the 1980s after a series of high-profile cases of scientific misconduct attracted the attention both of the US public and of the US Congress, which conducted a series of investigations into the matter. These included the misconduct cases regarding Robert Gallo, a prominent AIDS researcher, and Nobel Laureate David Baltimore. Even cases that were not found to be misconduct increased public and political interest in the behavior of researchers. This interest resulted in the development of federally prescribed definitions of scientific misconduct. Now there are requirements that federally funded institutions adopt policies for responding to allegations of research fraud and for protecting the whistle-blowers. This was followed by the current requirement that certain researchers be given ethics training with funding from federal research training grants.

This initial regulation was scandal-driven and was focused on preventing wrong or improper behavior. As these policies were implemented, it became apparent that this approach was not encouraging proper behavior. This new focus on fostering proper conduct by researchers led to the emergence of the field now generally referred to as the *responsible conduct of research*. This development is not the invention of the concept of scientific integrity, but it has significantly increased the attention bestowed on adherence to existing rules, regulations, guidelines, and commonly accepted professional codes for the proper conduct of research. It has been noted that much of what constitutes responsible conduct of research would be achieved if we all adhered to the basic code of conduct we learned in kindergarten: play fair, share, and tidy up.

The practice of evidence-based medicine requires high quality evidence. A primary source of such evidence is from scientifically based clinical research. To be able to use this evidence, one must be able to believe what one reads. For this reason it is absolutely necessary that the research be trustworthy. Research must be proposed, conducted, reported, and reviewed responsibly and with integrity. Research, and the entire scientific enterprise, are based upon trust. In order for that trust to exist, the consumer of the biomedical literature must be able to assume that the researcher has acted responsibly and conducted the research honestly and objectively.

The process of science and proper conduct of evidence-based medicine are equally dependent on the consumption and application of research findings being conducted with responsibility and integrity. This requires readers to be knowledgeable and open-minded in reading the literature. They must know the factual base and understand the techniques of experimental design, research, and statistical analysis. It is as important that the reader consumes and applies research without bias as it is that the research is conducted and reported without bias. Responsible use of the literature requires that the reader be conscientious in obtaining a broad and representative, if not complete, view of that segment. Building one's knowledge-base on reading a selected part of that literature, such as abstracts alone, risks incorporating incomplete or wrong information into clinical practice and may lead to bias in the interpretation of the work. Worse would be to act on pre-existing bias and selectively seek out only those studies in the literature that one agrees with or that support one's point of view, and to ignore those parts that disagree. In addition, it is essential that when one uses or refers to the work of others their contribution be appropriately referenced and credited.

Scientists conducting research with responsiblity and integrity constitutes the first line of defense in ensuring the truth and accuracy of biomedical research. It is important to recognize that the accuracy of scientific research does not depend upon the integrity of any single scientist or study, but instead depends on science as a whole. It relies on findings being reproduced and reinforced by other scientists, which is a mechanism that protects against a single finding or study being uncritically accepted as fact. In addition, the process of peer review further protects the integrity of the scientific record.

Research misconduct

Research or **scientific misconduct** represents events in which error is introduced into the body of scientific knowledge knowingly, through deception and misrepresentation. Research misconduct does not mean honest error or differences in opinion. Errors occurring as the result of negligence in the way the experiment is conducted are also not generally considered research misconduct. However, negligence in the experiment does fall outside the scope of responsible conduct of science guidelines.

In many respects, research misconduct is a very tangible concept. This contrasts to other areas within the broad scope of responsible conduct of research. Both the agencies sponsoring research and the institutions conducting research develop policies to deal with research misconduct. These policies require that a specific definition of research misconduct be developed. This effort has been fraught with controversy and resulted in a proliferation of similar, but not identical, definitions from various government agencies that sponsor research. Nearly all definitions agree that three basic concepts underlie scientific misconduct. These include **fabrication, falsification,** and **plagiarism**. In a nutshell, definitions agree that scientists should not lie, cheat, or steal. These ideas have now been included in a new single federal definition (Federal Register: November 2, 2005 [Volume 70, Number 211]).

The previous definition of research misconduct from the National Institutes of Health, the agency sponsoring most US government funded biomedical research, also included a statement prohibiting "other serious deviations from accepted research practices." This statement is difficult to define specifically but reflects the belief that there are other behaviors besides fabrication, falsification, and plagiarism that constitute research misconduct. A government-wide definition has been developed and approved. According to this policy "research misconduct is defined as fabrication, falsification, or plagiarism in proposing, performing, or reviewing research, or in reporting research results." (Federal Register: November 2, 2005 (Volume 70, Number 211]).

These three types of misconduct are defined as follows:

Fabrication is making up data and recording or reporting them.

Falsification is manipulating research materials, equipment, or processes, or changing or omitting data such that the research is not accurately represented in the research record.

Plagiarism is the appropriation of another person's ideas, processes, results, or words without giving appropriate credit.

It is likely that the vast majority of scientists, and people in general, know that it is wrong to lie, cheat, or steal. This probably includes those who engage in such behavior. There are clearly numerous motivations that lead people to engage in such practices. These may include, but are not limited to, acting on personal or political biases, having personal financial incentives, personal and professional ambition, and fear of failure. In our system of research, the need for financial support and desire for academic advancement as measures of financial and professional success are dependent upon the productivity of a research program. Until there are some fundamental changes in the way research is funded, these questionable incentives are likely to remain in place.

Many people believe that a substantial amount of research misconduct goes unreported because of concerns that there will be consequences to the whistle-blower. All institutions in the United States that engage in federally supported research must now have in place formal policies to prevent retaliation against whistle-blowers. Unfortunately, it is unlikely that someone will be able to recognize scientific misconduct simply by reading a research study unless the misconduct is plagiarism of work they did or is very familiar to them. Usually such misconduct, if found at all, is discovered locally or during the review process prior to publication and may never be disclosed to the general scientific community.

Conflict of interest

Conflicts of interest may provide the motivation for researchers to act outside of the boundaries of responsible conduct of research. Webster's dictionary defines **conflict of interest** as "A conflict between the private interests and professional responsibilities of a person in a position of trust." A useful definition in the context of biomedical research and patient care was stated by D. F. Thompson who stated that "a conflict of interest is a set of conditions in which professional judgement concerning a primary interest (such as patient welfare or the validity

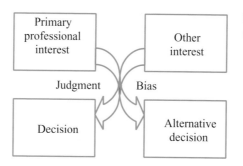

Fig. 16.1 Conflict of interest schematic.

of research) tends to be unduly influenced by secondary interest (such as financial gain)."[1] These relationships are diagrammed in Fig. 16.1. It is very important to recognize that conflicts of interest per se are common among people with complex professional careers. Simply having conflict of interest is not necessarily wrong and is often unavoidable. What is wrong is when one is inappropriately making decisions founded on these conflicts or when one accepts a new responsibility over a previous professional interest. An example of this would be a physician becoming a part owner of a lab, to which he or she sends patients for bloodwork, at the cost of the physician's previous priority of patient care. Decisions that are made based upon the bias produced by these interests are especially insidious when they result in the compromise of patient care or in research misconduct.

Many of the rules regarding conflict of interest focus on financial gain, not because it is the worst consequence, but because it is more objective and regulable. There is substantial reason for concern that financially based conflicts of interest have affected research outcomes. Recent studies of calcium channel blockers,[2] non-steroidal anti-inflammatory drugs,[3] and health effects of second-hand smoke[4] each found that physicians with financial ties to manufacturers were significantly less likely to criticize safety or efficacy. A study of clinical-trial publications[5] determined a significant association between positive results and pharmaceutical company funding. Analysis of the cost-effectiveness of six oncology drugs[6] found that pharmaceutical company sponsorship of economic analyses led to a reduced likelihood of reporting unfavorable results.

[1] D. F. Thompson. Understanding financial conflicts of interest. *N. Engl. J. Med.* 1993; 329: 573–576.
[2] H. T. Stelfox, G. Chua, K. O'Rourke & A. S. Detsky. Conflict of interest in the debate over calcium-channel antagonists. *N. Engl. J. Med.* 1998; 338: 101–106.
[3] P. A. Rochon, J. H. Gurwitz, R. W. Simms, P. R. Fortin, D. T. Felson, K. L. Minaker & T. C. Chalmers. A study of manufacturer-supported trials of nonsteroidal anti-inflammatory drugs in the treatment of arthritis. *Arch. Intern. Med.* 1994; 154: 157–163.
[4] R. M. Werner & T. A. Pearson. What's so passive about passive smoking? Secondhand smoke as a cause of atherosclerotic disease. *JAMA* 1998; 279: 157–158.
[5] R. A. Davidson. Source of funding and outcome of clinical trials. *J. Gen. Intern. Med.* 1986; 1: 155–158.
[6] M. Friedberg, B. Saffran, T. J. Stinson, W. Nelson & C. L. Bennett. Evaluation of conflict of interest in economic analyses of new drugs used in oncology. *JAMA* 1999; 282: 1453–1457.

Most academic institutions attempt to manage researcher's potential conflict of interest. This is justified as an attempt to limit the influence of those conflicts and protect the integrity of research outcomes and patient-care decisions. Surprisingly, some academicians have argued against such management on the grounds that it impugns the integrity of honest physicians and scientists. Some institutions have decided that limiting the opportunity for outside interests prevents recruitment and retention of the best faculty. The degree to which these activities are conflicts of interests remains an ongoing debate in the academic community.

Nearly all academic institutions engaging in research currently have policies to manage and/or limit conflicts of interest. Most of these focus exclusively on financial conflicts and are designed primarily to protect the institutions financially. Increased awareness of the consequences of conflict of interest will hopefully result in the development of policies that offer protection to research subjects and preserve the integrity of the research record.

There are several ways that institutions choose to manage conflict of interest. The most common is requiring disclosure of conflicts of interest with the rationale that individuals are less likely to act on conflicts if they are known. Other methods include limitations on the value of outside interests such as limiting the equity a researcher could have in a company with whom they work or limiting the amount of consultation fees they can collect. Recently some professional organizations have suggested that the only effective management for potential conflicts of interest is their complete elimination.

Some of the most difficult conflicts occur when physicians conduct clinical studies where they enroll their own patients as research subjects. This can place the performance of the research and patient care in direct conflict. Another common area of conflict is in studies funded by pharmaceutical companies. Often they desire a veto in all decisions affecting the conduct and publication of the results.

Research with human participants

In order to obtain definitive information on the pathophysiologic sequelae of human disease, as well as to assess risk factors, diagnostic modalities, and therapeutic interventions, it is necessary to use people as research subjects. After several instances of questionable practices in studies using human subjects, the US Congress passed the National Research Act in 1974. One outcome of this legislation was the publication of the Belmont Report that laid the foundation of ethical principles which govern the conduct of human studies and provide protection for human participants. These principles are respect for personal autonomy, beneficence, and justice.

The principle of respect for persons manifests itself in the practice of informed consent. **Informed consent** requires that individuals be made fully aware of the risks and benefits of the experimental protocol and that they be fully able to evaluate this information. Consent must be fully informed and entirely free of coercion.

The principle of beneficence manifests itself in the assessment of risk and benefit. The aim of research involving human subjects is to produce benefits to either the research subject, society at large, or both. At the same time, the magnitude of the risks must be considered. The nature of experimental procedures generally dictates that everything about them is not known and so risks, including some that are unforeseen, may occur. Research on human subjects should only take place when the potential benefits outweigh the potential risks. Another way of looking at this is the **doctrine of clinical equipoise**. At the onset of a study, the research aims, treatment and control, are equally likely to result in the best outcome. At the very least, the comparison group must be receiving a treatment consistent with the current standard of care. The application of this principle could render some placebo-controlled studies unethical.

The principle of justice manifests itself in the selection of research subjects. This principle dictates that the benefits and the risks of research be distributed fairly within the population. There should be no favoritism shown when enrolling patients into a study. For example, groups should be selected for inclusion into the research study based on characteristics of patients who would benefit from the therapy, and not because they are poor or uneducated.

The responsibilities for ensuring that these principles are applied rest with **Institutional Review Boards** (IRBs). These must include members of varying background, both scientific and non-scientific, who are knowledgeable of the institution's commitments and regulations, applicable law and ethics, and standards of professional conduct and practice. The IRB must approve both the initiation and continuation of each study involving human participants. The IRB seeks to ensure that risk is minimal and reasonable in relation to the anticipated benefit of the knowledge gained. The IRB evaluates whether selection of research subjects is equitable and ensures that consent is informed and documented, that provisions are included to monitor patient safety, and that privacy and confidentiality are protected.

One of the most difficult roles for the physician is the potential conflict between patient care responsibilities and the objectivity required of a researcher. Part of the duty of the IRB ought to be an evaluation of the methodology of the research study. Some researchers disagree with this role. But, it ensures that subjects, our patients, are not subjected to useless or incompetently done research.

Peer review and the responsible reporting of research

Peer review and the responsible reporting of research are two important and related subjects that impact directly on the integrity of the biomedical research record. Peer review is the mechanism used to judge the quality of research and is applied in several contexts. This review mechanism is founded on the premise that a proposal or manuscript is best judged by individuals with experience and expertise in the field.

The two primary contexts are the evaluation of research proposals and manuscript reviews for journals. This mechanism is used by the National Institutes of Health and nearly every other non-profit sponsor of biomedical research (e.g., American Heart Association, American Cancer Society, etc.) to evaluate research proposals. Almost all journals also use this mechanism. In general, readers should be able to assume that journal articles are peer-reviewed although it is important to be aware of those that are not. Readers should have a lower level of confidence in research reported in journals that are not peer-reviewed. In general, society-sponsored and high-profile journals are peer-reviewed. If there are doubts, check the information for authors section, which should describe the review process.

To be a responsible peer reviewer, one must be knowledgeable, impartial, and objective. It is not as easy as it might seem to meet all of these criteria. The more knowledgeable a reviewer is in the field of a proposal, the more likely they are to be a collaborator, competitor, or friend of the investigators. These factors, as well as potential conflicts of interest, may compromise their objectivity. Prior to publication or funding, proposals and manuscripts are considered privileged confidential communications that should not be shared. It is the responsibility of the reviewer to honor this confidentiality. It is similarly the responsibility of the reviewer not to appropriate any information gained from peer review into his or her own work.

As consumers and, perhaps, contributors to the biomedical literature, we need research to be reported responsibly. Responsible reporting of research also includes making each study a complete and meaningful contribution as opposed to breaking it up to achieve as many publications as possible. Additionally, it is important to make responsible conclusions and issue appropriate caveats on the limitations of the work. It is necessary to offer full and complete credit to all those who have contributed to the research, including references to earlier works. It is essential to always provide all information that would be essential to others who would repeat or extend the work.

17

Applicability and strength of evidence

Find out the cause of this effect, Or rather say, the cause of this defect, For this effect
defective comes by cause.

William Shakespeare (1564–1616): Hamlet

Learning objectives

In this chapter you will learn:

- the different levels of evidence
- the principles of applying the results of a study to a patient

The final step in the EBM process is the application of the evidence found in clinical studies to an individual patient. In order to do this, the reader of the medical literature must understand that all evidence is not created equal and that some forms of evidence are stronger than others. Once a cause-and-effect relationship is discovered, can it always be applied to the patient? What if the patient is of a different gender, socioeconomic, ethnic, or racial group than the study patients? This chapter will summarize these levels of evidence and help to put the applicability of the evidence into perspective. It will also help physicians decide how to apply lower levels of evidence to everyday clinical practice.

Applicability of results

The application of the results of a study is often difficult and frustrating for the clinician. Overall, one must consider the generalizability of study results to patients. A sample question would be; "Is a study of the risk of heart attack that was done in men applicable to a woman in your practice?" Answering this question involves inducing the strength of a presumed cause-and-effect relationship in that patient based upon uncertain evidence. This is the essence of the art of

Table 17.1. Criteria for application of results (in decreasing order of importance)

Strength of research design
Strength of result
Consistency of studies
Specificity (confounders)
Temporality (time–related)
Dose–response relationship
Biological plausibility
Coherence (consistency in time)
Analogous studies
Common sense

Source: After Sir Austin Bradford Hill. *A Short Textbook of Medical Statistics.* Oxford: Oxford University Press, 1977, pp. 309–323.

Fig. 17.1 The application of evidence to a particular clinical situation (from Chapter 2).

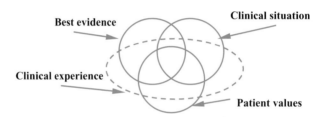

medicine and is a blend of the available evidence, clinical experience, the clinical situation, and the patient's preferences (Fig. 17.1).

One must consider the strength of the evidence for a particular intervention or risk factor. The stronger the study, the more likely it is that those results will be borne out in practice. A well-done RCT with a large sample size is the strongest evidence for the efficacy of a practice in a defined population. However, these are very expensive and difficult to perform, and physicians often must make vital clinical decisions based upon less stringent evidence.

Sir Austin Bradford Hill, the father of modern biostatistics and epidemiology, developed a useful set of rules to determine the strength of causation based upon the results of a clinical study. These are summarized in Table 17.1.

Levels of evidence

Strength of the research design

The strongest design for evaluation of a clinical question is a systematic review (SR) of multiple randomized clinical trials. Ideally, the studies in these reviews will be homogeneous and done with carefully controlled methodology. The process of data analysis of these meta-analyses is complex, and is the basis of the Cochrane Collaboration, a loose network of physicians who systematically review various topics and publish the results of their reviews. We will discuss these further in Chapter 33.

The randomized clinical trial (RCT) with human subjects is the strongest single research design capable of proving causation. It is least likely to have methodological confounders and is the only study design that can show that altering the cause alters the effect. Confounding variables both recognized and unrecognized, can and should be evenly distributed between control and experimental groups through adequate randomization, minimizing the likelihood of bias due to these differences. Ideally, the study should be double-blinded. In studies with strong results, those results should be accompanied by narrow confidence intervals. Clearly, the strongest evidence is the RCT carried out in the exact population that fits the patient in question. However, such a study is rarely available and physicians must use what evidence they can find, combined with their previous knowledge, to determine how the evidence produced by the study should be used. The n-of-1 RCT is another way of obtaining high quality evidence for a patient, but is difficult to perform and usually outside the scope of most medical practices at this time.

The next best level of evidence comes from observational studies. The results of such studies may only represent association and can never prove that changes in a cause can change the effect. The strongest observational-study research design supporting causation is a cohort study, which can be done with either a prospective or a non-concurrent design. Cohort studies can show that cause precedes effect but not that altering the cause alters the effect. Bias due to unrecognized confounding variables between the two groups might be present and should be sought and controlled for using multivariate analysis.

A case–control study is a weaker research design that can still support causation. The results of these studies can prove an association between the cause and the effect. Sometimes, the cause can be shown to precede the effect. However, altering the cause cannot be shown to alter the effect. A downside to these studies is that they are subject to many methodological problems that may bias the outcome. But, for uncommon and rare diseases, this may be the strongest evidence possible and can provide high-quality evidence if the study is done correctly.

Finally, case reports and descriptive studies including case series and cross-sectional studies have the lowest strength of evidence. These studies cannot prove cause and effect, they can only suggest an association between two variables and point the way toward further directions of research. For very rare conditions they can be the only, and therefore the best, source of evidence. This is true when they are the first studies to call attention to a particular disorder or when they are of the "all-or-none" type.

Hierarchies of research studies

There are several published hierarchies of classification for research studies. A system published by the Centre for Evidence-Based Medicine of Oxford University grades studies into levels from 1 through 5 and is an excellent grading scheme for clinical studies. This system grades studies by their overall quality and design. Level 1 studies are very large RCTs or systematic reviews. Level 2 studies are smaller RCTs with less than 50 subjects, RCTs with lower quality, or large high-quality cohort studies. Level 3 studies are smaller cohort or case–control studies. Level 4 evidence comes from case reports and low-level case–control and cohort studies. Finally, Level 5 is expert opinion or consensus based upon experience, physiology, or biological principles. Evidence-based medicine resources such as critically appraised topics (CATs) or Journal Club Banks must be evaluated on their own merits and should be peer-reviewed.

These levels of evidence are cataloged for articles of therapy or prevention, etiology or harm, prognosis, diagnosis, decision and economic analyses. This scheme, developed at the Centre for Evidence-Based Medicine at Oxford University is shown in Appendix 1.

Another classification scheme uses levels A through D to designate the strength of recommendations based upon the available evidence. Grade A is the strongest evidence and D the weakest. For studies of therapy or prevention, the following is a brief description of this classification of recommendations.

Grade A is a recommendation based on the strongest study design and consists of sublevels 1a to 1c. 1a is systematic reviews with homogeneity, free of worrisome variations, also known as heterogeneity, in the direction and degree of the results between individual studies. Heterogeneity, whether statistically significant or not, does not necessarily disqualify a study and should be addressed on an individual basis. Sublevel 1b is an individual randomized clinical trial with narrow confidence intervals. Studies with wide confidence intervals should be viewed with care and would not qualify as 1b level of evidence. Finally, the inclusion of the all-or-none case series as 1c evidence is somewhat controversial. These studies may be helpful for studying new, uniformly fatal, or very rare disorders, but should be viewed with care as they are incapable of proving any elements of contributory cause and are only considered preliminary findings.

Grade B is a recommendation based on the next level of strength of design and includes 2a, systematic reviews of homogeneous cohort studies; 2b, strong individual cohort studies or weak RCTs with less than 80% follow-up; and

2c, outcomes research. Also included are 3a, systematic reviews of homogeneous case–control studies, and 3b, individual case–control studies.

Grade C is a recommendation based on the weakest study designs and includes level 4, case series and lower-quality cohort and case–control studies. These studies fail to clearly define comparison groups, to measure exposures and outcomes in the same objective way in both groups, to identify or appropriately control known confounding variables, or carry out a sufficiently long and complete follow-up of patients.

Finally, grade D recommendations are not based upon any scientific studies and are therefore the lowest level of evidence. Also called level 5, they consist of expert opinion without explicit critical appraisal of studies. It is based solely upon personal experience, applied physiology, or the results of bench research.

These strength-of-evidence recommendations apply to average patients. Individual practitioners can modify them in light of a patient's unique characteristics, risk factors, responsiveness, and preferences about the care they receive. A level that fails to provide a conclusive answer can be preceded by a minus sign –. This may occur because of wide confidence intervals that result in a lack of statistical significance but fails to exclude a clinically important benefit or harm. This also may occur as a result of a systematic review with serious and statistically significant heterogeneity. Evidence with these problems is inconclusive and can only generate Grade C recommendations.

A new proposal for grading evidence is in the recently published GRADE scheme. This stands for the *Grading of Recommendations Assessment, Development and Evaluation* Working Group. Established in 2000, it consists of a group of EBM researchers and practitioners, many of whom had other quality of evidence schemes that they regularly used and which were often in conflict with each other. This group has created a uniform schema for classifying the quality of research studies based on the ability to prove the cause and effect relationship. The scheme is outlined in Table 17.2.[1] Software for the GRADE process is available as shareware on their website: www.gradeworkinggroup.org and through the Cochrane Collaboration.

Strength of results

The actual strength of association is the next important issue to consider. This refers to the clinical and statistical significance of the results. It is reflected in

[1] D. Atkins, D. Best, P. A. Briss, M. Eccles, Y. Falck-Ytter, S. Flottorp, G. H. Guyatt, R. T. Harbour, M.C. Haugh, D. Henry, S. Hill, R. Jaeschke, G. Leng, A. Liberati, N. Magrini, J. Mason, P. Middleton, J. Mrukowicz, D. O'Connell, A. D. Oxman, B. Phillips, H. J. Schunemann, T. T. Edejer, H. Varonen, G. E. Vist, W. R. Williams Jr. & S. Zaza; Grade Working Group. Grading quality of evidence and strength of recommendations. *BMJ*. 2004; 328: 1490.

Table 17.2. GRADE recommendations

High	Randomized Clinical Trial – Further research is unlikely to change our confidence in the estimate of the effects
Moderate	Further research is likely to have an important impact on our confidence in our estimate of the effects and may change the estimate
Low	Cohort studies – Further research is likely to have an important impact on our confidence in our estimate of the effects and is likely to change the estimate
Very low	Any other evidence – Any estimate of effect is uncertain

Decrease grade if:

1. Serious (−1) or very serious (−2) limitations to study quality
2. Important inconsistency
3. Some (−1) or major (−2) uncertainty about directness
4. Imprecise or sparse data (−1)
5. High probability of reporting bias (−1)

Increase grade if:

1. Strong evidence of association – significant relative risk >2 (< 0.5) based on consistent evidence from two or more observational studies with no plausible confounders (+1)
2. Very strong evidence of association – significant relative risk >5 (< 0.2) based on direct evidence with no major threats to validity (+1)
3. Evidence of a dose response gradient (+1)
4. All plausible confounders would have reduced the effect (+1)

the magnitude of the effect size or the difference found between the two groups studied. The larger the effect size and lower the P value, the more likely that the results did not occur by chance alone and there is a real difference between the groups. Other common measures of association are odds ratios and relative risk: the larger they are, the stronger the association. A relative risk or odds ratio over 5 or over 2 with very narrow confidence intervals should be considered strong. Confidence intervals (CI) quantify the precision of the result and give the potential range of this strength of association. Confidence intervals should be routinely given in any study.

Even if the effect size, odds ratio (OR), or relative risk (RR) is statistically significant, one must decide if this result is clinically important. There are a number of factors to consider when assessing clinical importance. First, lower levels of RR or OR may be important in situations where the baseline risk level is fairly high. However, if the CI for these measures is overly wide, the results are less precise and therefore less meaningful. Second, finding no effect size or one that was not statistically significant may have occurred because of lack of power. The skew of the CI may give a subjective sense of the power of a negative study. Last, other measures of strength of association include the number needed to treat to get benefit (NNTB), obtained from randomized clinical trials, and the number needed to screen to get benefit (NNSB) and number needed to treat to get harm (NNTH), obtained from cohort or case–control studies.

John Snow performed what is acknowledged as the first modern recorded epidemiologic study in 1854. Known as the Broad Street Pump study, he proved that the cause of a cholera outbreak in London was the pump on Broad Street. This pump was supplied by water from one company and was associated with a high rate of cholera infection in the houses it fed, while a different company's pump had a much lower rate of infection. The relative risk of death was 14, suggesting a very strong association between consumption of water from the tainted pump and death due to cholera. A modern-day example is the high strength of association in the connection between smoking and lung cancer. Here the relative risk in heavy smokers is about 20. With such high association, competing hypotheses for the cause of lung cancer are unlikely and the course for the clinician should be obvious.

Consistency of evidence

The next feature to consider when looking at levels of evidence is the consistency of the results. Overall, it is critical that different researchers in different settings and at different times should have done research on the same topic. The results of these comparable studies should be consistent, and if the effect size is similar in these studies, the evidence is stronger. Be aware that less consistency exists in those studies that use different research designs, clinical settings, or study populations. A good example of the consistency of evidence occurred with studies looking at smoking and lung cancer. For this association, prior to the 1965 Surgeon General's report, there were 29 retrospective and 7 prospective studies, all of which showed an association between smoking and lung cancer.

A single study that shows results that are discordant from many other studies suggests the presence of bias in that particular study. However, sometimes a single large study will show a discordant result compared with multiple small studies. This may be due to lack of power of the small studies and if this occurs, the reader must carefully evaluate the methodology of all the studies and use those studies with the best and least-biased methodology. In general, large studies result in more believable results. If a study is small, a change in the outcome status of one or two patients could change the entire study conclusion from positive to negative.

Specificity

The next characteristic to consider is the specificity of the results. This means making sure that the cause in the study is the actual factor associated with the effect. Often, the putative risk factor is confused with a confounding factor or a surrogate marker may produce both cause and effect.

Specificity can be a problematic feature of generalization as there are usually multiple sources of causation in chronic illness and multiple effects from one type of cause. For example, before the advent of milk pasteurization, there were multiple diverse diseases associated with the consumption of milk. A few of these were tuberculosis, undulant fever, typhoid, and diphtheria. To attribute the cause of all these diseases to the milk ignores the fact that what they have in common is that they are all caused by bacteria. The milk is simply the vehicle and once the presence of bacteria and their role in human diseases were determined, it could be seen that ridding milk of all bacteria was the solution to preventing milkborne transmission of these diseases. Then the next step was inspecting the cows for those same diseases and eradicating them from the herd.

We can relate this concept to cancer of the lung in smokers. Overall, the death rate in smokers is higher than in non-smokers. For most causes of death, the increase in death rate in smokers is about double (200%) that of nonsmokers. However, for lung cancer specifically, the increase in the death rate in smokers is almost 2000%, an increase of 20 times. This lung cancer death rate is more specific than the increased death rate for other diseases. In those other diseases, smoking is a less significant risk factor, since there are multiple other factors that contribute to the death rate for those diseases. However, it is still a factor! In lung cancer, smoking is a much more significant factor in the death rate.

Temporal relationship

The next characteristic that should be considered is the temporal relationship between the purported cause and effect. In order to have a temporal relationship, there should be an appropriate chronological sequence of events found by the study. The disease progression should follow a predictable path from risk-factor exposure to the outcome and that pattern should be reproducible from study to study. Be aware that it is also possible that the effect may produce the cause. For example, some smokers quit smoking just prior to getting sick with lung cancer. While they may attribute their illness to quitting, the illness was present long before they finally decided to quit. Is quitting smoking the cause and lung cancer the effect? In this case, the cancer may appear to be the cause and the cessation of smoking the effect. The causality may be difficult to determine in many cases, especially with slowly progressive and chronic diseases.

Dose–response

The dose–response gradient can help define cause and effect if there are varying concentrations of the cause and varying degrees of association with the effect. Usually, the association becomes stronger with increasing amounts of exposure to the cause. However, some cause-and-effect relationships show the opposite correlation, with increasing strength of association when exposure decreases. An example of this inverse relationship is the connection between vitamin intake and birth defects. As the consumption of folic acid increases in a population, the incidence of neural tube birth defects decreases. The direction and magnitude of the effect should also show a consistent dose–response gradient. This gradient can be demonstrated in randomized clinical trials and cohort studies but not in case–control or descriptive studies.

In general, we would expect that an increased dose or duration of the cause would produce an increased risk or severity of the effect. The more cigarettes smoked, the higher the risk of lung cancer. The risk of lung cancer decreases among former smokers as the time from giving up smoking increases. Some phenomena produce a J-shaped curve relating exposure to outcome. In these cases, the risk is highest at both increased and decreased rates of exposure while it is lowest in the middle. For example, a recent study of the effect of obesity on mortality showed a higher mortality among patients with the highest and lowest body mass index with the lowest mortality among people with the mid-range levels of body mass index.

Biological plausibility

When trying to decide on applicability of study results, biological plausibility should be considered. The results of the study should be consistent with what we know about the biology of the body, cells, tissues, and organs, and with data from various branches of biological sciences. There should be some basic science in-vitro bench or animal studies to support the conclusions and previously known biologic mechanisms should be able to explain the results. Is there a reason in biology that men and women smokers will have different rates of lung cancer? For some medical issues, gender, ethnicity, or cultural background has a huge influence while for other medical issues the influence is very little. To determine which areas fall into each category, more studies of gender and other differences for medical interventions are required.

Coherence of the evidence over time

In order to have strong evidence, there should be consistency of the evidence over varying types of studies. The results of a cohort study should be similar to those of case–control or cross-sectional studies done on the same cause-and-effect relationship. Studies that show consistency with previously known epidemiological data are said to evidence epidemiological consistency. Also, results should agree with previously discovered relationships between the presumed cause and effect in studies done on other populations around the world. An association of high cholesterol with increased deaths due to myocardial infarction was noted in several epidemiological studies in Scandinavian countries. A prospective study in the United States found similar results. As an aside, a potential confounding factor in this is the increase in cigarette smoking and related diseases in men after World War I and women following World War II.

Analogy

Reasoning by analogy is one of the weakest criteria allowing generalization. Knowing that a certain vitamin deficiency predisposes women to deliver babies with certain birth defects will marginally strengthen the evidence that another vitamin or nutritional factor has a similar effect. When using analogy, the proposed cause-and-effect relationship is supported by findings from studies using the same methods but different variables. For example, multiple studies using the same methodology have demonstrated that aspirin is an effective agent for the secondary prevention of myocardial infarction (MI). From this, one could infer that a potent anticoagulant like warfarin ought to have the same effect. However, warfarin may increase mortality because of the side effect of causing increased bleeding. How about suggesting that warfarin use decreases the risk of stroke in patients who have had transient ischemic attacks, or MI in patients with unstable angina? Again, although it is suggested by an initial study, the proposed new intervention may not prove beneficial when studied alone.

Common sense

Finally, in order to consider applying a study result to a patient, the association should make sense and competing explanations associating risk and outcome should be ruled out. For instance, very sick patients are likely to have a poor outcome even if given a very good drug, thus making the drug look less efficacious than it truly is. Conversely, if most patients with a disease do well without any therapy, it may be very difficult to prove that one drug is better than another for that disease. This is referred to as the Pollyanna effect. When dealing with this effect, an inordinately large number of patients would be necessary to prove a beneficial effect of a medication. There are a few consequences of not using common sense. It may lead to the overselling of potent drugs, and may result in clinical researchers neglecting more common, cheaper, and better forms of therapy. Similarly, patients thinking that a new wonder drug will cure them may delay seeking care at a time when a potentially serious problem is easily treated and complications averted.

Finally, it is up to the individual physician to determine how a particular piece of evidence should be used in a particular patient. As stated earlier, this is the art

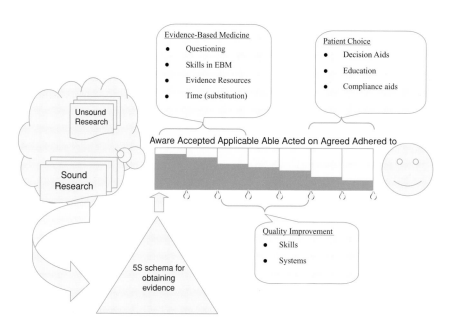

Fig. 17.2 Pathman's Pipeline of application of innovation from well done research to use in all appropriate patients (From P. Glasziou, used with permission).

of medicine. There are many people that decry the slavish use of EBM in patient-care decisions. There are also those who demand that we use only the highest evidence. There must be a middle ground. We must learn to use the best evidence in the most appropriate situations and communicate this effectively to our patients. There is a real need for more high-quality evidence for the practice of medicine; however, we must treat our patients now with the highest-quality evidence available.

Pathman's Pipeline

The Pathman 'leaky' pipeline is a model of knowledge transfer, taking the best evidence from the research arena into everyday practice. This model considers the ways that evidence will be lost in the process of diffusion into the everyday practice of medicine. It was developed by D.E. Pathman, a family physician in the 1970s, to model the reasons why physicians did not vaccinate children with routine vaccinations. It has been expanded to model the reasons that physicians don't use the best evidence (Fig. 17.2). Any model of EBM must consider the consequences of the constructs in this model on the behavior of practicing physicians and acceptability of evidence by patients.

Providers must be *aware* of the evidence through reading journals or getting notification through list services or other on-line resources or Continuing Medical Education (CME). They must then *accept* the evidence as being legitimate and useful. This follows a bell-shaped curve with the innovators followed by the early adopters, early majority, late majority, and finally the laggards. Providers must believe that the evidence is *applicable* to their patients, specifically the one in their clinic at that time. They must then be *able* to perform the intervention. This can be a problem in rural areas or less developed countries. Finally, the providers must *act* upon the evidence and apply it to their patients. However, it is still up to the patient to *agree* to accept the evidence and finally be compliant and *adhere* to the evidence. The next chapter will discuss the process of communication of the best evidence to patients.

18

Communicating evidence to patients

Laura J. Zakowski, M.D., Shobhina G. Chheda, M.D., M.P.H., and
Christine S. Seibert, M.D.

Think like a wise man but communicate in the language of the people.

William Butler Yeats (1865–1939)

Learning objectives

In this chapter you will learn:

- when to communicate evidence with a patient
- five steps to communicating evidence
- how health literacy affects the communication of evidence
- common pitfalls to communicating evidence and their solutions

When a patient asks a question, the health-care provider may need to review evidence or evidence-based recommendations to best answer that question. Once familiar with study results or clinical recommendations directed at the patient's question, communicating evidence to a patient occurs through a variety of methods. Only when the patient's perspective is known, can this advice be tailored to the individual patient. This chapter addresses both the patient's and the health-care provider's role in the communication of evidence.

Patient scenario

To highlight the communication challenges for evidence-based medicine, we will start with a clinical case. A patient in clinic asks whether she should take aspirin to prevent strokes and heart attacks. She is a 59-year-old woman who has high cholesterol (total cholesterol 231 mg/dL, triglycerides 74 mg/dL, HDL cholesterol 52 mg/dL, and LDL cholesterol 164 mg/dL), BMI 35 kg/m^2 and sedentary lifestyle. She has worked for at least a year on weight loss and cholesterol reduction through diet and is frustrated by her lack of results. She is otherwise healthy. Her family history is significant for stroke in her mother at age 75

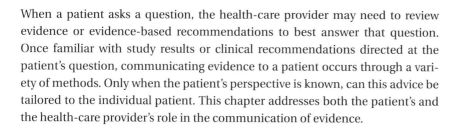

Table 18.1. Steps for communicating evidence with patients

1. Understand the patient's experience and expectations
2. Build partnerships
3. Provide evidence, including uncertainties
4. Present recommendations
5. Check for understanding and agreement

From: R. M. Epstein, B. S. Alper & T. E. Quill. Communicating evidence for participatory decision making. *JAMA.* 2004; 291: 2359–2366.

and heart attack in her father at age 60. She is hesitant to take medication, however, she wants to know if she should take aspirin to prevent strokes and heart attacks. Throughout the chapter, we will refer to this case and the dilemma that this patient presents.

Steps to communicating evidence

Questions like this do not have a simple yes or no answer; therefore more discussion between the provider and the patient is often needed. This discussion provides an opportunity for the provider to encourage the patient to be involved in the decision. Shared or participatory decision making is part of a larger effort toward patient-centered care, where neither the patient nor the provider makes the decision about what to do, rather both parties participate. The provider is responsible for getting the best available evidence to the patient, who must then be assisted in interpreting this evidence and putting it into the context of their life.

Very little evidence exists as to the best approach to communicate evidence to patients in either shared or physician-driven decision-making models. However, Epstein and colleagues have proposed a step-wise approach to this discussion using a shared decision model of communication that we have found helpful (Table 18.1). We use these steps as a basis for discussion about communication of evidence.

Step 1: Understand the patient's experience and expectations

Using the patient's query about aspirin as an example, first determine why the patient is asking, using a simple question such as "What do you know about how aspirin affects heart attacks and strokes?" This will help the provider understand if the patient has a rudimentary or more advanced understanding of the question. When communicating evidence, knowing the patient's baseline understanding of the question avoids reviewing information of which the patient is already aware. Finding the level of understanding is a sure way to acknowledge that the process of care is truly patient-centered.

This first step helps determine if it is necessary to communicate evidence. A patient with a question does not automatically trigger the need for a discussion of the evidence, since a patient may have already decided the course of action and asks the question as a means of validation of her knowledge. A patient may also ask a question that does not require a review of the evidence. For example, a patient may ask her physician's opinion about continuing her bisphosphonate for osteoporosis. When asking her further about her perspective, she tells you that she is concerned about the cost of the treatment. In this case, communication of the benefits of bisphosphonates will not answer her question directly. Rather, understanding her financial limitations is more appropriate. For some questions about therapy, there may be no need to discuss evidence, because the patient and the provider may be in clear agreement about the treatment. Our patient's question of aspirin as a preventive treatment against stroke and heart attacks is one that seems to require a discussion of the best available evidence.

Though typical office visits are short, taking time to understand the patient's perspective may help avoid cultural assumptions. For example, when seeing a patient who is culturally different from you, one might assume that the patient's values are different as well. On the other hand, it is easy to make false assumptions of shared values based on misperceived similarities of backgrounds between the provider and the patient. Understanding the patient's perspective comes from active questioning of the patient to determine their values and perspectives and avoids assumptions about similarities and differences.

Patients have varying levels of understanding of health-care issues, some with vast and others with limited previous health-care experience and levels of understanding. The patient's level of health literacy clearly affects her perspective on the question and how she will interpret any discussion of results and recommendations. During the initial phases of the discussion about her question, it is important to understand her health literacy and general literacy level. Asking the patient what she knows about the problem can provide an impression of health literacy. This may be adequate, but asking a question such as: "How comfortable are you with the way you read?" can provide an impression of general literacy.

This initial step also helps to frame a benefit and risk discussion. For example, if a patient wishes to avoid taking a medication because he or she is more concerned about the side effects of treatment than the benefits of treatment, focus the discussion on the evidence in this area.

Pitfalls to understanding the patient's experience and expectations

Some of the most well-designed studies, which have the highest potential to affect practice, are often time-limited and do not always address long-term effects, about which patients frequently have an interest. Also, many studies report major morbidity and mortality of treatment, yet, patients may be more concerned about the quality-of-life effects of treatment over many years. In other studies, the use of composite outcomes can make it difficult to directly answer a patient's question since some of these are more important to the patient than others. The patient in our example wishes to know whether aspirin reduces the risk of heart attack. Although one may find a study that shows a statistically significant reduction of myocardial infarction, if the result is only reported as a composite outcome along with other outcomes such as reduced incidence of angina and heart failure, the result will not directly address your patient's question. Since this type of presentation of data is used by authors when an individual outcome is not itself statistically significant, the combination of outcomes is used to achieve statistical significance and get the study published. But, the composite is often made up of various outcomes not all of which have the same value to the patient. The goal of a discussion with the patient is to explain the results of each of the composite components so that she can make up her mind about which of the outcomes are important to her.

Recommendations for understanding the patient's experience and expectations

The patient's perspective on the problem as well as the available evidence determines the true need to proceed with further steps to communicate evidence. It is possible that the patient's questions relate only to background information, which is clearly defined in the science of medicine and not dependent on your interpretation of the most recent research evidence for an answer. Then, if evidence is needed to answer a patient's question, first check to see whether it truly addresses the patients query about her desired outcomes rather than outcomes that are not important to the patient.

Step 2: Build partnerships

Taking time for this step is a way to build rapport with the patient. After discussing the patient's perspective, an impression will have developed of whether one generally agrees or disagrees with the patient. At this point in the discussion, it should be clear what, if any, existing evidence may be of interest to the patient. The physician will also have a good understanding of whether to spend a majority of their time discussing basic or more advanced information. Using phrases such as "Let me summarize what you told me so far" or "It sounds like you are not sure what to do next" can help to build partnership that will allow a transition to the third step in the process of communicating evidence. In the example, the patient who is interested in aspirin for prevention of strokes and heart attacks is frustrated by her lack of reduction of weight or cholesterol after implementing some lifestyle changes. Expressing empathy for her struggles will likely help the patient see you as partner in her care.

Step 3: Provide evidence

As health-care providers, numbers are an important consideration in our decision-making process. While some may want the results this way, many patients do not want results to be that specific or in numerical form. As a general rule, patients tend to want few specific numbers, although patients' preferences range from not wanting to know more than a brief statement or the "bottom line" of what the evidence shows to wanting to know as much as is available about the actual study results. Check the patient's preference for information by asking: "Do you want to hear specific numbers or only general information?" Many patients aren't sure about this, and many providers don't ask. Another way to start is by giving minimal information and allowing the patient to ask for more, or follow this basic information by asking the patient whether more specific information is desired. Previous experiences with the patient can also assist in determining how much information to discuss.

Presenting the information

There are a number of ways to communicate information to patients and understanding the patient's desires can help determine the best way to do this. The first approach is to use conceptual terms, such as "most patients" or "almost every patient" or "very few patients." This approach avoids the use of numbers when presenting results. A second approach is to use general numerical terms, such as "half the patients" or "1 in 100 patients." The use of numerical terms is more precise than conceptual terms, but can be more confusing to patients. While these are the most common verbal approaches, both conceptual and numerical representations can be graphed, either with rough sketches or stick figures. In a few clinical situations, more refined means of communicating evidence have been developed, such as decision aid programs available for prostate cancer screening. The patient answers questions at a computer about his preferences regarding prostate cancer screening and treatment. These preferences then determine a recommendation for that patient about prostate cancer screening using a decision tree similar to the ones that will be discussed in Chapter 30. Unfortunately, these types of programs are not yet widely developed for most decision making.

The quality of the evidence also needs to be communicated in addition to a discussion of the risks and benefits of treatment. For example, if the highest level of evidence found was an evidence-based review from a trusted source, the quality of the evidence being communicated is higher and discussions can be done with more confidence. If there is only poor quality of evidence, such as would be available only from a case series, the provider will be less confident in the quality of the evidence and should convey more uncertainty.

Pitfalls to providing the evidence

The most common pitfall when providing evidence is giving the patient more information than she wants or needs although often the most noteworthy pitfalls are related to the misleading nature of words and numbers. Consider this example: A patient who has a headache asks about the cause. The answer given to the patient is: "*Usually* headaches like yours are caused by stress. Only in *extremely rare* circumstances is a headache like yours caused by a brain tumor." How frequently is this type of headache caused by stress? How frequently is this type of headache caused by a brain tumor? In this example, expressing the common nature of stress headaches as "usually" can be very vague. When residents and interns in medicine and surgery were asked to quantify this term, they chose a range of percents between 50–95%. In this example stating that headaches due to a brain tumor occurred only in "extremely rare" circumstances is also imprecise. When asked to quantify "extremely rare" residents and interns chose a range of percents between 1–10%. Knowing that the disease is rare or extremely rare may be consoling, but if there is a 1 to 10% chance that it is present, this may not be very satisfactory for the patient. It is clear that there is a great potential for misunderstanding when converting numbers to words.

Unfortunately, using actual numbers to provide evidence is not necessarily clearer than words. Results of studies of therapy can be expressed in a variety of ways. For example in a study where the outcomes are reported in binary terms such as life or death, or heart attack or no heart attack, a physician can describe the results numerically as a relative risk reduction, an absolute risk reduction, a number needed to treat to benefit, length of survival or disease-free interval. When describing outcomes, results have the potential to sound quite different to a patient. The following example describes the same outcome in different ways:

- Relative risk reduction: This medication reduces heart attacks by 34% when compared to placebo.
- Absolute risk reduction: When patients take this medication, 1.4% fewer patients taking it experienced heart attacks compared to placebo.
- Number needed to treat to benefit (NNTB): For every 71 patients treated with this medication, one additional patient will benefit. This also means that for every 71 patients treated, 70 get no additional benefit from taking the medication.
- Calculated length of disease-free interval: Patients who take this medication for 5 years will live approximately 2 months longer before they get a heart attack.

When treatment benefits are described in relative terms such as a relative risk reduction, patients are more likely to think that the treatment is helpful. The description of outcomes in absolute terms such as absolute risk reduction, leads patients to perceive less benefit from the medications. This occurs because the relative changes sound bigger than absolute changes and are, therefore, more attractive. When the NNTB and length of disease-free survival are compared, a recent study showed that patients preferred treatment outcomes to be expressed as NNTB. The authors of this study suggested that patients saw the NNTB as an avoidance of a heart attack or as a gamble, thinking that "maybe I will be the one who won't have the heart attack," as opposed to a postponement of an inevitable event.

A patient's ability to understand study results for diagnostic tests may be hampered by using percentages instead of frequencies to describe those outcomes. Gigerenzer has demonstrated that for most people, describing results as 2% instead of 1 in 50 will more likely be confusing (see the Bibliography). Using these "natural frequencies" to describe statistical results can make it much easier to understand fairly complex statistics. When describing a diagnostic test using natural frequencies, give the sensitivity and specificity as the number who have disease and will be detected (True Positive Rate) and the number who don't have the disease and will be detected as having it (False Positive Rate). Then you can give the numbers who have the disease and a positive or negative test as a proportion of those with a positive or negative test. The concept of natural frequencies has been described in much more detail by Gerd Gigerenzer in his book about describing risk.

Patients' interpretations of study results are frequently affected by how the results of the study are presented, or framed. For example, if a study evaluated an outcome such as life or death, this can be presented in either a positive way by saying that 4 out of 5 patients lived or a negative way, that 1 out of 5 patients died. The use of positive or negative terms to describe study outcomes does influence a patient's decision and is described as **framing bias**.

A study of patients, radiologists, and business students illustrated this point. They were asked to imagine they had lung cancer and to choose between surgery and radiation therapy. When the same results were presented first in terms of death and then in terms of life, about one quarter of the study subjects changed their mind about their preference. To avoid confusion associated with use of either percentages or framing biases, using comparisons can be helpful. For example, if a patient is considering whether to proceed with a mammogram, using a statement such as "The effect of yearly screening is about the same as driving 300 fewer miles per year" is helpful, if known. This puts the risk into perspective with a common daily risk of living and helps the patient put it into perspective. We will discuss this further when talking about quantifying patient values in Chapter 30.

Recommendations about providing the evidence

The most important recommendation is to avoid overwhelming the patient with too much information. The key to avoiding this pitfall is to repeatedly check with the patient before and during delivery of the information to find out how much she understands. Using verbal terms such as "usually" instead of numbers is less precise, and may give unintended meaning to the information. If use of numbers is acceptable to the patient, we recommend using them. When numbers are used as part of the discussion present them in natural frequencies rather than percents. If familiar comparisons are available, this can be additionally helpful. To avoid the framing bias, results should be presented in both positive and negative terms.

Another recommendation is to use a variety of examples to communicate evidence. For our example patient who is interested in aspirin to prevent heart attacks and strokes, it may be most practical to use multiple modalities for presenting information including verbal and pictorial presentations, presenting the evidence in this way: "In a large study of women like you who took aspirin for 10 years, there was no difference in number of heart attacks between patients who took aspirin and those who didn't. Two out of 1000 fewer women who took aspirin had strokes. In that study, 1 out of 1000 women experienced excessive bleeding from the aspirin."

Step 4: Present recommendations

If a number of options exist and one is not clearly superior, the choices should be presented objectively. If one has a strong belief that one option is the best for the patient, state that with an explicit discussion of the evidence and how the option best fits with the patient's values. This step is closely connected to the strength of the evidence. When the evidence is less than robust from weak study designs or because there are no known studies available, you cannot give strong evidence-based recommendations and must mitigate this by presenting options. When the evidence is stronger, present a recommendation and explain how that recommendation may meet the patient's goals. In all cases, the physician has to be careful about differentiating evidence-based recommendations from those generated from personal experiences or biases regarding treatment.

For our patient interested in aspirin for prevention of strokes and heart attacks, we might say: "While I understand it has been hard to lose weight and reduce your cholesterol, taking an aspirin won't help you prevent heart attacks and is only very minimally helpful in preventing strokes. I do not recommend that you take aspirin."

Step 5: Check for understanding and agreement

Bringing the interview to a close should include checking for understanding by using questions such as "Have I explained that clearly?". This may not be enough. Instead ask the patient "How would you summarize what I said?" This is more likely to indicate whether the patient understands the evidence and your recommendations. Another important part of this step is to allow the patient time to ask questions. When the physician and the patient are both in agreement that the information has been successfully transmitted and all questions have been answered, then a good decision can be made.

19

Critical appraisal of qualitative research studies

Steven R. Simon, M.D., M.P.H.

> You cannot acquire experience by making experiments. You cannot create experience. You must undergo it.
>
> Albert Camus (1913–1960)

Learning objectives

In this chapter you will learn:
- the basic concepts of qualitative research
- process for critical appraisal of qualitative research
- goals and limitations of qualitative research

While the evidence-based medicine movement has espoused the critical appraisal and clinical application of controlled trials and observational studies to guide medical decision making, much of medicine and health care revolves around issues and complexities not ideally suited to quantitative research. Qualitative research is a field dedicated to characterizing and illuminating the knowledge, attitudes, and behaviors of individuals in the context of health care and clinical medicine. Whereas quantitative research is interested in testing hypotheses and estimating effect sizes with precision, qualitative research attempts to describe the breadth of issues surrounding a problem or issue, frequently yielding questions and generating hypotheses to be tested. Qualitative research in medicine frequently draws on expertise from anthropology, psychology, and sociology, fields steeped in a tradition of careful observation of human behavior. Unfortunately, some in medicine have an attitude that qualitative research is not particularly worthwhile for informing patient care. But, you will see that qualitative studies can be powerful tools to expose psychosocial issues in medicine and as hypothesis-generating studies about personal preferences of patients and health-care workers.

Types of qualitative research studies

Qualitative research studies usually involve the collection of a body of information, through direct observation, interviews, or existing documents. Researchers then apply one or more analytic approaches to sift through the available data to identify the main themes and the range of emotions, concerns, or approaches. In the medical literature, in-depth interviews with individuals such as patients or health-care providers and focus-group interviews and discussions among patients with a particular condition are the most common study designs encountered. Observations of clinical behavior and analyses of narratives found in medical documents (e.g., medical records) also appear with some frequency. Examples of the qualitative research studies are described in Table 19.1.

When is it appropriate to use qualitative research?

Qualitative research is an appropriate approach to answering research questions about the social, attitudinal, behavioral, and emotional dimensions of health care. When the spectrum of perspectives needs to be known for the development of interventions such as educational programs or technological implementations, qualitative research can characterize the barriers to and facilitators of change toward the desired practice. This can be the initial research to determine the barriers to adoption of new research results in general practice. When the research question is, "Why do patients behave in a certain way?" or "What issues drive a health-care organization to establish certain policies?", qualitative research methods offer a rigorous approach to data collection and analysis that can reduce the need to rely on isolated anecdote or opinion.

What are the methods of qualitative research?

Although qualitative research studies have more methodological latitude to accommodate the wide range of data used for analysis, readers of qualitative research reports can nevertheless expect to find a clear statement of the study objectives, an account of how subjects were selected to participate and the rationale behind that selection process, a description of the data elements and how they were collected, and an explanation of the analytic approach. Readers of qualitative studies should be able to critically appraise all of these components of the research methods.

Table 19.1. Examples of Qualitative Research Studies

In-depth interviews

In developing an intervention to improve the use of acid-reducing medications in an HMO, researchers carried out in-depth interviews with 10 full-time primary care physicians about their knowledge, attitudes, and practice regarding dyspepsia; the use of chronic acid-suppressing drugs; approaches to diagnosing and treating *Helicobacter pylori* infection; and the feasibility and acceptability of various potential interventions that might be used in a quality improvement program to explore the rationale underlying various medication decisions and the barriers to prescribing consistent with evidence-based guidelines. (Reference: S. R. Majumdar, S. B. Soumerai, M. Lee & D. Ross-Degnan. Designing an intervention to improve the management of Helicobacter pylori infection. *Jt. Comm. J. Qual. Improv.* 2001; 27:405–414.)

Focus-group interviews

To investigate the role of secrets in medicine, researchers conducted a series of eight focus groups among 61 primary care physicians in Israel with a wide variety of seniority, ethnic, religious, and immigration backgrounds. The authors' analysis revealed insights about definitions, prevalence, process, and content of secrets in primary care. (Reference: S. Reis, A. Biderman, R. Mitki & J. M. Borkan. Secrets in primary care: A qualitative exploration and conceptual model. *J. Gen. Intern. Med.* 2007; 22: 1246–1253.)

Observation of clinical encounters

In a study of patient–physician communication about colorectal cancer screening, researchers drew from an existing data set of videotaped primary care encounters to explore the extent to which colorectal cancer screening discussions occur in everyday clinical practice. The researchers transcribed the videotaped discussions and reviewed both the videotapes and the transcriptions, coding content related to the specific types of screening discussed, messages conveyed, and time spent. (Reference: M. S. Wolf, D. W. Baker & G. Makoul. Physician-patient communication about colorectal cancer screening. *J. Gen. Intern. Med.* 2007; 22: 1493–1499.)

Study objective

The study objective should be explicitly stated, usually in the Introduction section of the article. This objective is often framed as a research question and is the alternative or research hypothesis for the study. Unlike quantitative research studies, where the study objective is generally very specific and outcome-based, the objective or research question in qualitative studies frequently has a non-specific or general flavor. In fact, it is one of the strengths of qualitative research that the specific details surrounding the study objective often emerge through the data collection and the analytic processes can actually change the direction of the research. Nevertheless, it is important for readers to be able to assess what the researchers originally set out to accomplish.

Sampling

While quantitative research studies generally recruit participants through random selection or other similar approaches to minimize the potential for selection bias, qualitative research studies are not concerned with accruing a pool of individuals that resemble the larger population. Instead, qualitative studies use **purposive sampling**, the intentional recruitment of individuals with specific characteristics to encompass the broadest possible range of perspectives on the issue being studied. In qualitative research, a sample size is generally not pre-specified. Instead, researchers identify and recruit participants until it becomes apparent that all salient attitudes or perspectives have been identified. This approach is known variously as **theoretical saturation** or **sampling to redundancy**. Readers should assess the researchers' rationale for selecting and sampling the set of study participants, and that rationale should be consistent with the study objectives.

Data Collection

In assessing the validity of the results of quantitative studies, the reader can consider whether and how all relevant variables were measured, whether adequate numbers of study participants were included, and whether the data were measured and collected in an unbiased fashion. Similarly, in qualitative research studies, the reader should expect to find a credible description of how the researchers obtained the data and be able to assess whether the data collection approach likely yielded all relevant perspectives or behaviors being studied. This criterion is tricky for both researchers and readers, since determining the spectrum of relevant concepts likely comprises part of the study's objective. Researchers should describe the iterative process by which they collected information and used the data to inform continued data collection. The approach chosen for data collection should combine feasibility and validity. Readers should ask, and authors should articulate, whether alternative approaches were considered and, if so, why they were not taken.

Authors should also detail the efforts undertaken to ascertain information that may be sensitive for a variety of reasons. For example, there may be issues of privacy or social standing which could prevent individuals from revealing information relevant to the study questions. Researchers and readers must always be concerned about **social desirability bias** when considering the responses or comments that participants may provide when they know they are being observed. The extent to which researchers attempt to collect richly detailed perspectives from study subjects can help to reassure the reader that subjects at least had ample opportunity to express their knowledge, attitudes, or concerns.

Analysis

There is no single correct approach to analyzing qualitative data. The approach that researchers take will reflect the study question, the nature of the available data, and the preferences of the researchers themselves. This flexibility can be daunting for researcher and reader alike. Nevertheless, several key principles should guide all qualitative analyses, and readers should be able to assess how well the study adhered to these principles.

All data should be considered in the analysis. This point may seem obvious, but it is important that readers feel reasonably confident that the data collection not only captured all relevant perspectives but that the analysis did not disregard or overlook elements of data that should be considered. There is no sure-fire way to determine whether all data were included in the analysis, but readers can reasonably expect study authors to report that they used a systematic method for cataloguing all data elements. While not essential, many studies use computer software to manage data. Consider whether multiple observers participated in the analysis and whether the data were reviewed multiple times. The agreement between observers, also known as the inter-rater reliability, should be measured and reported.

The results of interviews or open-ended questions can be analyzed using an iterative technique of identification of common themes. First the answers to questions given by an initial group are reviewed and the important themes are selected by one observer. The responses are catalogued into these themes. A second researcher goes over those same responses with the list of themes and catalogues the responses, blinded from the results of the first researcher. Following this process, inter-rater reliability is assessed and quantified using a test such as the Kappa statistic. If the degree of agreement is substantial, one reviewer can categorize and analyze the remaining responses.

Studies of human subjects' attitudes or perspectives rarely yield a set of observations that unanimously signal a common theme or perspective. It is common in qualitative studies for investigators to come upon observations or sentiments that do not seem to fit what the preponderance of their data seem to be signaling. These discrepancies are to be expected in qualitative research and, in fact, are an important part of characterizing the range of emotions or behaviors among the study participants. Readers should be suspicious of the study's findings if the results of a qualitative study all seem to fall neatly in line with one salient emerging theory or conclusion.

Researchers should triangulate their observations. **Triangulation** refers to the process by which key findings are verified or corroborated through multiple sources. For example, researchers will frequently have subjective reactions to qualitative data, and these reactions help them to formulate conclusions and should lead to further data collection. Having multiple researchers independently analyzing the primary data helps to ensure that the findings are not unduly influenced by the subjective reactions of a single researcher. Another form of triangulation involves comparing the results of the analysis with external information, either from or about the study participants or from other studies. Theories or conclusions from one study may not be consistent with existing theories in similar fields, but when such similarities are observed, or when the results would seem to fit broader social science theories or models, researchers and readers may be more confident about the validity of the analysis.

Researchers frequently perform another form of triangulation known as **member-checking**. This approach involves taking the study findings back to the study participants and verifying the conclusions with them. Frequently, this process of member-checking will lead to additional data and further illumination of the conclusions. Since the purpose of qualitative research is, in large measure, to describe or understand the phenomena of interest from the perspective of the participants, member-checking is useful, because the participants are the only ones who can legitimately judge the credibility of the results.

Readers of qualitative articles will encounter a few analytic approaches and principles that are commonly employed and deserve mention by name. A **content analysis** generally examines words or phrases within a wide range of texts and analyzes them as they are used in context and in relationship with other language. An example of a content analytic strategy is **immersion-crystallization**. Using this approach, researchers immerse themselves repeatedly in the collected data, usually in the form of transcripts or audio or video recordings, and through iterative review and interaction in investigator meetings, coupled with reflection and intuitive insight, clear, consistent, and reportable observations emerge and crystallize.

Grounded theory is another important qualitative approach that readers will encounter. The self-defined purpose of grounded theory is to develop theory about phenomena of interest, but this theory must be grounded in the reality of observation. The methods of grounded theory research include **coding, memoing**, and **integrating**. Coding involves naming and labeling sentences, phrases, words, or even body language into distinct categories; memoing means that the researchers keep written notes about their observations during data analysis and during the coding process; and integration, in short, involves bringing the coded information and memos together, through reflection and discussion, to form a theory that accounts for all the coded information and researchers' observations. For grounded theory, as for any other qualitative approach, triangulation, member-checking and other approaches to ensuring validity remain relevant.

Applying the results of qualitative research

How do I apply the results?

Judging the validity of qualitative research is no easy task, but determining when and how to apply the results is even murkier. When qualitative research is intended to generate hypotheses for future research or to test the feasibility and acceptability of interventions, then applying the results is relatively straightforward. Whatever is learned from the qualitative studies can be incorporated in the design of future studies, typically quantitative, to test hypotheses. For example, if a qualitative research study suggests that patients prefer full and timely disclosure when medical errors occur, survey research can determine whether this preference applies broadly and whether there are subsets of the population for whom it does not apply. Moreover, intervention studies can test whether educating clinicians about disclosure results in greater levels of patient satisfaction or other important outcomes.

But when can the results of qualitative research be applied directly to the day-to-day delivery of patient care? The answer to this question is, as for quantitative research, that readers must ask, "Were the study participants similar to those in my own environment?" If the qualitative study under review included patients or community members, were they similar in demographic and clinical characteristics to patients in my own practice or community? If the study participants were clinicians, were their clinical and professional situations similar to my own?

If the answers to these questions are "yes," or even "maybe," then the reader can use the results of the study to reflect on his or her own practice situation. If the qualitative research study explored patients' perceived barriers to obtaining preventive health care, for example, and if the study population seems similar enough to one's own, then the clinician can justifiably consider these potential barriers among his or her own patients, and ask about them. Considering another example, if a qualitative study exploring patient–doctor interactions at the end of life revealed evidence of physicians distancing themselves from relationships with their patients, clinicians should reflect and ask themselves – and their patients – how they can improve in this area.

Qualitative research studies rarely result in landmark findings that, in and of themselves, transform the practice of medicine or the delivery of health care. Nevertheless, qualitative studies increasingly form the foundation for quantitative research, intervention studies, and reflection on the humanistic components of health care.

20

An overview of decision making in medicine

Nothing is more difficult, and therefore more precious, than to be able to decide.

Napoleon I (1769–1821)

Learning objectives

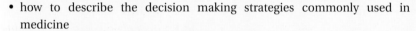

In this chapter you will learn:

- how to describe the decision making strategies commonly used in medicine
- the process of formulating a differential diagnosis
- how to define pretest probability of disease
- the common modes of thought that can aid or hinder good decision making
- the problem associated with premature closure of the differential diagnosis and some tactics to avoid that problem

Chapters 21 to 31 teach the process involved in making a diagnosis and thereby determining the best course of management for one's patient. First, we will address the principles of how to use diagnostic tests efficiently and effectively. Then, we will present some mathematical techniques that can help the health-care practitioner and the health-care system policy maker come to the most appropriate medical decisions for both individuals and populations of patients.

Medical decision making

Medical decision making is more complex now than ever before. The way one uses clinical information will affect the accuracy of diagnoses and ultimately the outcome for one's patient. Incorrect use of data will lead the physician away from the correct diagnosis, may result in pain, suffering, and expense for the patient, and may increase cost and decrease the efficiency of the health-care system.

Clinical diagnosis requires early hypothesis generation called the differential diagnosis. This is a list of plausible diseases from which the patient may be suffering, based upon the information gathered in the history and physical examination. Gathering more clinical data, usually obtained by performing diagnostic tests, refines this list. However, using diagnostic tests without paying attention to their reliability and validity can lead to poor decision making and ineffective care of the patient. Overall, we are trying to measure the ability of each element of the history, physical examination, and laboratory testing to accurately distinguish patients who have a given disease from those without that disease. The quantitative measure of this is expressed mathematically as the likelihood ratios of a positive or negative test. This tells us how much more likely it is that a patient has the disease if the test is positive or how much less likely the disease is if the test is negative.

Diagnostic-test characteristics are relatively stable characteristics of a test and must be considered in the overall process of diagnosis and management of a disease. The most commonly measured diagnostic-test characteristics are the sensitivity, which is the ability of a test to find disease when it is present, and specificity, defined as the ability of a test to find a patient without disease among people who are not diseased. A positive test's ability to predict disease when it is positive is the positive predictive value. Similarly, a negative predictive value is the test's ability to predict lack of disease when it is negative. These values both depend on the disease prevalence in a population, which is also called the pre-test probability. The likelihood ratios can then be used to revise the original diagnostic impression to calculate the statistical likelihood of the final diagnosis, the post-test probability. This can be calculated using a simple equation or nomogram.

The characteristics of tests can be used to find treatment and testing thresholds. The **treatment threshold** is the pretest probability above which we would treat without testing. The **testing threshold** is the pretest probability below which we would neither treat nor test for a particular disease. Finally, the **receiver operating characteristic** (ROC) curves are graphs that summarize sensitivity and specificity over a series of cutoff values. They are used to determine the overall value of a test, the best cutoff point for a test, and the best test when comparing two diagnostic tests.

More advanced mathematical constructs for making medical decisions involve the use of decision trees, which quantify diagnostic and treatment pathways using branch points to help choose between treatment options. Ideally, they will show the most effective care process. This is heavily influenced by patient values, which can be quantified for this process. Finally, the cost-effectiveness of a given treatment can be determined and it will help choose between treatment options when making decisions for a population.

Variation in medical practice and the justification for the use of practice guidelines

More than ever in the current health-care debate, physician decisions are being challenged. One major reason is that not all physician decisions are correct or even consistent. A recent study of managed care organization (MCO) physicians showed that only half of the physicians in the study treated their diabetic and heart-attack patients with proven lifesaving drugs. A recent estimate of medical errors suggested that up to 98 000 deaths per year in the United States were due to preventable medical errors. This leads to the perception that many physician decisions are arbitrary and highly variable.

Several studies done in the 1970s showed a marked geographic variation in the rate of common surgeries. In Maine, hysterectomy rates varied from less than 20% in one county to greater than 70% in another. This variation was true despite similar demographic patterns and physician manpower in the two counties. Studies looking at prostate surgery, heart bypass, and thyroid surgery show variation in rates of up to 300% in different counties in New England. Among Medicare patients, rates for many procedures in 13 large metropolitan areas varied by greater than 300%. Rates for knee replacement varied by 700% and for carotid endarterectomies by greater than 2000%.

How well do physicians agree among themselves about treatment or diagnosis? In one study, cardiologists reviewing angiograms could not reliably agree upon whether there was an arterial blockage. Sixty percent disagreed on whether the blockage was at a proximal or distal location. There was a 40% disagreement on whether the blockage was greater or less than 50%. In another study, the same cardiologists disagreed with themselves from 8% to 37% of the time when re-reading the same angiograms. Given a hypothetical patient and asked to give a second opinion about the need for surgery, half of the surgeons asked gave the opinion that no surgery was indicated. When asked about the same patient 2 years later, 40% had changed their mind.

Physicians routinely treat high intraocular pressure because if intraocular pressure is high it could lead to glaucoma and blindness. How high must the intraocular pressure be in order to justify treatment? In 1961, the ophthalmologic textbooks said 24 mmHg. In 1976, it was noted to be 30 mmHg without any explanation for this change based upon clinical trials.

There are numerous other examples of physician disagreement. Physician experts asked to give their estimate of the effect on mortality of screening for colon cancer varied from 5% to 95%. Heart surgeons asked to estimate the 10-year failure rates of implanted heart valves varied from 3% to 95%. All of these examples suggest that physician decision making is not standardized. Evidence-based decision making in health care, the conscientious application of the best possible evidence to each clinical encounter, can help us regain the confidence of the public and the integrity of the profession.

More standardized practice can help reduce second-guessing of physician decisions. This questioning commonly occurs with utilization review of physician decisions by managed care organizations or government payors. It can lead to rejection of coverage for "extra" hospital days or refusal of payment for recommended surgery or other therapies. This questioning also occurs in medical malpractice cases where an expert reviews care through a retrospective review of medical records. Second-guessing, as well as the marked variation in physician practices, can be reduced through the use of practice guidelines for the diagnosis and treatment of common disorders. When used to improve diagnosis, we refer to these guidelines as diagnostic clinical prediction rules.

A primary cause of physician variability lies in the complexity of clinical problems. Clinical decision making is both multifaceted and practiced on highly individualized patients. Some factors to consider with clinical decision making include patient expectations, changing reimbursement policies, competition, malpractice threat, peer pressure, and incomplete information. Overall, physicians are well-meaning and confront not only biological but also sociological and political variability. We can't know the outcomes of our decisions beforehand, but must act anyway.

There are some barriers to the process of using best evidence in medical decision making. The quality of evidence that one is looking for is often only fair or poor. Some physicians believe that if there is no evidence from well-done randomized control trials, then the treatment in questions should not be used. Be aware that lack of evidence is not equal to evidence of lack of effect. Most physicians gladly accept much weaker evidence, yet don't have the clinical expertise to put that evidence into perspective for a particular clinical encounter. They also may not be able to discern well-done RCTs or even observational studies from those that are heavily biased. This goes to show that there is a need for clinical expertise as part of the EBM process.

Some of the reasons for the high degree of uncertainty in physician decision making are noted in Table 20.1. Physicians want some certainty before they are willing to use an intervention, yet tend to do what was learned in medical school or learned from the average practitioner. The rationalization for this is that if everyone is doing the treatment, it must be appropriate. Some physician treatment decisions are based on the fact that a disease is common or severe. If a disease is common, or the outcome severe, they are more willing to use whatever treatment is available. There are even times when physicians feel the need simply to do something, and the proposed treatment is all they have. There is also a certain amount of fascination with new diagnostic or treatment modalities that results in wholesale increases in usage of those methods.

Table 20.1. Causes of variability in physician performance

(1)	**Complexity of clinical problem**	multiple factors influence actions
(2)	**Uncertainty of outcomes of decisions**	variability of outcomes in studies
(3)	**Need to act**	feeling on our part that we have to "do something"
(4)	**Large placebo effect**	spontaneous cures (sometimes doing nothing but educating is the best thing)
(5)	**Patient expectations**	expectation from patients and society that what we do will work
(6)	**Political expectations**	do what is cheapest and best
(7)	**Malpractice threat**	don't make any mistakes
(8)	**Peer pressure**	do things the same way that other physicians are doing them
(9)	**Technological imperative**	we have a new technology so let's use it

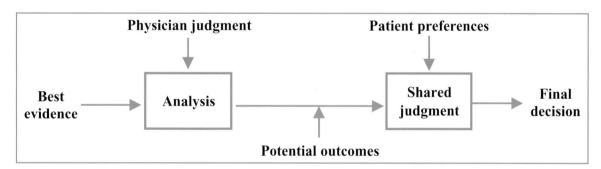

Fig. 20.1 Anatomy of a decision.

One way physicians can do better is by having better clinical research and improved quality of evidence for clinical decisions. Physicians must also increase their ability to use the available evidence through improving individual and collective reasoning and actions. Figure 20.1 shows the anatomy of a clinical decision, a simplified look at decision making in general and the factors that influence the process. Reduction of error in the decision-making process requires better training of physicians in all three parts of EBM: evaluating the evidence, understanding the clinical situation, and having good patient communications. Another way to reduce error is by "automating" the decision process. If there is good evidence for a certain practice, it ought to be done the best way known at all times. Practice guidelines are one way of automating part of the decision-making process for physicians.

In 1910, Abraham Flexner asked physicians and medical schools to stop teaching empiricism and rely on solid scientific information. In those days, empiric facts were usually based on single-case testimonials or poorly documented

Table 20.2. Components of the H&P (with a clinical example)

Chief complaint	Why the patient sought medical care (e.g., coughing up blood, hemoptysis)
History of present illness	Description of symptoms: what, when, where, how much, etc. (e.g., coughing up spots of bright red blood four or five times a day for 3 days associated with some shortness of breath, fever, poor appetite, occasional chest pain, and fatigue)
Past medical history	Previous illness and operations, medications and allergies, including herbal, vitamin, and supplement use (e.g., seizure disorder, on phenytoin daily, no operations or allergies)
Family and social histories	Hereditary illness, habits and activities, diet, etc. (e.g., iv drug abuser, homeless, poor diet, adopted and does not know about his or her family medical history)
Review of systems	Review of all possible symptoms of all bodily systems. (e.g., recent weight loss and night sweats for the past 3 weeks, occasional indigestion)
Physical examination	(e.g., somewhat emaciated male in minimal respiratory distress, cervical lymphadenopathy, dullness to percussion at right upper lobe area and few rales in this area, multiple skin lesions consistent with needle marks and associated sclerosis of veins, remainder of examination normal)

case presentations. He proposed teaching and applying the pathophysiological approach to diagnosis and treatment. The medical establishment endorsed this, and the modern medical school was born. Currently, we are in the throes of a paradigm shift. We want to see the empirical data for a particular therapy or diagnosis and ought to act only on evidence that is of high quality.

The clinical examination

In most cases in health care, a patient does not walk into the physician's office and present with a pre-made diagnosis. They arrive with a series of signs and symptoms that one must interpret correctly in order to make a diagnosis and initiate the most appropriate therapy. The process by which this occurs begins with the clinical examination. Traditionally, this consists of several components collectively called the history and physical or H&P (Table 20.2).

Table 20.3. OLDCARTS acronym for history of the present illness

O	Onset of symptoms and chronological description of change in the symptoms
L	Location of symptoms and radiation to other areas
D	Duration of individual episodes or from when symptoms started
C	Characteristics of the symptoms
A	Associated or aggravating factors
R	Relieving factors
T	Timing, when is it worse or better
S	Severity on a scale from 0 to 10

The chief complaint is the stated reason that the patient comes to medical attention. It is often a disorder of normal functioning that alarms the patient and tells the clinician in which systems to look for pathology.

The history of the present illness is a chronological description of the chief complaint. The clinician seeks to determine the onset of the symptoms, their quality, frequency, duration, associated symptoms, and exacerbating and alleviating factors. The acronym OPQRSTAAAA is often used to remind clinicians of the elements of the history of the present illness. OPQRSTAAAA stands for Onset, Position, Quality, Radiation, Severity, Timing, Aggravating, Alleviating, Associated factors, and Attribution. A brief review of the patient's symptoms seeks to find dysfunction in any other parts of the body that could be associated with the potential disease. It is important to include all the pertinent positives and negatives in reporting the history of the present illness. Another acronym for the history of the present illness, OLDCARTS is described in Table 20.3.

The past medical history, past surgical history, family history, social and occupational history, and the medication and allergy history are all designed to get a picture of the patient's medical and social background. This puts the illness into the context of the person's life and is an integral part of any medical history. The accuracy and adequacy of this part of the history is extremely important. Some experts feel that this is the most important part of the practice of holistic medicine, helping ensure that the physician looks at the whole patient and the patient's environment.

The review of systems gives the clinician an overview of the patient's additional medical conditions. These may or may not be related to the chief complaint. This aspect of the medical history helps the clinician develop other hypotheses as to the cause of the patient's problem. It also gives the clinician more insight into the patient's overall well-being, attitudes toward illness, and comfort level with various symptoms.

Finally, the physical examination is an attempt to elicit objective signs of disease in the patient. The physical exam usually helps to confirm or deny the clinician's suspicions based upon the history.

An old adage states that in 80% of patients, the final diagnosis comes solely from the history. In another 15% it comes from the physical examination, and only in the remaining 5% from additional diagnostic testing. This may appear to overstate the value of the history and physical, but not by much.

Clinical observation is a powerful tool for deciding what diseases are possible in a given patient, and most of the time the results of the H&P determine which additional data to seek. Once the H&P has been exhausted, the clinician must know how to obtain the additional required data in a reliable and accurate way by using diagnostic tests which can appropriately achieve the best outcome for the patient. For the health-care system, this must also be done at a reasonable cost not only in dollars, but also in patient lives, time, and anxiety if an incorrect diagnosis is made.

Hypothesis generation in the clinical encounter

While performing the H&P, the clinician develops a set of hypotheses about what diseases could be causing the patient's problem. This list is called the differential diagnosis and some diseases on this list are more likely than others to be present in that patient. When finished with the H&P, the clinician estimates the probability of each of these diseases and rank-orders this list. The probability of a patient having a particular disease on that list is referred to as the pretest probability of disease. It may be equivalent to the prevalence of that disease in the population of patients with similar results on the medical history and physical examination.

The numbers for pretest probability come from one's knowledge of medicine and from studies of disease prevalence in medical literature. Let's use the example of a 50-year-old North American alcoholic with no history of liver disease, who presents to an emergency department with black tarry stools that are suggestive of digested blood in the stool. This symptom is most likely caused by esophageal varices, by gastritis, or by a stomach ulcer. The prevalence of each of these diseases in this population is 5% for varices, 55% for ulcer, and 40% for gastritis. In this particular case, the probabilities add up to 100% since there are virtually no other diagnostic possibilities. This is also knows as *sigma p equals one*, and applies when the diseases on the list of differential diagnoses are all mutually exclusive. Rarely, a person fitting this description will turn out to have gastric cancer, which occurs in less than 1% of patients presenting like this and can be left off the list for the time being. If none of the other diseases are diagnosed, then one needs to look for this rare disease. In this case, a single diagnostic test, the upper gastrointestinal endoscopy, is the test of choice for detecting all four diagnostic possibilities.

There are other situations when the presenting history and physical are much more vague. In these cases, it is likely that the total pretest probability can add up to more than 100%. This occurs because of the desire on the part of the physician not to miss an important disease. Therefore, each disease should be considered by itself when determining the probability of its occurrence. This probability takes into account how much the history and physical examination of the patient resemble the diseases on the differential diagnosis. The assigned probability value based on this resemblance is very high, high, moderate, low, or very low. In our desire not to miss an important disease, probabilities that may be much greater than the true prevalence of the disease are often assigned to some diagnoses on the list. We will give an example of this shortly.

Physicians must take the individual patient's qualities into consideration when assigning pretest probabilities. For example, a patient with chest pain can have coronary artery disease, gastroesophageal reflux disease, panic disorder, or a combination of the three. In general, panic disorder is much more likely in a 20-year-old, while coronary artery disease is more likely in a 50-year-old. When considering this aspect of pretest probabilities, it becomes evident that a more realistic way of assigning probabilities is to have them reflect the likelihood of that disease in a single patient rather than the prevalence in a population. This allows the clinician to consider the unique aspects of a patient's history and physical examination when making the differential diagnosis.

Constructing the differential diagnosis

The differential diagnosis begins with diseases that are very likely and for which the patient has many of the classical symptoms and signs. These are also known as the leading hypotheses or working diagnoses. Next, diseases that are possible are included on the list if they are serious and potentially life- or limb-threatening. These are the active alternatives to the working diagnoses and must be ruled out of the list. This means that the clinicians must be relatively certain from the history and physical examination that these alternative diagnoses are not present. Put another way, the pretest probability of those alternative diseases is so vanishingly small that it becomes clinically insignificant. If the history and physical examination do not rule out a diagnosis, then a diagnostic test that can reliably rule it out must be performed. Diseases that can be easily treated can also be included in the differential diagnosis and occasionally, the diagnosis is confirmed by a trial of therapy, which if successful, confirms the diagnosis. Last to be included are diseases that are very unlikely and not serious, or are more difficult and potentially dangerous to treat. These diseases are less possible because they

Fig. 20.2 A 2 × 2 table view of pretest probabilities.

	Common presentation	Rare presentation
Common disease	90%	9%
Rare disease	0.9%	0.09%

have already been ruled out by the history and physical, but ought to be kept in mind for future consideration if necessary or if any clues to their presence show themselves during the evaluation. A good example of this would be a patient with chest pain and no risk factors for pulmonary embolism who has a low transcutaneous oxygen saturation. Now one should begin to look more closely for the diagnosis of pulmonary embolism in this patient.

When considering a diagnosis, it is helpful to have a framework for considering likelihood of each disease on one's list. One schema for classifying this is shown in Fig. 20.2, which describes the overall probability of diseases using a 2 × 2 table. This only helps to get an overview and does not help one determine the pretest probability of each disease on the differential diagnosis. In this schema, each disease is considered as if the total probability of disease adds up to 100%. One must tailor the probabilities in one's differential diagnosis to the individual patient. Bear in mind that a patient is more likely to present with a rare or unusual presentation of a common disease, than a common presentation of a rare disease.

As stated earlier, the first step in generating a differential diagnosis is to systematically make a list of all the possible causes of a patient's symptoms. This skill is learned through the intensive study of diseases and reinforced by clinical experience and practice. When medical students first start doing this, it is useful to make the list as exhaustive as possible to avoid missing any diseases. Think of all possible diseases by category that might cause the signs or symptoms. There are several helpful mnemonics that can help get a differential diagnosis started. One is VINDICATE (Table 20.4). Initially, list all possible diseases for a chief complaint by category. Then assign a pretest probability for each disease on the differential list. The values of pretest probability are relative and can be assigned according to the scale shown in Table 20.5. Physicians are more likely to agree with each other on prioritizing diagnoses if using a relative scale like this, rather than trying to assign a numerical probability to each disease on the list. One must consider the ramifications of missing a diagnosis. If the disease is immediately life- or limb-threatening, it needs to be ruled out, regardless of the probability assigned. If the likelihood of a disease is very very low, the diagnostician should look for evidence that the disease might be present, such as an abberrent element of the history, physical examination or diagnostic tests to suggest that the

Table 20.4. Mnemonic to remember classification of disease for a differential diagnosis

V   Vascular
I   Inflammatory/Infectious
N   Neoplastic/Neurologic and psychiatric
D   Degenerative/Dietary
I   Intoxication/Idiopathic/Iatrogenic
C   Congenital
A   Allergic/Autoimmune
T   Trauma
E   Endocrine & metabolic

Table 20.5. Useful schema for assigning pretest (a-priori) probabilities

Pretest probability		Action	Interpretation
	<1%	Off the list – for now. But, must consider if other diseases later are found not to be present.	**Rare disease** (rare presentation)
	1%	Can't exclude, but very unlikely (effectively **ruled out**)	**Rare disease** (common presentation)
Low	10%	Should be **ruled out**	**Common disease** (rare presentation)
	25%	Possible	
Moderate	50%	50–50 (toss-up)	
	75%	Probable	
High	90%	Very likely	**Common disease** (common presentation)
	99%	Almost certain – **ruled in**	
	99.9%	**Pathognomonic** – there is no other disease which will present like this. This is a unique presentation of this disease, and therefore the patient can only have this disease.	

disease is more likely. We will use this schema for selecting pretest probabilities for the rest of the book.

For example, if a 21-year-old man came in to the Emergency Department complaining of chest pain, a physician would first perform a complete history and physical examination. Following this, one might suspect that anxiety or a pectoralis muscle strain are the cause of his pain. These would have very high pretest probabilities (50–90%). One should also consider slightly less likely and more serious causes which are easily treatable, such as pericarditis, spontaneous pneumothorax, pneumonia, or esophageal spasm secondary to acid reflux. These would have variably lower pretest probabilities (1–50%). Next, there are hypotheses that are much less likely, such as myocardial infarction, dissecting thoracic aortic aneurysm, and pulmonary embolism. The pretest probabilities of these are all much less than 1%. Finally, one must consider some disorders, such as lung cancer, that are so rare and not immediately life- or limb-threatening that they are ruled out because of the patient's age.

If a 39-year-old man presented with the same complaint of chest pain, but not the typical sqeezing, pressure-like pain of angina pectoris, one could look up the pretest probability of coronary artery disease in population studies. This can be found in an article by Patterson, which states that the probability that this patient has angina pectoris is about 20%.[1] This means that about 1/5 of all 39-year-old men with this presentation will have significant coronary artery disease. These data would change one's list and put myocardial infarction higher up on the differential. Since this is a potentially dangerous disease, additional testing is required to rule it out.

Making the differential diagnosis means considering diseases from three perspectives: probability of the disease, severity of the disease, and ease of treatment of the disease. The differential diagnosis is a complex interplay between these factors and the patient's signs and symptoms.

Narrowing the differential

Here is a more common, everyday example. A physician is examining a 7-year-old child who is sick with a sore throat. The pysician suspects that this child might have strep throat, which is a common illness in children and thus assigns it a high pretest probability of disease. This is the working diagnosis. The differential diagnosis also includes another common disease, viral pharyngitis. Also included are uncommon diseases like epiglottitis, which is severe and life-threatening, and mononucleosis. Finally, extremely rare diseases are included such as diphtheria and gonorrhea. For this patient's workup, the more serious and uncommon diseases must be actively ruled out. In this case, that can almost certainly be done with an accurate history disclosing lack of sexual abuse and oral–genital contact to rule out gonorrhea. A history of diphtheria immunization and a physical examination without the typical pseudomembrane in the

---

[1] R. E. Patterson & S. F. Horowitz. Importance of epidemiology and biostatistics in deciding clinical strategies for using diagnostic tests: a simplified approach using examples from coronary artery disease. *J. Am. Coll. Cardiol.* 1989; 13: 1653–1665.

Table 20.6. Differential diagnosis of sample patient

Disease	Pretest probability of disease	
Streptococcal infection	50%	Likely, common, and treatable
Viruses	50%	Likely, common, and self-limiting
Mononucleosis	1%	Unlikely, uncommon, and self-limiting
Epiglottitis	<1%	Unlikely and uncommon
Gonorrhea	<<1%	Rare
Diphtheria	<<<1%	Very rare

hypopharynx can rule out diphtheria. Lack of physical signs of epiglottitis such as difficulty swallowing, drooling, and stridor would rule out epiglottitis, and lack of symptoms of fatigue and physical signs like cervical adenopathy would rule out mononucleosis.

If there are no characteristic signs and symptoms of epiglottitis, mononucleosis, gonorrhea, or diphtheria, then the differential diagnosis narrows down to strep throat and viral pharyngitis. The physician can then apply a published decision rule to differentiate strep throat from viral pharyngitis. If it is positive, then treat for strep throat with antibiotics; if negative, then treat symptomatically for viral pharyngitis. If the rule comes up inconclusive, then the physician must consider doing a diagnostic test. In that case, in order to make a final diagnosis, one must do a throat culture.

In this case, the physician believes that doing this test will make a difference. In addition to deciding to perform a diagnostic test, he or she must also decide what kind of culture to take, since the type of culture that will demonstrate strep is different from one that will grow gonorrhea. Since we know that gonorrhea is extremely rare in children, especially when there is no historical evidence of sexual abuse, the physician should decide against culturing the child for gonorrhea bacteria and do a bacterial culture for strep.

Throughout this example, several decisions were made about this child's illness. First, we set up a differential diagnosis in descending order of likelihood and assigned a pretest probability to each disease on that list (Table 20.6). None of the diseases on the list had a pretest probability of 100%, so we decided to do some tests to determine which diagnosis was most likely. The tests vary in their cost – in dollars, ease of performance, patient discomfort, potential complications, and many other factors. For our example of a sore throat, these are listed in Table 20.7.

One must determine which of all these tests is worth doing in order to make the diagnosis most efficiently. This is determined by the cost of the test, the ability of the test to accurately identify the clinical disease, and whether identifying with

Table 20.7. Relative costs of tests

Disease	Test	Cost	Relative ease to treat
Streptococcal infection	Rapid strep antigen or throat culture	$	Easy and safe
Viruses	Viral culture	$$$	Easy and safe
Epiglottitis	Neck x-ray	$$	Difficult
Mononucleosis	Epstein–Barr antigen test	$$	Easy
Diphtheria	Culture or diphtheria serology	$$$$	Difficult
Gonorrhea	Gonorrhea culture	$$	Difficult

the test will make a difference for the patient. In the previous example, if the diagnosis of strep throat was in question, a rapid strep antigen would be the test of choice to rule it in or out. We usually don't do viral cultures since the treatment is the same whether the patient is known to have a particular virus or not.

For our 39-year-old man with chest pain, the differential diagnosis would initially include anxiety, musculoskeletal, coronary artery disease, aneurysm, and pneumothorax. For anxiety and musculoskeletal causes, the pretest probability is high, as these are common in this age group. In fact, as previously discussed, the most likely cause of chest pain in a 39-year-old is going to be pain of musculoskeletal origin. For some of the other diseases on the list, their pretest probabilities would be approximately similar to that of coronary artery disease. However, because of the potential severity of heart disease and most of the other diseases on the differential, it is necessary to do some diagnostic testing to rule out those possibilities. For some of diseases such as pneumothorax, dissecting aortic aneurysm, and pneumonia, a single chest x-ray can rule them out if the image is normal. For others such as coronary artery disease or pulmonary embolism, a more complex algorithmic scheme is necessary to rule in or rule out the diseases.

Strategies for making a medical diagnosis

There are several diagnostic strategies that clinicians employ when using patient data to make a diagnosis. These are presented here as unique methods even though most clinicians use a combination of them to make a diagnosis.

Pattern recognition is the spontaneous and instantaneous recognition of a previously learned pattern. It is usually the starting point for creating a differential diagnosis and determines those diagnoses that will be at the top of the list. This method is employed by the seasoned clinician for most patients. Usually, an experienced clinician will be able to sense when the pattern is not characteristic of the disease. This occurs when there is a rare presentation of common disease or common presentation of a rare disease. An experienced doctor knows when to look beyond the apparent pattern and to search for clues that the patient is presenting with an unusual disease. Premature closure of the differential diagnosis is a pitfall of pattern recognition that is more common to neophytes and will be discussed at the end of this chapter.

The **multiple branching strategy** is an algorithmic approach to diagnosis using a preset path with multiple branching nodes that will lead to a correct final conclusion. Examples of this are diagnostic clinical guidelines or decision rules. These are tools to assist the clinician in remembering the steps to make a proper diagnosis. If they are simple and easily memorized, they can be very useful. More complex diagnostic decision tools can be of greater help when used with a computer.

The **strategy of exhaustion,** also called diagnosis by possibility, involves "the painstaking and invariant search for but paying no immediate attention to the importance of all the medical facts about the patient."[2] This is followed by carefully sifting through the data for a diagnosis. Although, more often than not, this technique will usually come up with the correct diagnosis, the process is time consuming and not cost-effective. A good example of this can be found in the Case Records of the Massachusetts General Hospital feature found in each issue of the *New England Journal of Medicine*. This strategy is most helpful in diagnosing very uncommon diseases or very uncommon presentations of common diseases.

The **hypothetico-deductive strategy,** also called diagnosis by probability, involves the formulation of a short list of potential diagnoses from the earliest clues about the patient. Initial hypothesis generation is based on pattern recognition to suggest certain diagnoses. This basic differential diagnosis is followed by the performance of clinical maneuvers and diagnostic tests that will increase or decrease the probability of each disease on the list. Further refinement of the differential results in a shortlist of diagnoses and the further testing or the initiation of treatment will lead to the final diagnosis. This is the best strategy to use and will lead to a correct diagnosis in most cases. A good example of this can be found in the Clinical Decision Making feature found frequently and irregularly in the *New England Journal of Medicine*.

Heuristics: how we think

Heuristics are cognitive shortcuts used in prioritizing diagnoses. They help to deal with the magnitude and complexity of clinical data. Heuristics are not

---

[2] D. L. Sackett, R. B. Haynes, P. Tugwell & G. H. Guyatt. *Clinical Epidemiology: A Basic Science for Clinical Medicine.* 2nd edn. Boston: Little Brown, 1991.

always helpful, but physicians should recognize the way they use them in order to solve problems effectively and prevent mistakes in clinical diagnosis. There are three important heuristics that are used in medical diagnosis. They are representativeness, availability, and competing hypotheses heuristics.

Representativeness heuristic. The probability that a diagnosis is thought of is based upon how closely its essential features resemble the features of a typical description of the disease. This is analogous to the process of pattern recognition and is accurate if a physician has seen many typical and atypical cases of common diseases. It can lead to erroneous diagnosis if one initially thinks of rare diseases based upon the patient presentation. For example, because a child's sore throat is described as very severe, a physician might immediately think of gonorrhea, which is particularly painful. The severity of the pain of the sore throat represents gonorrhea in diagnostic thinking. To ignore or minimize the more common causes of sore throat, thinking of a rare disease more often than a common one, is incorrect. Remember that unusual or rare presentations of common diseases such as strep throat, occur more often than common presentations of rare diseases such as pharyngeal gonorrhea.

Availability heuristic. The probability of a diagnosis is judged by the ease with which the diagnosis is remembered. The diagnoses of patients that have been most recently cared for are the ones that are brought to the forefront of one's consciousness. This can be thought of as a form of recall bias. If a physician recently took care of a patient with a sore throat who had gonorrhea, he or she will be more likely to look for that as the cause of sore throat in the next patient even though this is a very rare cause of sore throat. The availability heuristic is much more problematic and likely to occur if a recently missed diagnosis was of a rare and serious disease.

Anchoring and adjustment. This heuristic refers to the reality that special characteristics of a patient are used to estimate the probability of a given diagnosis. A differential diagnosis is initially formed and additional information is used to increase or decrease the probability of disease. This technique is the way we think about most diagnoses, and is also called the **competing hypotheses heuristic**. For example, if a patient presents with a sore throat, the physician should think of common causes of sore throat and come up with diagnoses of either a viral pharyngitis or strep throat. These are the anchors. After getting more history and doing a physical examination the physician decides that the characteristics of the sore throat are more like a viral pharyngitis than strep throat. This is the adjustment, and as a result, the other diagnoses on the differential diagnosis list are considered extremely unlikely. The adjustment is based on diagnostic information from the history and physical examination and from diagnostic tests. The process is shown in Fig. 20.3. Throughout the patient encounter, new information

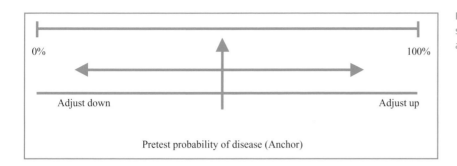

Fig. 20.3 Hypothetico-deductive strategy using anchoring and adjustment.

is compared against all diagnoses being considered, which subsequently changes the probability estimates for each diagnosis and reorders the differential.

The problem of premature closure of the differential diagnosis

One of the most common problems novices have with diagnosis is that they are unable to recognize atypical patterns. This common error in diagnostic thinking occurs when the novice jumps to the conclusion that a pattern exists when in reality, it does not. There is a tendency to attribute illness to a common and often less serious problem rather than search for a less likely, but potentially more serious illness. This is called premature closure of the differential diagnosis. It represents removal from consideration of many diseases from the differential diagnosis list because the clinician jumped to a too early conclusion on the nature of the patient's illness.

Sadly, this phenomenon is not limited to neophytes. Even experienced clinicians can make this mistake, thinking that a patient has a common illness when, in fact, it is a more serious but less common one. No one expects the clinician always immediately to come up with the correct diagnosis of a rare presentation or a rare disease. However, the key to good diagnosis is recognizing when a patient's presentation or response to therapy is not following the pattern that was expected, and revisiting the differential diagnosis when this occurs.

Premature closure of the differential diagnosis can be avoided by following two simple rules. The first is to always include a healthy list of possibilities in the differential diagnosis for any patient. Don't be seduced by an apparently obvious diagnosis. When one finds oneself commonly diagnosing a patient within the first few minutes of initiating the history, step back and look for other clues that could dismiss one diagnosis and add other diagnoses to the list. Then ask oneself whether those other diseases can be excluded simply through the history and physical examination. Since most common diseases do occur commonly, the disease that was first thought of will often turn out to be correct. However, it is more likely to miss important clues of the presence of another less common disease if a physician focuses only on that first diagnosis.

The second step is to avoid modifying the final list until all the relevant information has been collected. After completing the history, make a detailed and objective list of all the diseases for consideration and determine their relative probabilities. The formal application of such a list will be invaluable for the novice student and resident, and will be done in a less and less formal way by the expert.

21

Sources of error in the clinical encounter

Here is my secret, it is very simple: it is only with the heart that one can see rightly; what is essential is invisible to the eye.

Antoine de Saint-Exupéry (1900–1944): The Little Prince

Learning objectives

In this chapter you will learn:

- the measures of precision in clinical decision making
- how to identify potential causes of clinical disagreement and inaccuracy in the clinical examination
- strategies for preventing error in the clinical encounter

The clinical encounter between doctor and patient is the beginning of the medical decision making process. During the clinical encounter, the physician has the opportunity to gather the most accurate information about the nature of the illness and the meaning of that illness to the patient. If there are errors made in processing this information, the resulting decisions may not be in the patient's best interests. This can lead to overuse, underuse, or misuse of therapies and increased error in medical practice.

Measuring clinical consistency

Precision is the extent to which multiple examinations of the same patient agree with one another. In addition, each part of the examination should be accurately reproducible by a second examiner. **Accuracy** is the proximity of a given clinical observation to the true clinical state. The synthesis of all the clinical findings should represent the actual clinical or pathophysiological derangement possessed by the patient.

If two people measure the same parameter several times, for instance the temperature of a sick child, we can determine the consistency of this measurement. In this example, different observers can obtain different results when they measure the temperature of a child using a thermometer because they use slightly different techniques such as varying the time that the thermometer is left in the patient or reading the mercury level differently. The **kappa statistic** is a statistical measurement of the precision of a clinical finding and measures inter-observer consistency between measurements and intra-observer consistency, the ability of the same observer to reproduce a measurement. The kappa statistic is described in detail in Chapter 7 and should be calculated and reported in any study of the usefulness of a diagnostic test.

We often assume that all diagnostic tests are precise. Many studies have demonstrated that most non-automated tests have some some degree of subjectivity in their interpretation. This has been seen in commonly used x-ray tests such as CT scan, mammography, and angiography. It is also present in tests commonly considered to be the gold standard such as the interpretation of tissue samples from biopsies or surgery.

There are many potential sources of error and clinical disagreement in the process of the clinical examination. If the examiner is not aware of these, they will lead to inaccurate data. A broad classification of these sources of error includes the examiner, the examinee, and the environment.

The examiner

Tendencies to record inference rather than evidence

The examiner should record actual findings including both the subjective ones reported by the patient and objective ones detected by the physician's senses. The physician should not make assumptions about the meaning of exam findings prior to creating a complete differential diagnosis. For example, a physician examining a patient's abdomen may feel a mass in the right upper quadrant and record that he or she felt the gall bladder. This may be incorrect, and in fact the mass could be a liver cancer, aneurysm, or hernia.

Ensnarement by diagnostic classification schemes

Jumping to conclusions about the nature of the diagnosis based on an incorrect coding scheme can lead to the wrong diagnosis through premature closure of the differential diagnosis. If a physician hears wheezes in the lungs and assumes that the patient has asthma when in fact they have congestive heart failure, there will be a serious error in diagnosis and lead to incorrect treatment. The diagnosis of heart failure can be made from other features of the history and clues in the physical exam.

Entrapment by prior expectation

Jumping to conclusions about the diagnosis based upon a first impression of the chief complaint can lead to the wrong diagnosis due to lack of consideration of other diagnoses. This, along with incorrect coding schemes, is called premature closure of the differential diagnosis, and discussed in Chapter 20. If a physician examines a patient who presents with a sore throat, fever, aches, nasal congestion, and cough and thinks it is a cold, he or she may miss hearing wheezes in the lungs by only doing a cursory examination of the chest. This occurs because the physician didn't expect the wheezes to be present in a cold, but in fact, the patient may have acute bronchitis which will present with wheezing. In any case, the symptoms can be easily and effectively treated, but the therapy will be ineffective if the diagnosis is incorrect.

Bias

Everyone brings an internal set of biases with them, which are based upon upbringing, schooling, training, and experiences. These biases can easily lead to erroneous diagnoses. If a physician assumes, without further investigation, that a disabled man with alcohol on his breath is simply a drunk who needs a place to stay, a significant head injury could easily be missed. Denying pain medication to someone who may appear to be a drug abuser can result in unnecessary suffering for the patient, incorrect diagnosis, and incorrect therapy.

Biologic variations in the senses

Hearing, sight, smell, and touch will vary between examiners and will change with age of the examiner. As one's hearing decreases, it becomes harder to hear subtle sounds like heart murmurs or gallop sounds.

Not asking

If you don't ask, you won't find out! Many clinicians don't ask newly diagnosed cancer patients about the presence of depression, although at least one-third of cancer patients are depressed and treating the depression may make it easier to treat the cancer. Treatment for depression will make the patient feel more in control, thus less likely to look for other methods of therapy such as alternative or complementary medicine to the exclusion of proven chemotherapy. Other typical examples involve asking difficult questions. Many physicians don't ask about sexual history, alcohol use, or domestic violence because they may be afraid of opening Pandora's box. On the other hand, most patients are reluctant to give important information spontaneously about these issues, and need to be asked in a non-threatening way. When asked in an honest and respectful manner, almost all patients are pleased that these difficult questions are being asked and will give accurate and detailed information. This is part of the art of medicine.

Simple ignorance

Physicians have to know what they are doing in order to be able to do it well. Poor history and physical examination skills will lead to incorrect diagnoses. For example, if a physician doesn't know the significance of the straight leg raise test in the back examination, he or she won't do it or will do it incorrectly. This can lead to a missed diagnosis of a herniated lumbar disc and continued pain for the patient.

Level of risk

Physicians must be aware of their own level of risk taking. This will directly affect the amount of risk projected onto the patient. If the physician doesn't personally like taking risks, then he or she may try to minimize risk for the patient. On the other hand, if the physician doesn't mind taking risks, he or she may not try to minimize risk for the patient. Physicians can be classified by their risk-taking behavior into *risk minimizers* or *test minimizers*. Risk-taking physicians are less likely to admit patients with chest pain to the hospital than physicians who are risk averse or risk minimizers.

   Risk minimizers tend to order more tests than test minimizers. They may order more tests than would be necessary in order to reduce the risk of missing the diagnosis. They are more likely to order tests or recommend treatments even when the risk of missing a diagnosis or the potential benefit from the therapy is small. Test minimizers may order fewer tests than might be necessary and thereby increase the risk of missing a diagnosis in the patient. They are less likely to recommend certain tests or treatments, thinking that their patient would not want to take the risk associated with the test or therapy, but will be willing to take the risk associated with an error of omission in the process of diagnosis or treatment. The test minimizer projects that the patient is willing to take the risk of missing an unlikely diagnosis and would not want any additional tests performed.

To minimize the bias associated with risk-taking behavior, physicians must ask themselves what they would do if this patient were their loved one. Then, the physician should do that for his or her patient. Additionally, use the communications techniques discussed in Chapter 18 to maximize understanding, informed consent, and shared decision making with the patient. Scrupulous honesty and open communications with the patient are a must here.

Know when you are having a bad day

Everyone has off days. If things aren't working right because of personal issues, such as a fight with your spouse, kids, or partners, problems paying your bills, or other issues, don't take it out on patients. Physicians must learn to overcome their own feelings and not let them get in the way of good and empathic communications with patients. If this is not possible, it is better to reschedule for a different day.

The examinee

Biologic variation in the system being examined

The main source of random error in medicine is biologic variation. People are complex biological organisms and all physiological responses vary from person to person, or from time to time in the same person. For example, some patients with chronic bronchitis will have audible wheezes and rhonchi while others won't have wheezes and will only have a cough on forced expiration. Some people with heart attacks have typical crushing substantial chest pain while others have a fainting spell, weakness, or shortness of breath as their only symptom. Understanding this will lead to better appreciation of subtle variations in the history and physical examination.

Effects of illness and medication

Ignoring the effect of medication or illness on the physiologic response of the patient may result in an inaccurate examination. For instance, patients who take beta-blocker drugs for hypertension will have a slowing of the pulse, so they may not have the expected physical exam findings like tachycardia even if they are in a condition such as shock.

Memory and rumination

Patients may remember their medical history differently at different times, which results in a form of recall bias. This explains the commonly observed phenomenon that the attending seems to obtain the most accurate history. The intern or medical student will usually obtain the first history from a patient. When the attending gets the history later, the patient will have had time to reconsider their answers to the questions and may give a different and more accurate history. They may have recalled things they did not remember or thought were not important during the first questioning. A way to reduce this is by summarizing the history obtained several times during the initial encounter.

Filling in

Sometimes patients will invent parts of the history because they cannot recall what actually happened. This commonly occurs with dementia patients and alcoholics during withdrawal. In most of these cases, orientation to time and place is also lost. In some instances, otherwise oriented patients will be unable to recall an event because they were briefly impaired and actually don't know what happened. This is common in the elderly who fall as a result of a syncopal episode. These patients may fill in a plausible explanation for their fall such as "I must have tripped." In a case like this, try to get an explicit description of the entire event step by step before simply attributing their fall to tripping over something.

Toss-ups

Some questions can be answered correctly in many different ways, and because of this, the way a question is worded may result in the patient giving apparently contradictory answers. Descriptors of pain and discomfort are notoriously vague in their presentation and will change from telling to telling by the patient. Asking "do you have pain" could be answered no by the patient who describes their pain as pressure and doesn't equate that with pain. The examiner will not find out that this person has chest pain without asking more specific questions using other common descriptors of chest pain such as aching, burning, pressure, or discomfort.

Patient ignorance

The patient may not be able to give accurate and correct answers due to lack of understanding of the examiner's questions. The average patient understands at the level of a tenth-grade student, meaning that half of patients are below the tenth-grade level. They may not understand the meaning of a word as simple as congestion, and answer no, when they have a cough and stuffed nose. To avoid this error, avoid using complex medical or non-medical terminology.

Patient speaks different language

Situations in which the patient and physician cannot understand each other often lead to misinterpretation of communication. Federal law requires US hospitals to have translators available for any patient who cannot speak or understand spoken English including deaf persons. In situations where a translator is not immediately available, a translation service sponsored by AT&T is available by phone. This is especially important because patients who do not speak English are more likely to be admitted to the hospital from the Emergency Department, and to have additional and often unnecessary diagnostic testing performed.

Patient embarrassment

Patients will not usually volunteer sensitive information although they may be very anxious to discuss these same topics when asked directly. This includes questions about sexual problems, domestic violence, and alcohol or drug abuse. For example, even though teenagers are engaged in sexual activity, they may not know how to ask about protection from pregnancy or sexually transmitted diseases. It is better to assume that most patients will not feel comfortable asking questions about these awkward subjects, thus the physician should ask about these issues directly in an empathetic and non-judgmental manner.

Denial

Some patients will minimize certain complaints because they are afraid of finding out they have a bad disease. They may say that their pain is really not so bad and that the tests or treatments the physician is proposing are not necessary. The physician's job is to determine the patient's fear, educate the patient about the nature of the illness, and help him or her make an informed decision.

Patient assessment of risk and level of risk taking

Some patients will reject the physician's interpretation of the nature of their complaint because of their own risk-taking behavior. They may be more willing or less willing to take a risk than the physician thinks is reasonable. The physician must follow the precept of patient autonomy here. The physician's job is to educate the patient about the nature of their illness and the level of risk they are assuming by their behavior, and then help them make an informed decision. In the end, if the patient decides to refuse the physician's suggestions for evaluation and treatment after being fully informed of the risks and benefits, they have the capacity to refuse care and should be treated with therapies that they will accept.

Lying

Finally, there are occasions when a patient will simply lie to the physician. Questions about alcohol or drug abuse, child abuse, and sexual activity are common areas where this occurs. The physician may detect inconsistencies in the history or pick up secondary clues that give an idea that this may be happening. The best way to handle this situation is to get corroborating evidence from the family, current and previous physicians, and medical records. Sometimes, the physician must simply believe them and treat them anyway.

The environment

Disruptive environments for the examination

Excess noise or interruptions, including background noise or children in the examination room, make it hard to be accurate in examination. This may be unavoidable in some circumstances like in the Emergency Department with its chaotic environment and constant noise from disruptive patients. If it is impossible to remove the noise, make sure it is compensated for in some other way. It may take longer to gather information in these circumstances, but the physician will be rewarded with increased accuracy.

Disruptive interactions between the examiner and the examined

Patients who are uncooperative, delirious, agitated, or in severe pain, as well as crying children are in this category. In this circumstance, the physician must simply try his or her best to do a competent examination over the interruptions. Providing pain relief for patients with severe pain early in the encounter will usually help to obtain a better history and more accurate examination. Occasionally in the Emergency Department, patients have to be sedated in order to examine them properly.

Reluctant co-workers

As a physician, nurses, residents, and other physicians may disagree with your evaluation. If you believe that your evaluation is correct and evidence-based, their opinions should not stand in the way. For instance, if a patient comes to the Emergency Department with the worst headache of their life, the correct medical action is to rule out a subarachnoid hemorrhage. This is done with a CT scan and, if that is negative, a spinal tap. The fact that this occurs at two o'clock in the morning should not make a difference in the decision to order the CT scan. This is true even if the radiologist asks to wait until morning to do the procedure or if the nurses say that the spinal tap is unnecessary since it takes more nursing time. The physician must know when to stand his or her ground and stick up for the patient.

Incomplete function or use of diagnostic tools

Diagnostic instruments and tools should be functioning properly and the examiner should be an expert in their use. One should know how the stethoscope, blood pressure cuff, ophthalmoscope, otoscope, reflex hammer, and tuning fork are correctly used and check on them before use. Practice using these tools before seeing patients. This would also apply to more technological tools such as x-rays and other imaging devices, electrocardiograms, transcutaneous oxymetry measuring devices, just to name a few of the common diagnostic tools in common usage.

Strategies for preventing or minimizing error in the clinical examination

The following suggestions will help to avoid making errors in the clinical examination. The examination is a tool for making an accurate final diagnosis. In order to serve this purpose, the examination must be done in a meticulous and systematic way.

(1) **Match the diagnostic environment to the diagnostic task**. It is necessary to make sure the environment is user friendly to the physician and the patient. Wherever possible, get rid of noisy distractions.

(2) **Repeat key elements of the examination**. Physicians should review and summarize the history with patients to make sure the data are correct. Make sure the physical examination findings are accurate by repeating them and observing how they change with time and treatment.

(3) **Corroborate important elements of the patient history with documents and witnesses**. Physicians need to ensure that all the information is gathered personally, without relying on secondhand information. If the patient does not speak English or is deaf, get a translator. Overall, physicians should not make clinical decisions based on an incomplete history due to the inability to accurately understand the patient, or based on secondhand history that is not corroborated.

(4) **Confirm key clinical findings with appropriate tests**. The physician should determine which tests are most useful in order to refine the diagnosis.

Table 21.1. Problem-oriented medical record: the SOAP format

S **Subjective** information gathered directly from the patient – the history.
O **Objective** information gathered during the patient examination and from diagnostic tests.
A **Assessment** of the patient's problem including a differential diagnosis and the likelihood of each disease on the list, as well as other psycho-social problems that may affect the diagnostic process or therapeutic relationship. This is where inference should be noted. Make a determination of the nature of the patient's problem and the interpretation of that problem, the diagnosis. Initially this will be a provisional diagnosis, differential diagnosis, or just a summary statement of the problem.
P **Plan** of treatment or further diagnostic testing.

This aspect of medical decision making is the basis of the next several chapters.

(5) **Ask blinded colleagues to examine the patient**. Physicians should corroborate findings to make sure that they are accurate. This will occur more often during medical school and residency training, and may be difficult to do in private practice. However, even experienced physicians will occasionally ask colleagues to check part of their clinical examination when things don't quite add up. Obtaining reasonable and timely consultation with a specialist is another way of double checking examination findings.

(6) **Report evidence as well as inference, making a clear distinction between the two**. Initially, the physician should record the facts only. When this is done, it is then appropriate to clearly note clinical interpretations in the record by using the problem-oriented medical record and the SOAP format (Table 21.1).

(7) **Use appropriate technical tools**. Physicians need to make sure that physical examination tools are working properly and that they know how to use them well.

(8) **Blind the assessment of raw diagnostic test data**. The physician should look at the results of diagnostic tests objectively, applying the principles of medical decision making contained in the next several chapters. The physician should not be overly optimistic or pessimistic about the value of a single lab test, and should apply rigorous methods of decision making in determining the meaning of the test results.

(9) **Apply social sciences, as well as biologic sciences of medicine**. The physician should remember that the patient is functioning within a social context. Emotional, cultural, and spiritual components of health are important

in getting an accurate picture of the patient. These can easily affect the interpretation of the information gathered.

(10) **Write legibly**. Physicians must realize that others will read their notes and prescriptions. If the handwriting is not legible, mistakes will occur. If this is a serious problem, individual physicians could consider dictating charts or using a computer for medical charting.

The use of diagnostic tests

Learning objectives

In this chapter you will learn:
- the uses and abuses of diagnostic tests
- the hierarchical format to determine the usefulness of a diagnostic test

The Institute of Medicine has determined that error in medicine is due to overuse, underuse, and misuse of medical resources – resources such as diagnostic tests. In order to understand the best way to use diagnostic tests, it is helpful to have a hierarchical format within which to view them.

The use of medical tests in making a diagnosis

Before deciding on ordering a diagnostic test, physicians should have a good reason for doing the test. There are four general reasons for ordering a diagnostic test.

(1) To establish a diagnosis in a patient with signs and symptoms. Examples of this are a throat culture in a patient with a sore throat to look for hemolytic group A streptococcus bacteria or a mammogram in a woman with a palpable breast mass to look for a cancer.

(2) To screen for disease among asymptomatic patients. Examples of this are the phenylketonuria test in a healthy newborn to detect a rare genetic disorder, a mammogram in a woman without signs or symptoms of a breast mass, or the prostate specific antigen test in a healthy asymptomatic man to look for prostate cancer. Screening tests will not directly benefit the majority of people who get them, since they don't have the disease, but the result can be

reassuring if it is negative. In general there are five criteria that must be met for a successful screening test – burden of suffering, early detectability, test validity, acceptability, and improved outcome – and unless all these are met, the test should not be recommended. We will discuss these in Chapter 28.

(3) To provide prognostic information on patients with established disease. Examples of this are a CD-4 count or viral load in a patient with HIV infection to look for susceptibility to opportunistic infection, or a CA-27.29 or 15.3 in a woman with breast cancer to look for disease recurrence.

(4) To monitor ongoing therapy, maximize effectiveness, and minimize side effects. One example of this is monitoring the prothrombin time in patients on warfarin therapy. This checks the patient's level of anticoagulation and prevents levels from being either too low, thus leading to new clotting, or too high, and leading to excess bleeding. Another example is therapeutic gentamycin level in patients on this antibiotic to reduce the likelihood of toxic levels causing renal failure.

Important features to determine the usefulness of a diagnostic test

There are several ways of looking at the usefulness of diagnostic tests. This hierarchical evaluation uses six possible endpoints to determine a test's utility. The more criteria in the schema that are fulfilled, the more potentially useful the test will be. On the contrary, tests that fulfill fewer criteria have more limited usefulness. These criteria are based on an article by Pearl.[1]

(1) **Technical aspects**. What are the technical performance characteristics of the test? How easy and cheap is it to perform and how reliable are the results?

  (a) **Reliable and precise** – results should be reproducible, giving the same result when the test is repeated on the same individual under the same conditions. This is usually a function of the instrumentation or operator reliability of the test. While precision used to be assumed to be present for all diagnostic tests, many studies have demonstrated that with most non-automated tests, there is some degree of subjectivity in test interpretation. This has been seen in x-ray tests such as CT scan, mammography, and angiography. It is also present in tests commonly considered to be the "gold standard" such as the interpretation of tissue samples from autopsies, biopsies, or surgery.

  (b) **Accurate** – the test should produce the correct result or the actual value of the variable it is seeking to measure all of the time. The determination of accuracy depends upon the ability of the instrument's result to be the same as the result determined using a standardized specimen and

[1] W. S. Pearl. A hierarchical outcomes approach to test assessment. *Ann. Emerg. Med.* 1999; 33: 77–84.

an instrument that has been specially calibrated to always measure the same result.

(c) **Operator dependence** – test results may depend on the skill of the person performing the test. A person with more experience, better training, or more talent will get more precise and accurate results on many tests.

(d) **Feasibility and acceptability** – how easy is it to do the test? Is there a large and expensive machine that must be bought? Is the test invasive or uncomfortable to perform? For example, many patients cannot tolerate being in an MRI machine because they have claustrophobia. For this subset of patients, an MRI would be an unacceptable test. If a test is very expensive and not covered by health insurance, the patient may not be able to pay for it, making it a useless test for them.

(e) **Interference and cross-reactivity** – are there any substances such as bodily components, medications, or foods that will interfere with the results? These substances may create false positive test results. The substances may also prevent the test from picking up true positives and thereby make them false negatives. An example of this if a person eats poppyseed bagels, they will give a false positive urine test for opiates.

(f) **Inter-observer and intra-observer reliability** – previously discussed in the section on the kappa statistic (Chapter 7), this concept is related to operator dependence.

(2) **Diagnostic accuracy**. How well does the test help in making the diagnosis of the disease? This includes the concepts of validity, likelihood ratios, sensitivity, specificity, predictive values, and area under the ROC curve. These concepts will be discussed in the next several chapters.

(a) **Validity** – the test should discriminate between individuals with and without the disorder in question. How does the test result compare to that obtained using the gold standard? **Criterion-based validity** describes how well the measurement agrees with other approaches for measuring the same characteristic, and is a very important measurement in studies of diagnostic tests.

(b) **The gold standard** – this is also known as the **reference standard**. The result of a gold-standard test defines the presence or absence of the disease (i.e., all patients with the disease have a positive test and all patients without the disease have a negative test). All other diagnostic tests must be compared to a gold standard for the disease. There are very few true gold standards in medicine and some are better or scientifically more pure than others. Some typical gold standards are:

(i) Surgical or pathological specimens. These are traditionally considered to be the ultimate gold standard, but their interpretations can vary with different pathologists.

(ii) Blood culture for bacteremia. Theoretically, all bacteria that are present in the blood should grow on a suitable culture medium. Sometimes, for technical reasons, the culture does not grow bacteria even though they were present in the blood. This can occur because the technician doesn't plate the culture properly, it is stored at an incorrect temperature, or there just happened to be no bacteria in the particular 10-cc vial of blood that was sampled.

(iii) Jones criteria for rheumatic fever. This is a set of fairly objective criteria for making a diagnosis of rheumatic fever. Factors that could decrease the accuracy of these criteria are that a component of the criteria, such as temperature, may be measured incorrectly in some patients, or another criterion like arthritis may be interpreted incorrectly by the observer.

(iv) DSM IV criteria for major depression. These criteria are objective, yet depend on the clinician's interpretation of the patient's description of their symptoms.

(v) X-rays. As mentioned previously, x-rays are open to variation in the reading, even by experienced radiologists.

(vi) Long-term follow-up. The ultimate fall-back or de-facto gold standard. If we are ultimately interested in finding out how well a test works to separate the diseased patients from the healthy patients, we can follow everyone who received the test for a specified period of time and see which outcomes they all have. This technique works as long as the time period is long enough to see all the possible disease outcomes, yet short enough to study realistically.

(3) **Diagnostic thinking**. Does the result of the test cause a change in diagnosis after testing is complete? This includes concepts of incremental gain and confidence in the diagnosis. If we are almost certain that a patient has a disease based upon one test result or the history and physical exam, we don't need a second test to confirm that result. Diagnostic thinking only considers how the test performs in making the diagnosis in a given clinical setting, and is therefore closely related to diagnostic accuracy. The setting within which this thinking operates is dependent on the prevalence of the disease in the patient population being tested.

(4) **Therapeutic effectiveness**. Is there a change in management as a result of the outcome of the test? Also, is the test cost-effective in the management of the particular disease? For example, the venogram is the gold-standard test in the diagnosis of deep venous thrombosis. It is an expensive and invasive test that can cause some side effects, although these side effects are rarely lethal. Is this test worth it if an ultrasound is almost as accurate? Part of the art of medicine is determining which patients with one negative ultrasound can safely wait for a confirmatory ultrasound 3 days later, and which patients

need to have an immediate venogram or initiation of anticoagulant medication therapy.

(5) **Patient outcomes**. Does the result of the test mean that the patient will feel or be better? This considers biophysiological parameters, symptom severity, functional outcome, patient utility, expected values, morbidity avoided, mortality change, and cost-effectiveness of outcomes. We will discuss some of these issues in the chapter on decision trees and patient values (Chapter 31).

(6) **Societal outcomes**. Is the test effective for the society as a whole? Even a cheap test, if done excessively, may result in prohibitive costs to society. Outcomes include the additional cost of evaluation or treatment of patients with false positive test results and the psychosocial cost of these results on the patient and community. Other outcomes are the risk of missing the correct diagnosis in patients who are falsely negative and may suffer negative outcomes as a result of the diagnosis being missed. Again, physicians may need to also consider a cost analysis for evaluating the test. Interestingly, the perspective of the analysis can be the patient, the payor, or society as a whole. Overall, patient or societal outcomes ultimately determine the usefulness of a test as a screening tool.

23

Utility and characteristics of diagnostic tests: likelihood ratios, sensitivity, and specificity

It seems to me that science has a much greater likelihood of being true in the main than any philosophy hitherto advanced.

Bertrand Russell (1872–1970): The Philosophy of Logical Atomism, 1924

Learning objectives

In this chapter you will learn:

- the characteristics and definitions of normal and abnormal diagnostic test results
- how to define, calculate, and interpret likelihood ratios
- the process by which diagnostic decisions are modified in medicine and the use of likelihood ratios to choose the most appropriate test for a given purpose
- how to define, calculate, and use sensitivity and specificity
- how sensitivity and specificity relate to positive and negative likelihood ratios
- the process by which sensitivity and specificity can be used to make diagnostic decisions in medicine and how to choose the most appropriate test for a given purpose

In this chapter, we will be talking about the utility of a diagnostic test. This is a mathematical expression of the ability of a test to find persons with disease or exclude persons without disease. In general, a test's utility will depend on two factors. These are the likelihood ratios and the prevalence of disease in the target population. Additional test characteristics that will be introduced are the sensitivity and specificity. These factors will tell the user how useful the test will be in the clinical setting. Using a test without knowing these characteristics will result in problems that include missing correct diagnoses, over-ordering tests, increasing health-care costs, reducing trust in physicians, and increasing discomfort and side effects for the patient. Once one understands these properties of diagnostic tests, one will be able to determine when to best order them.

Why order a diagnostic test?

The indications for ordering a diagnostic test can be distilled into two simple rules. They are:

(1) When the characteristics of that test give it validity in the clinical setting. Will a positive or negative test be a true positive or a true negative result? Will that result help in correctly identifying a diseased patient from one without disease?

(2) When the test result will change the probability of the disease leading to a change of clinical strategy. What will a positive or negative test result tell me about this patient that I don't already know and that I need to know? Will the test results change my treatment plan for this patient?

If the test that is being considered does not fall into one of these categories, it should not be done!

What do diagnostic tests do?

Diagnostic tests are a way of obtaining information that provides a basis for revising disease probabilities. When a patient presents with a clinical problem, one first creates a differential diagnosis. One attempts to reduce the number of diseases on this list by ordering diagnostic tests. Ideally, each test will either rule in or rule out one or more of the diseases on the differential diagnosis list. Diseases which are common, have serious sequelae such as death or disability, or can be easily treated are usually the ones which must initially be ruled in or out.

We rule in disease when a positive test for that disease increases the probability of disease, making its presence so likely that we would treat the patient for that disease. This should also make all the other diseases on the differential diagnosis list so unlikely that we would no longer consider them as possible explanations for the patient's complaints. We rule out disease when a negative test for that disease reduces the probability of that disease, making it so unlikely that we would no longer look for evidence that our patient had that disease.

After setting up a list of possible diseases, we can assign a **pretest probability** to each disease on the differential. This is the estimated likelihood of disease in the particular patient before any testing is done. As we discussed earlier, it is based on the history and physical examination as well as on the prevalence of the disease in the population. It is also called the **prior** or **a-priori probability** of disease in that patient.

Post-test probability	$\propto$	Pretest probability	$\times$	Test factor
What we know after doing the test	=	What we knew before doing the test	$\times$	How much the test results change the likelihood of what we knew before

Fig. 23.1 Bayes' theorem.

After doing a diagnostic test, we are able to calculate the **post-test probability** of disease. This is the estimated likelihood of the disease in a patient after testing is done. This is also called the **posterior** or **a-posteriori probability** of disease. We can do this when the test result is either positive or negative. A positive test tends to rule in the disease while a negative test tends to rule out the disease. We normally think of a test as being something done by a lab or radiologist. However, the test can be an item of history, part of the physical examination, a laboratory test, a diagnostic x-ray, or any other diagnostic maneuver. Common examples of this are pulmonary function testing, psychological testing, EEG, or EKG.

Mathematically, the pretest probability of the disease is modified by the application of a diagnostic test to yield a post-test probability of the disease. This revision of the pretest disease probabilities is done using a number called the likelihood ratio (LR). Likelihood ratios are stable characteristics of a diagnostic test and give the strength of that test. The likelihood ratio can be used to revise disease probabilities using a form of Bayes' theorem (Fig. 23.1). We will return to Bayes' theorem in Chapter 24. Before fully looking at likelihood ratios, it is useful to look at the definitions of normality in diagnostic tests.

Types of test results

Dichotomous test results can have only two possible values. Typical results are yes or no, positive or negative, alive or dead, better or not. A common dichotomous result is x-ray results which are read as either normal or abnormal and showing a particular abnormality. There is also the middle ground, or gray zone, in these tests as sometimes they will be unreadable because of poor technical quality. In addition, there are many subtle gradations that can appear on an x-ray and lead to various readings, but they may not pertain to the disease for which the patient is being evaluated.

Continuous test results can have more than two possible values. The serum sodium level or the level of other blood components is an example of a continuous test. A patient can have any of a theoretically infinite number of values for the test result. In real life, serum sodium can take any value from about 100

Fig. 23.2 Gaussian results of a
diagnostic test.

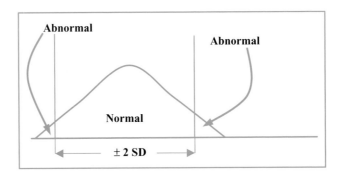

to 170, although at the extremes the person is near death. In practice, we often take continuous tests and select a set of values for the variable that will be considered normal (135–145 mEq/dL for serum sodium) thereby turning this continuous test into a dichotomous test, which is reported as normal or abnormal. Values of the serum sodium below 135 mEq/dL, called hyponatremia, or above 145 mEq/dL, called hypernatremia, are both abnormal. Clearly, the farther from the normal range, the more serious the problem.

Definitions of a normal test result

There are many mathematical ways to describe the results of a diagnostic test as normal or abnormal. In the method of percentiles, cutoffs are chosen at preset percentiles of the diagnostic test results. These preset percentiles are chosen as the upper and lower limits of normal. All values above the upper limit or below the lower limit of the normal percentiles are abnormal. This method assumes that all diseases have the same prevalence. A special case of this method is the **Gaussian** method. In this method, normal is 95%, which is plus or minus two standard deviations (± 2 SD) of the values observed of all tests done (Fig. 23.2). Results are only specific to the population being studied and cannot be generalized to other populations.

In reality, there are two normal distributions of test results (Fig. 23.3). One is for patients who are afflicted with the disease and the other is for those free of disease. There is usually an overlap of the distributions of test values for the sick and not-sick populations. The goal of the diagnostic test is to differentiate between the two groups. Some disease-free patients will have abnormal test results while some diseased patients will have normal results, thus setting any single value of the test as the cutoff between normal and abnormal will usually misclassify some patients. The ideal test, the gold standard, will have none of this overlap between diseased and non-diseased populations and will therefore be able to differentiate between them perfectly at all times.

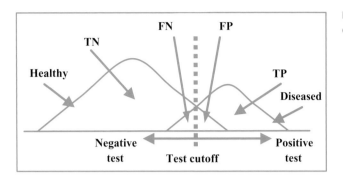

Fig. 23.3 The "real-life" results of a diagnostic test.

For almost all tests that are not a gold standard, there are four possible outcomes. True positives (TP) are those patients with disease who have a positive or abnormal test result. True negatives (TN) are those without the disease who have a negative or normal test result. False negatives (FN) are those with disease who have a negative or normal test result. False positives (FP) are those without disease who have a positive or abnormal test result. We can see this graphically in Fig. 23.3.

Ideally, when a research study of a diagnostic test is done, patients with and without the disease are all given both the diagnostic test and the gold-standard test. The results will show that some patients with a positive gold-standard test, and who have the disease, will have a positive diagnostic test and some will have a negative diagnostic test. The ones with a positive test are the true positives and those with a negative test are false negatives. A similar situation exists among patients who have a negative gold-standard test and therefore, are all actually disease-free. Some of them will have a negative diagnostic test result and are called true negatives and some will have a positive test result and are called false positives.

Strength of a diagnostic test

The results of a clinical study of a diagnostic test can determine the strength of the test. The ideal diagnostic test, the gold standard, will always discriminate diseased from non-diseased individuals in a population. This is another way of saying that the test is 100% accurate. The diagnostic test we are comparing to the gold standard is a test that is easier, cheaper, or safer than the gold standard, and we want to know its accuracy. That tells us how often it is correct, yielding either a true positive or true negative result and how often it is incorrect yielding either a false positive or false negative result.

From the results of this type of study, we can create a 2 × 2 table that divides a real or hypothetical population into four groups depending on their disease

Fig. 23.4 Results of a study of a
diagnostic test.

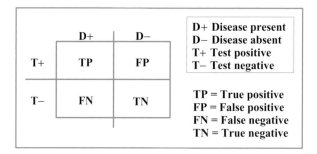

Fig. 23.5 Positive likelihood
ratio (LR+) calculations.

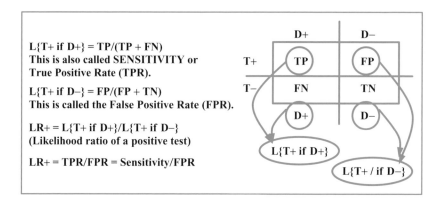

status (D+ or D–) and test results (T+ or T–). Patients are either diseased (D+)
or free of disease (D–) as determined by the gold standard test. The diagnostic
test is applied to the sample, and patients have either a positive (T+) or negative
(T–) diagnostic test. We can then create a 2 × 2 table to evaluate the mathematical characteristics of this diagnostic test. This 2 × 2 table (Fig. 23.4) is the conceptual basis for almost all calculations made in the next several chapters.

We can calculate the likelihood or probability of finding a positive test result if
a person does or does not have the disease. Similarly, we can calculate the likelihood of finding a negative test result if a person does or does not have the disease.
Comparing these likelihoods can give a ratio that shows the strength of the test.
Likelihoods are calculated for each of the four possible outcomes. They can be
compared in two ratios and are analogous to the relative risk in studies of risk or
harm. These are called the **positive** and **negative likelihood ratios**. In studies of
diagnostic tests, we are looking at the probability that a person with the disease
will have a positive test. Compare that to the probability that a person without
the disease has a positive test and the likelihood ratio of a positive test can be
calculated (LR+ in Fig. 23.5).

The LR+ tells us by how much a positive test increases the likelihood of disease
in a person being tested. We start with the likelihood of disease, do the test, and
as a result of a positive test that likelihood increases. The LR+ tells us how much

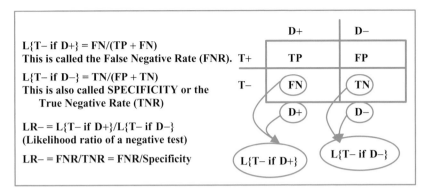

Fig. 23.6 Negative likelihood ratio (LR–) calculations.

of an increase in this likelihood we can expect. We can do the same thing for a negative test. In this case, we are looking at the likelihoods of having a negative test in people with and without the disease. The LR– or likelihood ratio of a negative test tells us by how much a negative test decreases the likelihood of disease in persons who are having the test done. Figure 23.6 describes these calculations.

Likelihood ratios are called stable characteristics of a test. This means that they do not change with the prevalence of the disease. Their values are determined by clinical studies against a gold standard, therefore, published reports of likelihood ratios are only as good as the gold standard against which they are based and the quality of the study that determined their value.

The likelihood ratios are the strength of the diagnostic test. The larger the value of LR+, the more a positive test will increase the probability of disease in a patient to whom the test is given and who then has a positive result. In general, one would like the likelihood ratio of a positive test to be very high, ideally greater than 10, to maximally increase the probability of disease after doing the test and getting a positive result. Similarly, one would want the likelihood ratio of a negative test to be very low, ideally less than 0.1 to maximally decrease the probability of disease after doing the test and getting a negative result. A qualitative list of LRs has been devised to show the strength of a test based upon LR values. These are listed in Table 23.1.

Table 23.1. Strength of test by likelihood ratio

Qualitative strength	LR+	LR–
Excellent	10	0.1
Very good	5	0.2
Fair	2	0.5
Useless	1	1

The likelihood that a patient with the disease has a positive test is also known as the sensitivity or the true positive rate (TPR). This tells the reader how sensitive the test is for finding those persons with disease when only looking at those with disease. It displays how often the result is a true positive compared to a false negative as it is the fraction of people with the disease who test positive. *It is important to note that sensitivity can only be calculated from among people who have the disease.* Probabilistically, it is expressed as $P[T+ \mid D+]$, the probability of a positive test if the person has disease.

If the result of a very sensitive test is negative, it tells us that the patient doesn't have the disease and the test is Negative in Health (NIH). This is because in a very sensitive test, there are very few false negatives, therefore virtually all negative tests must occur in non-diseased people. In addition, if the clinician has properly reduced the number of diagnostic possibilities, it would be even more unlikely that the patient has the disease in question. As a general rule, when two or more tests are available, the most sensitive one should be done to minimize the number of false negatives. This is especially true for serious diseases that are easily treated. An example of a very sensitive test is the thyroid simulating hormone (TSH) test for hypothyroidism. A normal TSH makes it extremely unlikely that the patient has hypothyroidism, thus with a normal TSH, hypothyroidism is ruled out. A sensitive test rules out disease – and the mnemonic is SnOut (**Sensitive** = ruled **Out**).

Similarly, the likelihood that a patient without disease has a positive test is also known as the false positive rate (FPR). It is equal to one minus the specificity. It tells us how often the result is a false positive compared to a true negative. FPR = FP/(FP + TN). This is the proportion of non-diseased people with a positive test.

The likelihood that a patient without the disease has a negative test is also known as the specificity or the true negative rate (TNR). It tells the reader how specific the test is for finding those persons without disease, when only looking at those without disease. It demonstrates how often the result is a true negative compared to a false positive, as it is the fraction of people without the disease who test negative. *It is important to realize that specificity can only be calculated from among people who do not have the disease.* Probabilistically, it is expressed as $P[T- \mid D-]$, the probability of a negative test if the person does not have disease.

If the result of a very specific test is positive, it tells us that the patient has the disease and the test is Positive in Disease (PID). This is because there are very few false positives, therefore any positive tests must occur in diseased people. If the clinician has properly reduced the number of diagnostic possibilities, then it would be even more likely that the patient does have the disease in question. When two or more tests are available, the most specific should be done to minimize the number of false positives. This is especially true for diseases that are

Table 23.2. Mnemonics for sensitivity and specificity

---

(1) SeNsitive tests are Negative in health (**NIH**)
 SPecific tests are Positive in disease (**PID**)
(2) Sensitivity: **SnOut** – sensitive tests rule out disease
 Specificity: **SpIn** – specific tests rule in disease
(3) SeNsitivity includes False Negatives
 SPecificity includes False Positives

---

not easily treated or for which the treatment is potentially dangerous. An example of a very specific test is the ultrasound for deep venous thrombosis of the leg. If the ultrasound is positive, it is extremely likely that there is a clot in the vein. Thus, a deep vein thrombosis is ruled in. A specific test rules in disease – and the mnemonic is SpIn (**Sp**ecificity = ruled **In**).

Similarly, the likelihood that a patient with disease has a negative test is also known as the false negative rate (FNR). It is equal to one minus the sensitivity. It tells the reader how often the result is a false negative compared to a true positive. FNR = FN/(FN + TP). This is the proportion of diseased people with a negative test.

Using sensitivity and specificity

The sensitivity and specificity are the mathematical components of the likelihood ratios. They are the characteristics that are most often measured and reported in studies of diagnostic tests in the medical literature. Three mnemonics can help to remember the difference between sensitivity and specificity. These are listed in Table 23.2. Like likelihood ratios, true positive rate, false positive rate, true negative rate, and false negative rate are also intrinsic characteristics of a diagnostic test. From the study results, we can use our 2 × 2 table (Fig. 23.7) that divided a real or hypothetical population into four groups depending on their disease status (D+ or D−) and test results (T+ or T−) as a starting point to evaluate these characteristics of the diagnostic test.

We have previously noted the mathematical relationship between sensitivity and specificity and the likelihood ratios. Likelihood ratios can be calculated from sensitivity and specificity. The formulas are as follows:

LR+ = sensitivity/(1 − specificity)
LR− = (1 − sensitivity)/specificity

Fig. 23.7 Sensitivity and
specificity calculations.

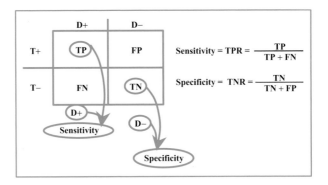

Fig. 23.8 The effect of changing
the cutoff point for a diagnostic
test.

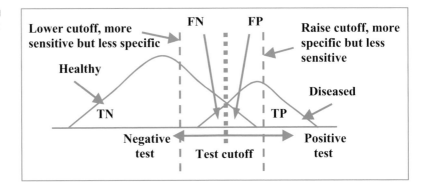

There is also a dynamic relationship between sensitivity and specificity. As the sensitivity of a test increases, the cutoff point moves to the left in Fig. 23.8. The number of true positives increases compared to the number of false negatives. At the same time, the number of false positives will increase compared to the number of true negatives. This will result in a decrease in the specificity. Notice what happens to the sensitivity and specificity in Fig. 23.8 when the test cutoff moves to the right. Now the sensitivity decreases as the specificity increases. We will see this dynamic relationship better when we discuss receiver operating characteristic curves in Chapter 25.

Sample problem

Diarrhea in children is usually caused by viral infection. However in some cases, bacterial infection causes the diarrhea and these cases should be treated with antibiotics. A study was done in which 156 young children with diarrhea had stool samples taken. All of them were tested for the presence of white blood cells in the stool, and a positive test was defined as one in which there were

	D+	D−	Totals
T+	23 (TP)	16 (FP)	39
T−	4 (FN)	113 (TN)	117
Totals	27	129	156 (N)

Fig. 23.9 A 2 × 2 table using data from the study of the use of fecal leukocytes in the diagnosis of bacterial diarrhea in children. The prevalence of disease is $27/156 = 0.17$. From: T. G. DeWitt, K. F. Humphrey & P. McCarthy. Clinical predictors of acute bacterial diarrhea in young children. *Pediatrics* 1985; 76: 551–556.

>5 white blood cells per high power field. All the children had a stool culture done, which was the gold standard. There were 27 children who had positive cultures and 23 of these had smears that were positive for fecal white blood cells. Of the 129 who had a negative stool culture, 16 had smears that were positive for fecal white blood cells. What are the likelihood ratios of the stool leukocyte test?

First make your 2 × 2 table (Fig. 23.9). From this you can tell that the prevalence is $27/156 = 0.17$.

$$L\{T+ \,|D+\} = \text{sensitivity or TPR} = TP/(TP + FN) = 23/(23 + 4) = 0.85$$

$$L\{T+ \,|D-\} = 1 - \text{specificity} = FPR = FP/(TN + FP) = 16/(113 + 16) = 0.12$$

From these we can calculate the likelihood ratio of a positive test:

$$LR+ = L\{T+ \,|D+\}/L\{T + \,|D-\} = 0.85/0.12 = 7.08$$

Doing the same for a negative test leads to the following results:

$$L\{T- \,|D+\} = 1 - \text{sensitivity} = FNR = FN/(TP + FN) = 4/(23 + 4) = 0.15$$

$$L\{T- \,|D-\} = \text{specificity or TNR} = TN/(TN + FP) = 113/(113 + 16) = 0.88$$

$$LR- = L\{T- \,|D+\}/L\{T- \,|D-\} = 0.15/0.88 = 0.17$$

These likelihood ratios are pretty good and this is a fairly good test since the $LR+ = 7.08$ and the $LR- = 0.17$ are very close to a strong test ($LR+ > 10$ and $LR- < 0.1$). This is a test that will increase the likelihood of disease by a lot if the test is positive and decrease the likelihood of disease by a lot if the test is negative. We will talk about applying these numbers in a real clinical situation in a later chapter.

It is always necessary to be aware of biases in a study, and this example is no different. The following are the potential biases in this study. It was done on 156 children who presented to an emergency department with severe diarrhea and were entered into the study. This meant that someone, either the resident or attending physician on duty at the time, thought that the child had infectious or bacterial diarrhea. Therefore, they were already screened before any testing was done on them and the study is subject to filter or selection bias. This simply means that the population in the study may not be representative of the population of all children with diarrhea like the ones being seen in a pediatric or family-practice office. The next chapter will deal with this problem and how to generalize the results of this study to real patients.

24

Bayes' theorem, predictive values, post-test probabilities, and interval likelihood ratios

As far as the laws of mathematics refer to reality, they are not certain; and as far as they are certain, they do not refer to reality.

Albert Einstein (1879–1955)

Learning objectives

In this chapter you will learn:

- how to define predictive values of positive and negative test results and how they differ from sensitivity and specificity
- the difference between odds and probability and how to use each correctly
- Bayes' theorem and the use of likelihood ratios to modify the probability of a disease
- how to define, calculate, and use interval likelihood ratios for a diagnostic test
- how to calculate and use positive and negative predictive values
- how to use predictive values to choose the appropriate test for a given diagnostic dilemma
- how to apply basic test characteristics to solve a clinical diagnostic problem
- the use of interval likelihood ratios in clinical decision making

In this chapter, we will be talking about the application of likelihood ratios, sensitivity, and specificity to a patient.

Introduction

Likelihood ratios, sensitivity, and specificity of a test are derived from studies of patients with and without disease. They are stable and essential characteristics of the test that give us the probabilities of a positive or negative test if the patient does or does not have disease. This is not the information a clinician needs to know in order to apply the test to a single patient.

What the clinician needs to know is: if a patient has a positive test, what is the likelihood that patient has the disease? The clinician is interested in how the test result relates to the patient. For a given patient, how will the probability of disease change given a positive or negative test result? Applying likelihood ratios or sensitivity and specificity to a selected pretest probability of disease will give the post-test probability to answer this question. There are two methods for doing this calculation. The first uses Bayes' theorem, while the second calculates the predictive values of a positive and negative test directly from sensitivity, specificity, and prevalence using the 2×2 table.

Predictive values

The positive predictive value (PPV) is the proportion of patients with the disease among all those who have a positive test. If the test comes back positive, it shows the probability that this patient really has the disease. Probabilistically, it is expressed as $P[D+ |T +]$, the probability of disease if a positive test occurs. It is also called the post-test or posterior probability of a positive test. A related concept is the false alarm rate (FAR), which is equal to 1 – PPV. That is the proportion of people with a positive test who do not have disease and will then be falsely alarmed by a positive test result.

The negative predictive value (NPV) is the proportion of patients without the disease among all those who have a negative test. If the test comes back negative, it shows the probability that this patient really does not have the disease. Probabilistically, it is expressed as $P[D– | T –]$, the probability of not having disease if a negative test occurs. It is also called the post-test or posterior probability of a negative test. A related concept is the false reassurance rate (FRR), which is equal to 1 – NPV. That is the proportion of people with a negative test who have disease and will be falsely reassured by a negative test result.

Bayes' theorem

Thomas Bayes was an English clergyman with broad talents. His famous theorem was presented posthumously in 1763. In eighteenth-century English, it said: "The probability of an event is the ratio between the value at which an expectation depending on the happening of the event ought to be computed and the value of the thing expected upon its happening." Now, that's not so easy to understand is it? In simple language, the theorem was an updated way to predict the odds of an event happening when confronted with new information. In statistics, this new information is that gained in the research process. In making diagnoses in clinical medicine, this new information is the likelihood ratio. Bayes' theorem is a way of using likelihood ratios (LRs) to revise disease probabilities.

Bayes' theorem was put into mathematical form by Laplace, the discoverer of his famous law. Its use in statistics was supplanted at the start of the twentieth century by Sir Ronald Fisher's ideas of statistical significance, the use of $P < 0.05$ for statistical significance. It was kept in the dark until revived in the 1980s. We won't get into the actual formula in its usual and original form here because it only involves another very long and useless formula. A derivation and the full mathematical formula for Bayes' theorem are given in Appendix 5, if interested. In it's simplest and most useful form, it states:

Post-test odds = pretest odds × LR

Odds and probabilities

In order to use Bayes' theorem and likelihood ratios, one must first convert the probability of disease to the odds of disease. Odds describe the chance that something will happen against the chance it will not happen. Probability describes the chance that something will happen against the chance that it will or will not happen. The odds of an outcome are the number of people affected divided by the number of people not affected. In contrast, the probability of an outcome is the number of people affected divided by the number of people at risk or those affected plus those not affected. Probability is what we are estimating when we select a pretest probability of disease for our patient. We next have to convert this to odds.

Let's use a simple example to show the relationship between odds and probability. If we have 5 white blocks and 5 black blocks in a jar, we can calculate the probability or odds of picking a black block at random and of course, without looking. The odds of the outcome of interest, picking a black block, are 5/5 = 1. There are equal odds of picking a white and black block. For every one black block that is picked, on average, one white block will be picked. The probability of the outcome of interest or picking a black block is 5/10 = 0.5. Half of all the picks will be a black block. Figure 24.1 shows this relationship.

In our society, odds are usually associated with gambling. In horse racing or other games of chance, the odds are usually given backward by convention. For example, the odds against Dr. Disaster winning the fifth race at Saratoga are 7 : 1. This means that this horse is likely to lose 7 times for every eight races he enters. In usual medical terminology, these numbers are reversed. We put the outcome we want on top and the one we don't want on the bottom. Therefore, the odds of him winning would be 1 : 7, or 1/7 or 0.14. He will win one time in eight.

The probability of Dr. Disaster winning is different. Here we answer the question of how many times will he have to race in order to win once? He will have to race eight times in order to have one win. The probability of him winning any

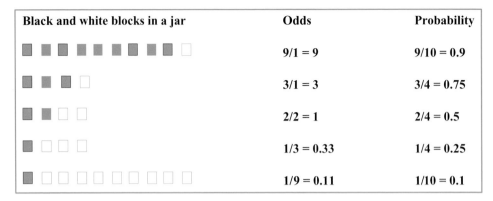

Black and white blocks in a jar	Odds	Probability
■ ■ ■ ■ ■ ■ ■ ■ □	9/1 = 9	9/10 = 0.9
■ ■ ■ □	3/1 = 3	3/4 = 0.75
■ ■ □ □	2/2 = 1	2/4 = 0.5
■ □ □ □	1/3 = 0.33	1/4 = 0.25
■ □ □ □ □ □ □ □ □	1/9 = 0.11	1/10 = 0.1

Fig. 24.1 Relationship between odds and probability. As the odds and probabilities get smaller, they also approximate each other. As they get larger, they become more and more different.

Fig. 24.2 Converting odds to probability (and back).

> **To convert odds to probability:**
>   Probability = Odds/(1 + Odds)
>
> **To convert probability to odds:**
>
>   Odds = Probability/(1 − Probability)

one race is 1 in 8 or 1/8 or 0.125. Since the odds and probabilities are small numbers, they are very similar. If he were a better horse and the odds of him winning were 1 : 1, or one win for every loss, the odds could be expressed as 1/1 or 1.0. Here the probability would be that he would win one race in every two he starts. The probability of winning is 1/2 or 0.5.

The language for odds and probabilities differs. Odds are expressed as one number to another: for example, odds of 1 : 2 are expressed as "one to two" and equal the fraction 0.5. This is the same as saying the odds are 0.5 to 1. Probability is expressed as a fraction. The same 1 : 2 odds would be expressed as "one in three" = 0.33. These two expressions and numbers are the same way of saying that for every three attempts, there will be one successful outcome.

There are mathematical formulas for converting odds to probability and vice versa. They are listed in Fig. 24.2.

Using likelihood ratios to revise pretest probabilities of disease

Likelihood ratios (LRs) can be used to revise disease pretest probabilities when test results are dichotomous, using Bayes' theorem. This says post-test odds of

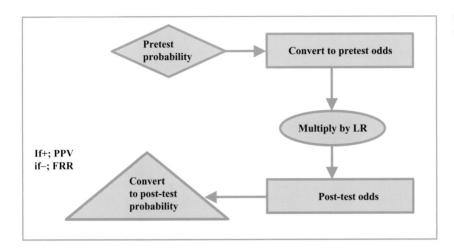

Fig. 24.3 Flowchart for Bayes' theorem.

disease equal pretest odds of disease times the likelihood ratio. We get the pretest probability of disease from our differential diagnosis list and our estimate of the possibility of disease in our patient. The pretest probability is converted to pretest odds and multiplied by the likelihood ratio. This results in the post-test odds, which are converted back to a probability, the post-test probability.

The end result of using Bayes' theorem when a positive test occurs is the post-test probability of disease. This is also called the positive predictive value (PPV). For a negative test, Bayes' theorem calculates the probability that the person still has disease even if a negative test occurs. This is called the false reassurance rate (FRR). From this, one can calculate the negative predictive value (NPV), which is the probability that a person with a negative test does not have the disease. Mathematically it is 1 minus the FRR. The process is represented graphically in Fig. 24.3.

We will demonstrate this with an example. A study was done to evaluate the use of the urine dipstick in testing for urinary tract infections (UTI) in children seen in a pediatric emergency department.[1] A positive leukocyte esterase and nitrite test on a urine dipstick was defined as being diagnostic of a UTI. In this case, a urine culture was done on all the children and therefore was the gold standard. A positive test on both indicators, the leukocyte esterase and nitrite, had a positive likelihood ratio (LR+) of 20 but a negative likelihood ratio (LR–) of 0.61. In the study population, the probability of a urinary tract infection in the children being evaluated in that setting was 0.09 (9%).

Suppose you are in a practice and estimate that a particular child whom you are seeing for fever has a pretest probability of 10% of having a UTI. This is equivalent to a low pretest probability of disease. If you want to find out what

[1] From K. N. Shaw, D. Hexter, K. L. McGowan & J. S. Schwartz. Clinical evaluation of a rapid screening test for urinary tract infections in children. *J. Pediatr.* 1991; 118: 733–736.

the post-test probabilities of a urinary tract infection are after using the dipstick test, use Bayes' theorem and do the following steps:

(1) **Convert probability to odds.** Pretest probability = 0.1, therefore, Pretest odds = 0.1/(1 − 0.1) = 0.11. (Remember, for low values, the same number could be used and get results that are close enough.)

(2) **Apply Bayes' theorem.** Multiply pretest odds by the likelihood ratio for a positive test (LR+). In this case, LR+ = 20, a very high LR+, so the test is very powerful if positive. Post-test odds = pretest odds × LR+ = 0.11 × 20 = 2.2.

(3) **Convert odds back to probability.** Post-test probability = odds/(odds + 1) = 2.2/3.2 = 0.69. (Here we have to do the formal calculation back to probability to get a reasonable result.)

(4) **Interpret the result.** Post-test probability or positive predictive value of disease is 69%. In other words, a positive urine dipstick has increased the probability of a urinary tract infection from 0.1 to 0.69. This is a big jump! Most tests have much less ability to jump the patient's pretest probability.

Using the same example for a negative test:

(1) Pretest probability and odds of disease are unchanged. Pretest odds = 0.11.

(2) LR− = 0.61, and post-test odds = 0.11 × 0.61 = 0.067.

(3) Post-test probability = 0.067/1.067 = 0.063.

In other words, a negative urine dipstick has reduced the probability of urinary tract infection from 0.1 to 0.06. This is the false reassurance rate (FRR), and tells us how many children we will falsely tell not to worry, in this case 6 out of 100. We can also calculate the negative predictive value, which is 1 − FRR, or 1 − 0.06. The NPV is, therefore, 0.94, or 94% of children with a negative test are free of disease. Of course, it is important to recognize that the pretest probability of not having a urinary tract infection before doing any test was estimated at 90%.

When we get a negative test result, we have to make a clinical decision. Should we do the urine culture or gold standard test for all children who have a negative dipstick test in order to pick up the 6% who actually have an infection? Or, should we just reassure them and repeat the test if the symptoms persist? This conundrum must be accurately communicated to the patient, and in this case the parents, and plans made for all contingencies. Choosing to do the urine culture on all children with a negative test will result in a huge number of unnecessary cultures. They are expensive and will result in a large expenditure of effort and money for the health-care system. Whether or not to do the urine culture depends on the consequences of not diagnosing an infection at the time the child presents with their initial symptoms. In the office, it is not known if these undetected children progress to kidney damage. The available evidence suggests that there is no significant delayed damage, that the majority of these infections will spontaneously clear or the child will show up with persistent symptoms and be treated at a later time.

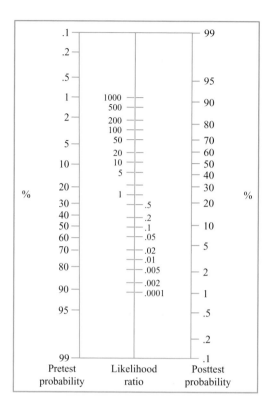

Fig. 24.4 Nomogram for Bayes'
theorem. From T. J. Fagan.
[letter.] *N. Engl. J. Med.* 1975;
293: 257. Used with permission.

The nomogram

A nomogram to calculate post-test probability using likelihood ratios was developed in 1975 by Fagan (Fig. 24.4). Begin by marking the LR and pretest probability on the nomogram. Connect these two points, and continue the line until the post-test probability is reached. This obviates the need to calculate pretest odds and post-test probability. For our example of a child with signs and symptoms of a urinary tract infection, the plot of the post-test probability for this clinical situation is shown in Fig. 24.5.

Calculating post-test probabilities using sensitivity and specificity directly

The other way of calculating post-test probabilities uses sensitivity and specificity directly to calculate the predictive values. Not only are positive and negative predictive values of the test related to the sensitivity and specificity, but they are also dependent on the prevalence of disease. The prevalence of disease is the

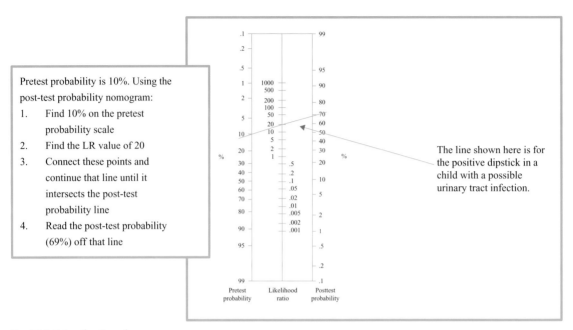

Pretest probability is 10%. Using the post-test probability nomogram:

1.   Find 10% on the pretest probability scale
2.   Find the LR value of 20
3.   Connect these points and continue that line until it intersects the post-test probability line
4.   Read the post-test probability (69%) off that line

The line shown here is for the positive dipstick in a child with a possible urinary tract infection.

Fig. 24.5 Using the Bayes' theorem nomogram in the example of UTI in children.

pretest probability of disease that has been assigned to the patient or the prevalence of disease in the population of interest. The history and physical exam give an estimate of the pretest probability. Simply knowing the sensitivity and specificity of a test without knowing the prevalence of the disease in the population from which the patient is drawn will not help to differentiate between disease and non-disease in your patient. Go back to Table 20.5 in Chapter 20 and look at the table of pretest probabilities again. This ought to help it make more sense.

Clinicians can use pretest probability for disease and non-disease respectively along with the test sensitivity and specificity to calculate the post-test probability that the patient has the disease (post-test probability = predictive value). This is shown graphically in Fig. 24.6.

Calculating predictive values step by step

(1) Pick a likely pretest probability (P) of disease using the rules we discussed in Chapter 20. Moderate errors in the selection of this number will not significantly affect the results or alter the interpretation of the result.

(2) Set up a cohort of 1000 (N) patients or use a similarly convenient number to make the math as easy as possible and divide them into diseased (D+ = P × N) and non-diseased (D− = (1 − P) × N) groups based on the estimated pretest probability or prevalence (P). Use the 2 × 2 table.

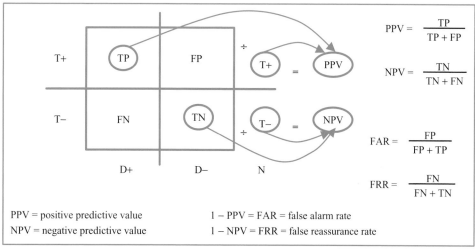

Fig. 24.6 Predictive values calculations.

(3) Multiply the D+ and D− by the sensitivity and specificity respectively to get the contents of the boxes TP and TN:

Sensitivity × D+ = TP

Specificity × D− = TN

(4) Fill in the remaining boxes, FN and FP. FN = (D+) − TP and FP = (D−) − TN.

(5) Calculate predictive values using the formulas

PPV = TP/(TP + FP)

NPV = TN/(TN + FN).

Let's go back to the 156 young children with diarrhea whom we met at the end of Chapter 23.[2] Recall that we calculated the sensitivity and specificity of the stool sample test for fecal white blood cells with > 5 cells/high power field defining a positive test and got 85% and 88%, respectively. We have already decided that this study population does not represent all children with diarrhea who present to a general pediatrician's office. In this setting, the pediatrician estimates the prevalence of bacterial diarrhea is closer to 0.02 than 0.17 as it was in the study: 27/156. How does the lower prevalence change the predictive values of the test? What is the likelihood of disease in a child with a positive or negative test?

(1) First, use 1000 patients (N) to set up the 2 × 2 table using the new estimated clinical prevalence of bacterial diarrhea of 0.02 or 20 out of 1000 (Fig. 24.7).

[2] T. G. Dewitt, K. F. Humphrey & P. McCarthy. Clinical predictors of acute bacterial diarrhea in young children. *Pediatrics* 1985; 76: 551–556.

Fig. 24.7 Set up the 2 × 2 table using a population of 1000 patients (N) and an estimated clinical prevalence (P) of bacterial diarrhea of 0.02.

	D+	D−	
T+	TP	FP	TP + FP
T−	FN	TN	FN + TN
	20	980	1000 (N)

Fig. 24.8 Multiply the number with disease (D+ = P × N) by the sensitivity and the number without disease (D− = (1 − P) × N) by the specificity to get the values of TP and TN.

	D+	D−	
T+	20 × 0.85 = 17	FP	
T−	FN	980 × 0.88 = 862	
	20	980	1000 (N)

Fig. 24.9 Subtract TP from D+ and TN from D− to get the values of FP and FN, and add the lines across.

	D+	D−	
T+	17	118	135
T−	3	862	865
	20 (P)	980 (N − P)	1000 (N)

(2) Next, multiply the number with disease by the sensitivity and without disease by the specificity to get the values of TP and TN. Round off decimals (Fig. 24.8).

(3) Fill in the FP and FN boxes and add the lines across (Fig. 24.9).

(4) Calculate PPV, NPV, FAR, and FRR:

$$PPV = TP/T+ = 17/135 = 0.13$$

$$NPV = TN/T- = 862/865 = 0.996$$

$$FAR = FP/T+ = 1 - PPV = 0.87$$

$$FRR = FN/T- = 1 - NPV = 0.004$$

(5) Interpret the results and decide how to use them.

Compared to the original population with a prevalence of 17.3%, we can see that the PPV drops significantly when the prevalence decreases. This is a general rule of the relationship between PPV and prevalence.

PPV of 13% means that most positives are not true positives but, in fact, they are children who do not have bacterial diarrhea. For every seven children treated with antibiotics thinking they had bacterial diarrhea, only one really needed it. The others got no benefit from any kind of antibacterial treatment. Clinicians have to decide whether it is better to treat six children without bacterial diarrhea in order to treat the one with the disorder, to treat no one with antibiotics, or to order another test to further eliminate the false positives. The upside to antibiotics is that bacterial diarrhea will get better faster with antibiotics. The downsides of antibiotic use include rare side effects such as allergic reactions and problems that are removed from the individual like increased bacterial resistance with high rates of antibiotic usage in the population. So, if a clinician decides this is not a serious problem and treatment is a reasonable trade-off then he or she will use antibiotics. If, on the other hand, a clinician decides that antibiotic resistance is a real and significant problem, and treatment will not change the course of the illness in a dramatic manner and not significantly alleviate much suffering, then he or she would choose not to treat. In that case, the clinician would decide to not do the fecal white blood cell test since even with a positive result, the patient would not be treated with antibiotics.

An NPV of 99.6% means that if the test is negative, only 4 in 1000 children with true bacterially caused infectious diarrhea will be missed, so the physician can safely avoid treating the patient with antibiotics. This is especially true since the result of non-treatment is simply prolonging the diarrhea by a day. The physician's treatment would be different if the results of non-treatment were serious, resulting in prolonged disease with significant morbidity or mortality. In that case, even 4 out of 1000 could be too many to miss, and the physician should do the gold standard test on all the children.

Predictive values are the numbers that clinicians need in order to determine the likelihood of disease in a patient with a positive or negative test result and a given pretest probability. These numbers will modify the differential diagnosis and change the pretest probabilities assigned to the patient.

Finally, we can do the same problem with likelihood ratios. The calculations are as follows:

LR+ = sensitivity/(1 − specificity) = 0.85/0.12 = 7.08
LR− = (1 − sensitivity)/specificity = 0.15/0.88 = 0.17

Using a pretest probability of 2%, the probability and odds are the same: 0.02. Applying Bayes' theorem, post-test odds = LR+ × 0.02 = 7.08 × 0.02 = 0.14, and post-test probability = 0.124. Compare this to the PPV of 0.13.

Similarly for a negative test: post-test odds = LR− × 0.02 = 0.17 × 0.02 = 0.0034. Compare this to the FRR of 0.004.

In summary, we now have two ways of calculating the post-test probability of disease given the operating characteristics of the tests. One is to use Bayes' theorem and likelihood ratios to modify pretest odds and calculate post-test odds. The other way is to use prevalence, sensitivity, and specificity in a 2 × 2 table to calculate predictive values.

Finally, we must think about accuracy. This term has been used more in the past to designate the strength of a diagnostic test. In this instance, it is the true positives and true negatives divided by the total population to whom the test was applied. However, this can be a grossly misleading number. If there are many people without the disease compared to with disease, a very specific test with few false positives will be accurate even with poor sensitivity. Thus, this says nothing about the sensitivity and should not be used as the measure of a test's performance. The same holds true for a population with very high prevalence of disease and high sensitivity.

Fig. 24.10 Interval likelihood ratio (iLR).

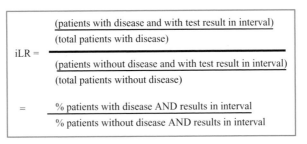

Interval likelihood ratios (iLR)

Likelihood ratios allow us to calculate post-test probabilities when continuous rather than just dichotomous test results are used. Single cutoff points of tests with continuous variable results set potential "traps" for the unwary clinician. Often in studies where the outcome variable of interest is a continuous variable, a single dichotomous cutoff point is selected as the best single-point cutoff between normal and abnormal patients. Valuable data are disregarded if the results of such a test are considered only "positive" or "negative." We can obviate this problem using interval likelihood ratios.

The "interval" LR (iLR) is the probability of a test result in the interval under consideration among diseased subjects, divided by the probability of a test result within the same interval among non-diseased subjects. Simply put, the interval likelihood ratio is the percentage of patients with disease who have test results in the interval divided by the percentage of patients without disease with test results in the interval (Fig. 24.10). If the iLR associated with an interval is less

Table 24.1. Distribution of white blood cell count in patients with and without appendicitis

WBC/μL	With appendicitis (% of 59)	Without appendicitis (% of 145)	iLR+ (95% CI)
4000–7000	1 (2%)	30 (21%)	0.1 (0–0.39)
7000–9000	9 (15%)	42 (29%)	0.52 (0–1.57)
9000–11000	4 (7%)	35 (24%)	0.29 (0–0.62)
11000–13000	22 (37%)	19 (13%)	2.8 (1.2–4.4)
13000–15000	6 (10%)	9 (6%)	1.7 (0–3.6)
15000–17000	8 (14%)	7 (5%)	2.8 (0–6.0)
17000–19000	4 (7%)	3 (2%)	3.5 (0–10)
19000–22000	5 (8%)	0 (0%)	Infinite (NA)
Total	59 (100%)	145 (100%)	

Example: For WBC from 4000 to 7000, iLR = (1/59)/(30/145) = 2%/21% = 0.1. From S. Dueholm, P. Bagi & M. Bud. Laboratory aid in the diagnosis of acute appendicitis. A blinded prospective trial concerning diagnostic value of leukocyte count, neutrophil differential count, and C-reactive protein. *Dis. Colon Rectum* 1989; 32: 855–859.

than 1 the probability of disease decreases and if greater than 1 the probability of disease increases.

When data are gathered for results of a continuous variable, predetermined cutoff points should be set. Then the number of people with and without disease in each interval can be determined. Many authorities believe that these results are more accurate and represent the true state of things better than a single cut-off point. The following illustration with the white cell count in appendicitis will illustrate this issue.

A 16-year-old girl comes to the emergency department complaining of right-lower-quadrant abdominal pain for 14 hours and a decreased appetite. Her physical examination reveals right-lower-quadrant tenderness and spasm and the clinician thinks that she might have appendicitis. A white blood count (WBC) is obtained and the result is a level of 10 200 cells/μL. The "normal" range is 4 500–11 000 cells/μL. Although this test result is "normal," it is just below the cutoff for an elevated WBC count. You know that a mildly elevated WBC count has a different implication than a highly elevated WBC count of 17 000 cells/μL. Interval likelihood ratios can help attack this question quantitatively.

Table 24.1 represents the distribution of WBC count results among 59 patients with confirmed appendicitis and 145 patients without appendicitis. For each interval, the probabilities for results within the interval were used to calculate an iLR.

Note that in this study the interval likelihood ratio is lower for the third interval (9k–11k) than for the second interval (7k–9k), and similarly for the intervals 11k–13k and 13k–15k. The 95% CIs overlap in each case and include the point estimate of the other group's iLR. Therefore the iLR differences found for these intervals are not statistically different. This is the result of the small sample size in this study, and probably represents a Type II error. This value of LR+ would more likely be in line and show a positive dose–response relationship if there were more patients. But the inconsistency of these results points up the need for more research to be done in this area.

Ideally, 95% CI should always be given for each LR. This allows the reader to determine the statistical significance of the results. In initial studies, researchers often "data dredge" by using several different cutoff points to see which gives the best LR or iLR and which are statistically significant. These results must be verified in a second study on a different population called a validation study.

Given this girl's symptoms and physical findings, we estimate that her pretest probability of appendicitis before obtaining results of WBC count is about 0.50. This says that we're not sure and it is a toss-up. What is the probability of appendicitis if our patient had a WBC count of 10 200? We will demonstrate how to determine this using Bayes' theorem.

Start with the pretest probability of 50% and calculate the odds. These are $0.5/(1 - 0.5)$. Pretest odds (appendicitis) $= 0.5/0.5 = 1$ and iLR $= 0.29$. Therefore post-test odds (appendicitis) $= 1 \times 0.29 = 0.29$, and post-test probability (appendicitis) $= 0.29/1.29 = 0.22$. This is less than before, but not low enough to rule out the diagnosis. We must therefore decide either to do another test or to observe the patient.

What happens if her white cell count is 7 500 (iLR $= 0.52$)? The pretest odds are unchanged and the post-test odds (appendicitis) $= 1 \times 0.52 = 0.52$. Post-test probability (appendicitis) $= 0.52/1.52 = 0.33$, leading to the same problem as with a white-cell count of 10 200.

What if her white-cell count is 17 500 (iLR $= 3.5$)? Again, the pretest odds are unchanged and the post-test odds (appendicitis) $= 1 \times 3.5 = 3.5$. Post-test probability (appendicitis) $= 3.5/4.5 = 0.78$. This is much higher, but far from good enough to immediately treat her for the suspected disease. In this case, treatment requires an operation on the appendix. This is major surgery and although pretty safe in this day and age, it is still more risky than not operating if the patient does not have appendicitis. Most surgeons want the probability of appendicitis to be over 85% before they will operate on the patient. This is called the treatment threshold.

Therefore, even with the white cell count this high, we have not crossed the treatment threshold of 85%. This value was adopted based upon previous studies and prevailing surgical practice when it was considered important to have a negative operative rate of 15% in order to prevent missing appendicitis and

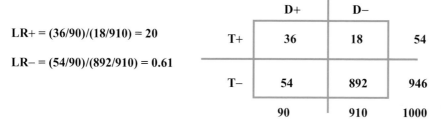

	D+	D−	
WBC > 9K T+	49	73	
WBC < 9K T−	10	72	
Totals	59	145	

Fig. 24.11 The 2 × 2 table for the use of a white blood cell count of greater than 9000 as a cutoff for diagnosing appendicitis. Data from S. Dueholm, P. Bagi & M. Bud. *Dis. Colon Rectum* 1989; 32: 855–859.

LR+ = (36/90)/(18/910) = 20

LR− = (54/90)/(892/910) = 0.61

	D+	D−	
T+	36	18	54
T−	54	892	946
	90	910	1000

Fig. 24.12 The 2 × 2 table to calculate the post-test probability of a urinary tract infection using the dipstick results on urine testing for UTI. Data from K. N. Shaw, D. Hexter, K. L. McGowan & J. S. Schwartz. *J. Pediatr.* 1991; 118: 733–736.

risking rupture of the appendix. Therefore, if the probability of appendicitis is greater than 0.85, the patient should be operated upon.

Let's see what will happen if we lump the test results together and consider a white blood cell count of 9 000 as the upper limit of normal. Now use likelihood ratios to calculate predictive values and apply them to a population with a prevalence of 50%. For the original study patients, LR+ = 1.66 and LR− = 0.34 (Fig. 24.11). For the patient in our example, post-test odds = 1 × 1.66 = 1.66 and the post-test probability = 1.66/2.66 = 0.62. This is slightly different from the results using the interval likelihood ratio, but is still below the treatment threshold.

For the study on the use of urine-dipstick testing for UTI which we discussed earlier in this chapter, the 2 × 2 table is shown in Fig. 24.12. In the original study, the prevalence was 0.09. Using the 2 × 2 table allows you to visualize the number of patients in each cell, and gives an idea of the usefulness of the test.

The probability of disease if a positive test occurs is 36/54 = 0.67, and the probability of disease if the test is negative is 54/946 = 0.057. These are very similar to the values calculated using the LRs. Remember, for our population we used a prevalence of 10% (not 9%).

Comparing tests and using ROC curves

Learning objectives

In this chapter you will learn:

- the dynamic relationship between sensitivity and specificity
- how to construct and interpret an ROC curve for a diagnostic test

Analysis of diagnostic test performance using ROC curves

ROC is an acronym for Receiver Operating Characteristics. It is a concept that originated during the early days of World War II when radar was a newly developed technology. The radar operators had to learn to distinguish true signals, approaching enemy planes, from noise, usually flocks of birds like geese or clouds. The ROC curve let them decide which signals were most likely to be which. In medicine, an ROC curve tells you which test has the best ability to differentiate healthy people from ill ones.

The ROC curve plots sensitivity against specificity. The convention has been to plot the sensitivity, the true positive rate against 1 – specificity, the false positive rate. This ratio looks like the likelihood ratio, doesn't it? The ROC curve for a particular diagnostic test tells which cutoff point maximizes sensitivity, specificity, and both. ROC curves for two tests can also tell you which test is best.

By convention, when drawing ROC curves the x-axis is the false positive rate, 1 – specificity, going from 0 to 1 or 0% to 100%, and the y- axis is the sensitivity or true positive rate, also going from 0 to 1 or 0% to 100%. The best cutoff point for making a diagnosis using a particular test would be the point closest to the (0,1) point, the point at which there is perfect sensitivity and specificity. It is by

Table 25.1. Sensitivity and specificity for each cutoff point of WBC count in appendicitis

WBC/µL	Sensitivity (95% CI)	Specificity (95% CI)	1 – specificity (95% CI)
>4000	100 (95–100)	0 (0–3)	100 (97–100)
>7000	98 (91–100)	21 (15–29)	79 (71–85)
>9000	83 (71–92)	50 (42–59)	50 (41–58)
>11000	76 (63–86)	74 (62–84)	26 (16–38)
>13000	39 (27–53)	87 (73–98)	13 (2–27)
>15000	29 (18–47)	93 (78–100)	7 (0–22)
>17000	15 (7–27)	98 (80–100)	2 (0–20)
>19000	6 (3–19)	100 (85–100)	0 (0–15)

Source: From S. Dueholm, P. Bagi & M. Bud. *Dis. Colon Rectum* 1989; 32: 855–859.

definition, the gold standard. This point has 0% false positive rate and 100% true positive rate, sensitivity.

Look at the data from the study about the usefulness of the white-blood-cell count in the diagnosis of appendicitis in the example of the girl with right-lower-quadrant pain (Table 25.1) and draw the ROC curve for the results (Fig. 25.1). The sensitivity and specificity was calculated for each cutoff point as a different dichotomous value. This has now created a curve of the sensitivity and specificity for different cutoff points of the white blood cell count in diagnosing appendicitis.

Comparing diagnostic tests

ROC curves can help determine which of two tests is better for a given purpose. First, examine the ROC curves for the two tests. Is one clearly better by virtue of being closer to the upper left corner than the other? For the hypothetical tests A and B depicted in Fig. 25.2(a) it is clear that test A outperforms test B over the entire range of lab values. This means that for any given cutoff point, the sensitivity and specificity of test A will always be better than for the corresponding point of test B.

Tests can also be compared even if their ROC curves overlap. This is illustrated in Fig. 25.2(b), where the curves for tests C and D overlap. One option is to chose a single cutoff value for the point closest to the (0,1) point on the graph, which will always be the best single cutoff point for making the diagnosis.

Another approach uses the concept of the area under the curve (AUC). A test whose ROC curve is the diagonal from the upper right (point 1,1) to the lower left

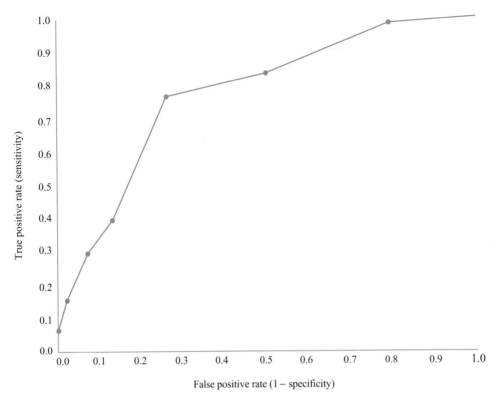

Fig. 25.1 ROC curve for white
blood cell count in appendicitis,
based on data in Table 25.1.

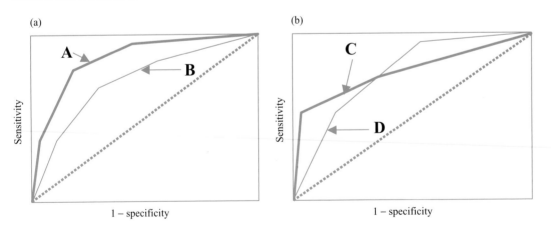

Fig. 25.2 ROC curves of four
hypothetical tests A, B, C, and D.

(point 0,0) is a worthless test. At any given point, it's sensitivity and false positive rate are equal, making diagnosis using this test a coin toss for all cutoff points. Think of the Likelihood Ratio as being one for any point on that curve. The AUC for this curve is 0.5 and is the same a flipping a coin. Similarly the gold standard test will be perfect and have an AUC of one (1.0). Ideally, look for an AUC that is as close to one as possible.

ROC curves that are close to the imaginary diagonal line are poor tests. For these tests, we can say that the AUC is only slightly greater than 0.5. Obviously, ROC curves that are under this line are such poor tests that they are worse than flipping a coin. We can use the AUC to statistically compare the area under two ROC curves.

The AUC has an understandable meaning. It answers the "two alternative-forced choice (2AFC) problem." This means that "given a normal patient chosen at random from the universe of normal patients, and an abnormal patient, again chosen at random, from the universe of abnormal patients, the AUC describes the probability that one can identify the abnormal patient using this test alone."[1]

There are several ways to measure the AUC for an ROC curve. The simplest is to count the blocks and calculate the percentage under the curve, the medical student level. A slightly more complex method is to calculate the trapezoidal area under the curve by approximating each segment as a regular geometric figure, the high-school-geometry level. The most complex way is to use the technique known as the "smoothed area using maximum likelihood estimation techniques," which can be done using a computer. There are programs written to calculate these areas under the curve.

A study looked at the usefulness of the CAGE questionnaire as a screening diagnostic tool for identifying alcoholism among adult patients in the outpatient medical practice of a university teaching hospital. In this population, the sensitivity of an affirmative answer to one or more of the CAGE questions (Table 25.2) was about 0.9 and the specificity was about 0.8. Although one could consider the CAGE "positive" if a patient has one or more answers in the affirmative, in reality the CAGE is more "positive" given more affirmative answers on the four component questions. In this test, each answer is given one point to make a total score from zero to four.

Have you ever felt you should **Cut down** on your drinking?
Have people **Annoyed** you by criticizing your drinking?
Have you ever felt bad or **Guilty** about your drinking?
Have you ever had a drink first thing in the morning to steady your nerves or get rid of a hangover (**Eye-opener**)?

---

[1] Michigan State University, Department of Internal Medicine. *Power Reading: Critical Appraisal of the Medical Literature.* Lansing, MI: Michigan State University, 1995.

Table 25.2. Results of CAGE questions using different cutoffs

Numbers of questions answered affirmatively	Alcoholic	Non-alcoholic	Sensitivity (TPR)	1 – specificity (FPR)
>3	56/294	56/527	0.19	0.00
>2	130/294	516/327	0.44	0.02
>1	216/294	482/527	0.73	0.09
>0	261/294	428/527	0.89	0.19

Source: Data from D. G. Buchsbaum, R. G. Buchanan, R. M. Centor, S. H. Schnoll & M. J. Lawton. Screening for alcohol abuse using CAGE scores and likelihood ratios. *Ann. Intern. Med.* 1991; 115: 774–777.

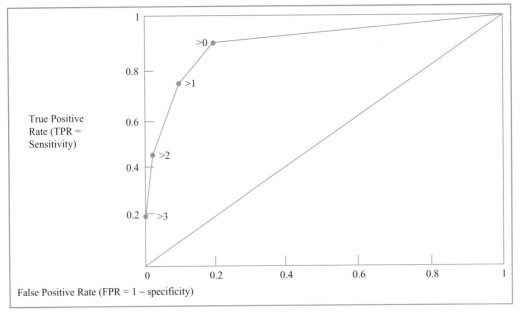

Fig. 25.3 ROC curve of CAGE question data from Table 25.2.

One has the choice of considering the CAGE questionnaire "positive" if the patient answers all four, three or more, two or more, or one or more of the component questions in the affirmative. Moving from a more stringent to a less stringent cutoff tends to sacrifice specificity (1 – FPR) for sensitivity (TPR).

By convention the ROC curves start at the FPR = 0 and TPR = 0 point. The CAGE here is always considered negative regardless of patients' answers. There are no false positives, but no alcoholics are detected. The ROC curves end at the

FPR = 1.0 and TPR = 1.0 point. The CAGE is always considered positive regardless of patients' answers. The test has perfect sensitivity but all non-alcoholics are falsely identified as positives.

When the ROC is plotted, the area under this curve is 0.89 units with a standard error of 0.13 units so we'd expect a randomly selected alcoholic patient from the sample population to have a higher CAGE score than a randomly selected non-alcoholic patient about 89% of the time. Computers can be used to compare ROC curves by calculating the AUCs and determining the statistical variance of the result. Another study of the CAGE questionnaire was done by Mayfield[2] on psychiatric inpatients whereas Buchsbaum's study (Table 25.2 and Fig. 25.3) used general-medicine outpatients. The Mayfield study had an AUC of 0.9 with a standard error of 0.17. Using a statistical test, these two study results are not statistically different, validating the result.

---

[2] D. Mayfield, G. McLeod & P. Hall. The CAGE questionnaire: validation of a new alcoholism screening instrument. *Am. J. Psychiatry* 1974; 131: 1121–1123.

Incremental gain and the threshold approach to diagnostic testing

Science is the great antidote to the poison of enthusiasm and superstition.

Adam Smith (1723–1790): The Wealth of Nations, 1776

Learning objectives

In this chapter you will learn:

- how to calculate and interpret the incremental diagnostic gain for a given clinical test result
- the concept of threshold values for testing and treating
- the use of multiple tests and the effect of independent and dependent tests on predictive values
- how predictive values help make diagnostic decisions in medicine and how to use predictive values to choose the appropriate test for a given purpose
- how to apply basic test characteristics to solve a clinical diagnostic problem

Revising probabilities with sensitivity and specificity

Remember the child from Chapter 20 with the sore throat? Let's revisit our differential diagnosis list (Table 26.1). Since strep and viruses are the only strong contenders on this list, it would be hoped that a negative strep test would mean that the likelihood of viruses as the cause of the sore throat is high enough to defer antibiotic treatment for this child. One would only need to rule out strep to do this. Therefore, it would make sense to do a rapid strep test. It comes up positive. Looking up the sensitivity and specificity of this test shows that they are 0.9 and 0.9, respectively. Now the pretest probability is 0.5 (50%). There are two ways to solve this problem, either using likelihood ratios or sensitivity and specificity to get the predictive values.

Table 26.1. Pretest probability: sore throat

Streptococcal infection	50%
Viruses	75%
Mononucleosis	5%
Epiglottitis	<1%
Diphtheria	<1%
Gonorrhea	<1%

	D+	D−	
T+	TP	FP	
T−	FN	TN	
	500 (D+)	500 (D−)	1000 (N)

If: Sensitivity = 0.9
          Specificity = 0.9
Then:
TP = D+ × sens. = 500 × 0.9 = 450
TN = D− × spec. = 500 × 0.9 = 450

Fig. 26.1 Set up the 2 × 2 table using a population of 1000 patients and an estimated clinical prevalence of strep throat infection of 0.5. Calculate the values of TP and TN as shown.

	D+	D−	
T+	450	50	500
T−	50	450	500
	500 (D+)	500 (D−)	1000 (N)

PPV = 450/500 = 0.9

NPV = 450/500 = 0.9

FAR = 1 − PPV = 0.1

FRR = 1 − NPV = 0.1

Fig. 26.2 Write the values of TP, TN, FP, and FN into the 2 × 2 table. Calculate PPV, NPV, FAR, and FRR as shown.

Using likelihood ratios

LR+ = sensitivity/(1 − specificity) = 0.9/0.1 = 9

LR− = (1 − sensitivity)/specificity = 0.1/0.9 = 0.11

Pretest probability of disease is 50%, so the pretest odds are 1 (50%/50% = 1). Applying Bayes' theorem:

For a positive test, post-test odds = LR+ ×1 = 9, so post-test probability = 0.9 (9/10 = 0.9), the positive predictive value.

For a negative test, post-test odds = LR− ×1 = 0.11, so post-test probability (FRR) = 0.1 (0.11/1.11 ≈ 0.1) and the negative predictive value = 0.9 (1 − 0.1).

Using sensitivity and specificity in a 2 × 2 table

This method is shown in Figs. 26.1 and 26.2. Whichever way the calculations are done, the positive predictive value is 0.9 and the negative predictive value is

Fig. 26.3 Results of calculating the values of the 2 × 2 table for a population of 1000 patients (N) and a clinical prevalence of strep throat infection that is low or 0.1 (100 out of 1000). Calculations for PPV and NPV are shown.

	D+	D−	
T+	90	90	180
T−	10	810	820
	100	900	1000

PPV = 90/180 = 0.5

NPV = 810/820 = 0.987

also 0.9. Therefore, with a positive test result, it is reasonable to accept this diagnosis and realize that one might have over- or unnecessarily treated one out of every 10 children who were treated with antibiotics and who would actually not have strep throat. But the cost of that is low enough that it is reasonable not to worry. This is also based on the risks of antibiotic treatment causing rare allergy to antibiotics and occasional gastrointestinal discomfort and diarrhea. This balances against the benefit of treatment, a 1-day shorter course of symptoms and some decrease in the very rare sequellae of strep infection, tonsillar abscess, and acute rheumatic fever.

Similarly, if the test had come up negative, the likelihood of strep is extremely low and one could accept that there might be 10% or one out of every 10 children who would be falsely reassured when they could be treated with antibiotics for this type of sore throat. However, looking at the risks of not treating the patient, one realizes that in this case they are also small. Rheumatic fever, once a common complication of strep throat, is now extremely rare, with much less than 1% of strep infections leading to this and the rate is even lower in most populations.

Bacterial resistance from overuse of antibiotics is the only other problem left and for now it is reasonable to decide that this will not deter writing a prescription for antibiotics. That decision on when to treat in order to decrease overuse of antibiotics would be deferred to a high-level government policy panel. We vow to try to use antibiotics only when reasonably indicated for a positive strep test and not for things like a common cold. This simple decision-making process will do until there is a blue-ribbon panel that will look at all the evidence and make a clinical guideline, algorithm, or practice guideline on when to treat and when to test for strep throat.

If the pretest probability of strep based upon signs and symptoms was much lower (say 10%), this equation will change (Fig. 26.3). Use the likelihood ratios to get the same results by starting with the pretest probability of disease, which is now 10%. The pretest odds are 0.11 and applying Bayes' theorem for a positive test with LR+, results in post-test odds (= 9 × 0.11) of 0.99. This makes the post-test probability (0.99/1.99) = 0.497. This is the positive predictive value, which is pretty close to the 0.5 that was obtained using the 2×2 table. Similarly, for a negative test, using the LR–, the post-test odds ($= 0.11 \times 0.11$) are 0.0121. Therefore, the post-test probability if the test is negative, which is equivalent to the false reassurance rate or FRR is 0.0121 and the negative predictive value ($1 - \text{FRR}$) is 0.988.

The PPV for a positive test is now 50%. With the patient as a partner in shared decision making, it is now reasonable to decide that since 1 day less of symptoms is the major benefit of antibiotics, it is not worth the excess antibiotic use to treat one without strep throat for every one with strep throat, and it is reasonable to withhold treatment. In the case of a pretest probability of 10%, it is then reasonable to decide not to do the test in the first place. If practicing in a community with a high incidence of acute rheumatic fever after strep throat infections, it may still be reasonable to test since that could make it worthwhile to treat all the positives to prevent this more serious sequella even though one would overtreat half of the children. Over-treating one child for every one correctly treated is a small price to pay for the prevention of a disease as serious as acute rheumatic fever, which will leave its victims with permanent heart deformities.

Incremental gain

Incremental gain is the expected increase in diagnostic certainty after the application of a diagnostic test. It is the change in the pretest estimate of a given diagnosis. Mathematically it is PPV – P or positive predictive value minus pretest probability. For a negative test, the incremental gain would be NPV – ($1 - P$). For incremental gain of a negative test, begin with the prevalence of no disease ($1- P$) and go up to the NPV. The difference simply tells how much the test will increase the probability of disease or how much "bang for your buck" occurs when using a particular diagnostic test. This is one measure of the usefulness of a diagnostic test. By convention use absolute values so that all the incremental gains are positive numbers. They are all improvements on the previous level of probability.

For a given range of pretest probability, what is the diagnostic gain from doing the test? Using the example of strep throat in a child and beginning with a pretest probability of 50%, after doing the test the new probability of disease was 90%. This represents an incremental gain of 40% ($90 - 50$). For a negative test the incremental gain would also be 40% since the initial probability of no disease was 50% and the post-test probability of no disease was 90% ($50 - 90$). Doing the same calculations for a patient with a higher pretest probability of disease, but in whom there is still some uncertainty of strep on clinical grounds, say that the pretest probability was estimated to be between a coin toss (50%) and certainty (100%) so put it at about 75%. How would that change the incremental gain? Figure 26.4 shows the 2×2 table and the calculations based on predictive values.

	D+	D−	
T+	675	25	700
T−	75	225	300
	750	250	1000

PPV = 675/700 = 0.964

NPV = 225/300 = 0.750

FAR = 1 − PPV = 0.036

FRR = 1 − NPV = 0.250

	D+	D−	
T+	810	10	820
T−	90	90	180
	900	100	1000

PPV = 810/820 = 0.988

NPV = 90/180 = 0.50

FAR = 1 − PPV = 0.012

FRR = 1 − NPV = 0.50

Using likelihood ratios we start with the pretest probability of disease, which is now 75% making the pretest odds equal to 3. Now the post-test odds for a positive test using LR+ are 9 × 3, which is 27 making the post-test probability (27/28) = 0.964. Similarly, for a negative test, use the LR− to calculate the post-test odds of 0.11 × 3, which is 0.33. Therefore, the post-test probability if the test is negative is the FRR, which is 0.25 and the negative predictive value 1 − FRR, which is 0.75.

Now the post-test probability of disease is more certain (96.4%), but if the test is negative it will be wrong more often (25%). The incremental gain is now only 21.4% for a positive test (96.4 − 75) and up to 50% for a negative test (75 − 25).

Now do the same for a pretest probability of 90%. This represents almost certainty based on signs and symptoms (Fig. 26.5). Using likelihood ratios, the pretest probability of disease is now 90%, so the pretest odds are 9 and multiply that by the likelihood ration LR+ to get the post-test odds for a positive test. This is 9 × 9 = 81. The post-test probability is therefore 0.987 (81/82). For a negative test, the post-test odds are calculated using LR−, which is 0.11 × 9 = 1, so the post-test probability, the FRR, is 0.5 and the negative predictive value is 1 − FRR = 0.5.

The incremental gains are now:

Positive test: 98.8 − 90 = 8.8

 Negative test: 50 − 10 = 40

So little (8.8%) is gained if the test is positive and a lot (40%) is gained if the test is negative. In order to avoid the false negatives it would probably be best to choose not to do the test if one was this certain and gave a high pretest

Table 26.2. Incremental gains for rapid strep throat tests

Pretest probability	Incremental gain T+	FN	Incremental gain T–	FP
10%	40 (10 to 50)	10/1000	8.8 (90 to 98.8)	90/1000
50%	40 (50 to 90)	50/1000	40 (50 to 90)	50/1000
75%	21.4 (75 to 96.4)	75/1000	50 (25 to 75)	25/1000
90%	8.8 (90 to 98.8)	90/1000	40 (10 to 50)	10/1000

probability that the child had strep throat. Putting all of these results in a table (Table 26.2) makes it easy to compare the results.

In general, the greatest incremental gain occurs when the pretest probability is in an intermediate range, usually between 20% and 70%. Notice also that as the pretest probability increased the number of false negatives also increased and the number of false positives decreased. The opposite happens when the pretest probability is very low and there will be an increased number of false positives and lower number of false negatives. This last situation occurs when working with a screening test.

The question that must then be asked is at what level of clinical certainty or pretest probability should a given test be done? This depends on the situation and the test. The use of threshold values can assist the clinician in making this judgment.

Threshold values

Incremental gain tells how much a diagnostic test increases the value of the pretest probability assigned based upon the history and physical and modified by the characteristics of the test and the prevalence of disease in the population from which the patient is drawn. This simply tells the amount of certainty gained by doing the test. One can decide not to do the test if the incremental gain is very small since very little is gained clinically. The midrange of pretest probability yields the highest incremental gain, which is lost at the extremes of pretest probability range.

Another way to look at the process of deciding whether to do a test is using the method of threshold values. In this process find the probability of disease above which one should treat no matter what, and conversely the level below which one would never treat, and therefore shouldn't even do the test. These are determined using the test characteristics and incremental gain to decide if it will be worthwhile to do a particular diagnostic test.

Determine threshold values by calculating PPV and NPV for many different levels of pretest probability. At each step ask if one still wanted to treat based upon a positive result or would be willing to rule out based on a negative test result. Decision trees can also be used to determine the threshold values and these will be covered in Chapter 30. An alternative method uses a simple balance sheet to approximate the threshold values. An explanation for this can be found in Appendix 6.

In practice, clinicians use their clinical judgment to determine the threshold values for each clinical situation. This is part of the "art of medicine" or that part of EBM based upon clinical experience. Clinicians ask themselves "will I gain any additional useful clinical information by doing this test?" If the answer to this question is no, they shouldn't do the test. They already know enough about the patient and should either treat or not treat regardless of the test result, since no useful additional information is gained by performing the test.

The **treatment threshold** is the value at which the clinician asks "do I know enough about the patient to begin treatment and would treat regardless of the results of the test?" If the answer to this question is yes, the test shouldn't be done. This occurs at high values of pretest probability. If a test is done, it ought to be one with high specificity, which can be used to rule in disease. But if a negative test result is obtained a confirmatory test or the gold-standard test must be done to avoid missing a person with a false negative test. If a test with high specificity only is chosen, a positive test will rule in disease, but there are too many false negatives, which must be confirmed with a second or gold standard test.

The **testing threshold** is the value at which the clinician asks "is the likelihood of disease so low that even if I got a positive test I would still not treat the patient?" If the answer to this question is yes, the test shouldn't be done. This occurs at low values of pretest probability. If a test is done it ought to be one with high sensitivity, which can be used to rule out disease. But, if a positive test result is obtained a confirmatory test or the gold-standard test must be done to avoid over-treating a person with a false positive test. If a test with high sensitivity only is chosen, a negative test will rule out disease, but there are too many false positives, which must be confirmed with a second or gold standard test.

Both of these threshold levels depend not only on the test characteristic, the sensitivity and specificity, and prevalence of disease, but also on the risks and benefits associated with treatment or non-treatment. The values of probability of disease for the treatment and testing thresholds should be established before doing the test. The clinician selects a pretest probability of disease, and determines whether performing the test will result in placing the patient above the treatment threshold or below the testing threshold. If it won't, the test would not be worth doing.

At pretest probabilities above the treatment threshold, testing may produce an unacceptable number of false negatives in spite of a high PPV. Some patients

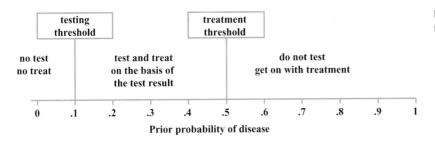

Fig. 26.6 Thresholds for strep throat example.

would be denied the benefits of treatment, perhaps more than would benefit from discovery of the disease and subsequent treatment. The pretest probability of disease is so great that treatment should proceed regardless of the results of the test. This is because if the test results are negative they are more likely to be a false negative and could miss someone with the disease. In that setting one must be ready to do a confirmatory test, possibly the gold standard test. In other words, one should be more willing to treat someone who does not have the disease and has a false positive test result, than to miss treating someone who is a false negative. This may not be true if treatment involves a lot of risk and suffering such as needing a major operation or taking potentially toxic medication.

At pretest probabilities below the testing threshold, testing would lead to an unacceptable number of false positives or a high FAR. Patients would be unnecessarily exposed to the side effects of further testing or treatment with very little benefit. The likelihood of disease in someone with a positive test is so small that treatment should not be done even if the test is positive since it is too likely that a positive test will be a false positive. Again one must be ready to do a confirmatory test. This approach is summarized in Fig. 26.6.

For the child in our example with a sore throat, this testing threshold is a pretest probability of strep throat below 10%. Below this level, applying the rapid strep antigen test and getting a positive result would still not increase the probability of disease enough to treat the patient and one can be certain enough that disease is not present that the benefit of treating is extremely small. Similarly, the treatment threshold is a pretest probability of strep throat above 50%. Above this level, applying the rapid strep antigen test and getting a negative result would still not decrease the probability of disease enough to refrain from treating the patient and one can be certain enough that disease is present so that the benefit of treatment is reasonably great. Between these values of pretest probability (from 10–50%) do the test first and treat only if the test is positive, since the post-test probability then increases above the treatment threshold. If the test is negative, the post-test probability is now below the testing threshold.

In this example of the child with a sore throat, almost all clinicians agree that if the pretest probability is 90% as would be present in a child with a severe sore throat, large lymph nodes, pus on the tonsils, bright red tonsils, fever, and no signs of a cold, the child ought to be treated without doing a test. There would still be a likelihood of incorrectly diagnosing about 10% of viral sore throats as strep throats with this estimate of disease. In general, as the probability of disease increases, the absolute number of missed strep throats will increase. In fact, most clinicians agree that if the post-test probability is greater than 50%, the child ought to be treated. This is the treatment threshold.

Similarly, if the probability of strep throat was 10% or less in a child with mild sore throat, slight redness, minimal enlargement of the tonsils, no pus, minimally swollen and non-tender lymph nodes, no fever, and signs of a cold, half of all positives will be false positives and too many children would be overtreated. There won't be much gain from a negative test, since almost all children are negative before we do the test. For a pretest probability of 10%, the PPV (as calculated before) is 50%, which is not above the treatment threshold value of 50%. The addition of the test is not going to help in differentiating the diagnosis of strep throat from that of viral pharyngitis. Therefore one should not do the test if this is the pretest probability of disease. This is the testing threshold.

If the pretest probability is between 10% and 50%, choose to do a test, probably the rapid strep antigen test that can be done quickly in the office and will give an immediate result. Choose to treat all children with a positive test result. Then decide what to do with a negative test. The options here are not to treat or to do the gold-standard test on all those children with a negative rapid strep test and with a moderately high pretest probability of about 50%. In this case one should do the throat-culture test. It is about five times more expensive and takes 2 days as opposed to 10 minutes for the rapid strep antigen test. However, there will still be a savings by having to do the gold-standard test on less than half of the patients, including all those with low pretest probability and negative tests and those with high pretest probability who have been treated without any testing.

In the example of strep throat, the "costs" of doing the relatively inexpensive test, of missing a case of uncommon complications and of treatment reactions such as allergies and side effects are all relatively low. Therefore the threshold for treatment would be pretty low, as will the threshold for testing.

This method is more important and becomes more complex in more serious clinical situations. Consider a patient complaining of shortness of breath. If one suspects a pulmonary embolism or a blood clot in the lungs, should an expensive and potentially dangerous test in which dye is injected into the pulmonary arteries, called a pulmonary angiogram and the gold standard for this disease, be done in order to be certain of the diagnosis? The test itself is very uncomfortable, has some serious complications of about 10% major bleeding at the site of injection and can cause death in less than 1% of patients.

Should one begin treatment based upon history, physical examination, and an "imperfect" diagnostic test such as a chest CT or ventilation–perfusion lung scan that came up positive? There are problems with treatment. Treating with anticoagulants or "blood thinners" can cause excess bleeding in an increasing number of patients as time on the drug increases and the patient will be falsely labeled as having a serious disease, which could affect their future employability and insurability. These are difficult decisions and must be made considering all the options and the patient's values. They are the ultimate combination of medical science and the physician's art.

Finally, 95% confidence intervals should be calculated on all values of likelihood ratios, sensitivity, specificity, and predictive values. The formulas for these are very complex. The best online calculator to do this can be found at the School of Public Health of the University of British Columbia website at http://spph.ubc.ca/sites/healthcare/files/calc/bayes.html. For very high or low values of sensitivity and specificity (FN or FP less than 5) use the rules for zero numerator to estimate the 95% CI. These are summarized in Chapter 13.

Multiple tests

The ideal test is capable of separating all normal people from people who have disease and defines the "gold standard." This test would be 100% sensitive and 100% specific and therefore, would have no false positive or false negative results. Few tests are both this highly sensitive and specific, so it is common practice to use multiple tests in the diagnosis of disease. Using multiple tests to rule in or rule out disease changes the pretest probability for each new test when used in combination. This is because each test performed should raise or lower the pretest probability for the next test in the sequence. It is not possible to predict a priori what happens to the probability of disease when multiple tests are used in combination and whether there are any changes in their operating characteristics when used sequentially.

This occurs because the tests may be dependent upon each other and measure the same or similar aspects of the disease process. One example is using two different enzyme markers to measure heart-muscle cell damage in a heart attack. Tests are independent of each other if they measure completely different things. An example of this would be cardiac muscle enzymes and radionuclide scan of the heart muscle. An overview of the effects of using multiple tests is seen in Fig. 26.7.

In many diagnostic situations, multiple tests must be used to determine the final diagnosis. This is required when application of an initial test does not raise the probability of disease above the treatment threshold. If a positive result on the initial test does not increase the post-test probability of disease above the treatment threshold, a second, "confirmatory" test must be done. The expectation in this case is that a positive result on the second test will

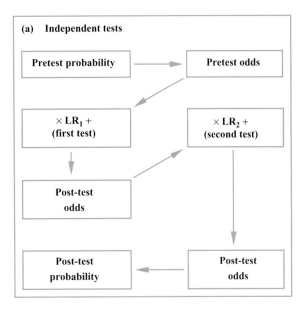
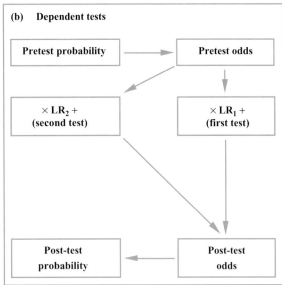

Fig. 26.7 Using multiple tests.

"clinch" the diagnosis by putting the post-test probability above the treatment threshold.

If the second test is negative this leads to more problems. This negative result must be considered in the calculations of post-test probability. If the post-test probability after the negative second test is below the testing threshold the diagnosis is ruled out. Similarly, if the second test is positive and the post-test probability after the second test is above the treatment threshold, the diagnosis is confirmed. If the second test is negative and the resulting post-test probability is not below the testing threshold, a third test must be done. If that is positive, more testing may still need to be done to resolve the discordant results on the three tests.

A complication in this process of calculation of post-test probability is that the two tests may not be independent of each other. If the tests are **independent**, they measure different things that are related to the same pathophysiological process. They both measure the same process but by different mechanisms. Another example of independent tests is in the diagnosis of blood clots in the legs, deep vein thrombosis or DVT. Ultrasound testing takes a picture of the veins and blood flow through the veins using sound waves and a transducer. The serum level of d-dimer measures the presence of a byproduct of the clotting process. The two tests are complementary and independent. A positive d-dimer test is very non-specific, and a positive test does not confirm the diagnosis of DVT. A subsequent positive ultrasound virtually confirms the diagnosis. The ultrasound is not as sensitive, but is very specific and a positive test rules in the disease.

Two tests are **dependent** if they both measure the same pathophysiological process in more or less the same way. An example would be the release of enzymes from damaged heart-muscle cells in an acute myocardial infarction, AMI. The release of creatine kinase (CK) and troponin I (TropI) both occur through related pathological mechanisms as infarcted myocardial muscle cells break down. Therefore they ought to have about the same characteristics of sensitivity and specificity. The two tests should give the same or similar results when they are consecutively done on the same patient. There is a difference in the time course of release of each enzyme. Both are released early but, TropI persists for a longer time than CK. This makes the two of them useful tests when monitored over time. If a patient has an increased serum level of CK, the diagnosis of AMI is confirmed. A negative TropI may cast doubt upon the diagnosis and a positive TropI will confirm the diagnosis.

The use of multiple tests is a more challenging clinical problem than the use of a single test alone. In general, a result that confirms the previous test result is considered confirmatory. A result that does not confirm the previous test result will most often not change the diagnosis immediately, and should only lead to questioning the veracity of the diagnosis. It then must be followed up with another test. If the pretest probability is high and the initial test is negative, the risk of a false negative is usually too great and a confirmatory test must be done. If the pretest probability is low and the initial test is positive, the risk of a false positive is usually too great and a confirmatory test must be done.

If the pretest probability is high, a positive test is confirmatory unless the specificity of that test is very low. If the pretest probability is low, a negative test excludes disease unless the sensitivity of that test is very low. Obviously if the pretest probabilities are either *very high* or *very low*, the clinician ought to consider not doing the test at all. In the case of very high pretest probability immediate initiation of treatment without doing the test should be considered as the pretest probability is probably above the treatment threshold. Similarly, in the case of very low pretest probability, the test ought not to be done in the first place since the pretest probability is probably below the testing threshold.

Real-life application of these principles

What happens in real life? Can these concepts be used clinically? It is relatively easy to learn to do the calculations necessary to determine post-test probability. However, in the clinical situation, "in the trenches," it is often not very helpful. Almost all clinicians will most often do what they always do and have been taught to do in a particular clinical situation when it is similar to other clinical encounters they have had in the past. Those actions should be based on these same principles of rational decision making, but are learned through training and continuing education. However, in difficult cases, one will sometimes need to think about these concepts and go through the process of application of diagnostic test characteristics and the use of Bayes' theorem to one's patient. There are some general rules that ought to be followed when using diagnostic tests.

If the pretest probability of a diagnosis is high and the test result is positive there should be no question but to treat the patient. Similarly, if the pretest probability is low and the test result is negative, there should be no question but not to treat the patient. However, if the suspected disease has a high pretest probability and the test is negative, additional tests must be used to confirm that the patient does not have the disease. If the second test is positive, that should lead to further investigation with additional tests, probably the gold standard to "break the tie." Similarly, if the disease has a low pretest probability and the test is positive, additional tests must be done to confirm that the patient actually has the disease. If the second test is negative, that should lead to further investigation with additional tests, probably the gold-standard test to "break the tie."

In patients with a medium pretest probability, it may not be possible for a single test to determine the need to treat, unless that test has a very high positive or very low negative likelihood ratio. In general, go with the results of the test if that result puts the post-test probability over the treatment threshold or under the testing threshold. The higher the LR+ of a positive test, preferably over 10 is best, the more likely it is to put the probability over the treatment threshold. The lower the LR− of a negative test, preferably under 0.1 is best, the more likely it is to put the probability under the testing threshold.

27

Sources of bias and critical appraisal of studies of diagnostic tests

It is a vice to trust all, and equally a vice to trust none.

Seneca (c.3 BC – AD 65): Letters to Lucilius

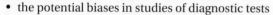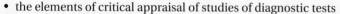

Learning objectives

In this chapter you will learn:

- the potential biases in studies of diagnostic tests
- the elements of critical appraisal of studies of diagnostic tests

Studies of diagnostic tests are unique in their design. Ideally they compare the tests in a sample of patients who have a diagnosis that we are certain is correct. The reader must be aware of potential sources of bias in evaluating these studies.

Overview of studies of diagnostic tests

In order to find bias in studies of diagnostic tests, it is necessary to know what these studies are intended to do. When evaluating studies of a diagnostic test, it is useful to use a structured approach. The first step is to formulate the four-part clinical question in the PICO format. In these cases, the question relates the diagnostic test, the intervention, to the gold standard, or the comparison. The patient population is those patients in whom the test would normally be done in a clinical setting and the target disorder is the disease that is attempting to be diagnosed.

A typical PICO question might be framed as follows. A blood clot in the lungs or a pulmonary embolism (PE) can be diagnosed with the new-generation x-ray-computed tomography scanners (CT) of the chest. Is this diagnostic tool as accurate as the gold-standard pulmonary angiogram obtained by squirting dye into the pulmonary artery and taking an x-ray and is it better than the old standard test, the ventilation–perfusion (V/Q) scan of the lungs? The clinical question asks: in patients suspected of having a PE (population), does the chest CT (intervention) diagnose PE (outcome as determined by angiogram) better than the V/Q scan (comparison)? This question asks what the sensitivity and specificity of the CT and V/Q scans are relative to the gold standard test, the angiogram, which is assumed to have perfect sensitivity and specificity.

Studies of diagnostic tests should begin with a representative sample of patients in whom the reasonable and average practitioner would be looking for the target disorder. This may not always be possible since studies done with different populations may result in different results of test characteristics, a result which cannot be predicted. Patient selection can easily limit the external validity of the test. In the ideal situation, the patients enrolled in the study are then all given the diagnostic test and the gold-standard tests without the researchers or the patient knowing the results of either test. The number of correct and incorrect diagnoses can then be computed.

As with any clinical study, there will be sources of bias in studies of diagnostic tests. Some of these are similar to biases that were presented in Chapter 8 on sources of bias in research, but others are unique to studies of diagnostic tests. You ought to look for three broad categories of bias when evaluating studies of diagnostic tests. These are selection bias, observer bias, and miscellaneous biases.

Selection bias

Filter bias

If the patients studied for a particular diagnostic test are selected because they possess a particular characteristic, the resulting operating characteristics found by this study can be skewed. The process of patient selection should be explicit in the study methods but it is often omitted. Part of the actual clinical diagnostic process is the clinician selecting or filtering out those patients who should get a particular diagnostic test done and those who don't need it. A clinician who believes that a particular patient does not have the target disorder would not order the test for that disease.

Suspect this form of bias when only a portion of eligible patients are given the test or entered into the study. The process by which patients are screened for having the testing should be explicitly stated in any study of a diagnostic test allowing the reader to determine the external validity of the study. Decide for yourself if a particular patient in actuality is similar enough to the patients in the study to have the test ordered and to expect results to be similar to those found in the study.

Using the example of a study of patients with suspected PE, what if only those patients who were strongly suspected of having a PE are enrolled in the study. If there is no clear-cut and reproducible way to deterimine how they were selected it would be difficult, if not impossible, to determine how to select patients to have the test done on them. It is possible that an unknown filter was applied to the process of patient selection for the study. Although this filter could be applied in an equitable and non-differential manner, it can still cause bias since its effect may be different in those patients with and without the target disease. This selection process usually makes the test work better than it would in the community situation. The community doctor, not knowing what that filter was, would not know which patients to select for the suggested test and would tend to be less selective of those patients to whom the test would be applied.

Spectrum and subgroup bias (case-mix bias)

A test may be more accurate when given to patients with classical forms of a disease. The test may be more likely to identify patients with the disease that is more severe or "well-developed" and less likely to accurately identify the disease in those patients who present earlier in the course of the disease or in whom the disease is occult or not obvious. This can be a reflection of real-life test performance. Most diagnostic tests have very little utility in the general and asymptomatic population, while being very useful in specific clinical situations. Most of that problem is due to a large percentage of false positives when the very low prevalence population is tested.

There are also cases for which the test characteristics, sensitivity and specificity, also increase as the severity of disease increases. Some patients with leaking cerebral aneurysms present with severe headaches. If only a small leak is present, the patient is more likely to present with a severe headache and no neurological deficits. In this case, the CT scan will miss the bleed almost 50% of the time. If there is a massive bleed and the patient is unconscious or has severe neurologic deficit, the CT is positive in almost 100% of cases. These are the sensitivity of the test in these two situations.

In the 1950s and 1960s, the yearly "executive physical examination," which included many laboratory, x-ray, and other tests was very popular, especially among corporate executives. The yield of these examinations was very low. In fact the results were most often normal and, when abnormal, were usually falsely positive. There is a similar phenomenon today with a proliferation of private CT scanners that are advertised as generalized screening tests for anyone who can pay for them. They are touted as being able to spot asymptomatic disease in early and curable stages with testimonials given on their usefulness. The correct use of screening tests will be discussed in Chapter 28.

Verification bias

Patients can be selected to receive the gold-standard test based upon the results of the diagnostic test being evaluated. But, sometimes those who have negative tests won't all have the gold-standard test done and have some other method for evaluating the presence or absence of disease in them. This will usually make the test perform better than it would if the gold standard were done on all patients who would be considered for the test in a real clinical situation. Frequently, patients with negative tests are followed clinically for a certain period of time instead of having the gold-standard test performed on them. This may be appropriate if no patients are lost to follow-up and if the presence of disease results in some measurable change in the patient over the time of follow-up. You cannot do this with silent diseases that become apparent only many years later unless you follow all of the patients in the study for many years.

Incorporation bias

This occurs if the diagnostic test being studied is used as or is part of the gold standard. One common way that this happens is that a diagnostic sign of interest becomes a reason that patients are enrolled into the study. This means that the final diagnosis of the disease is dependent on the presence of a positive diagnostic test. Ideally the diagnostic test and the gold standard should be independent of each other meaning that there is no mechanistic relationship between the diagnostic test and the gold standard.

A classic example of this type of bias occurs in studies of acute myocardial infarction (AMI). One criterion for diagnosis of AMI is the elevation of the creatine kinase enzyme (CK) in the blood of patients with AMI as a result of muscle damage from the infarction. Another criterion is characteristic changes on the electrocardiogram. Studies of the usefulness of CK as a serum marker for making the diagnosis of AMI will be flawed if it is used as part of the definition of AMI. It will be increased in all AMI patients since it is both the diagnostic test being investigated and the reference or gold-standard test. This will make the diagnostic test look better or more accurate in the diagnosis of AMI resulting in higher sensitivity and specificity than it probably has in real-life diagnosis.

In another example, patients with suspected carpal tunnel syndrome have certain common clinical signs of carpal tunnel syndrome such as tenderness over the carpal tunnel. The presence of this sign gets them into a study looking at the validity and usefulness of common signs of carpal tunnel syndrome, which are important diagnostic criteria in patients referred for specialty care. This bias makes that sign look better than it actually is in making a positive diagnosis since patients who might not have this sign, and who likely have milder disease, were never referred to the specialist and were therefore excluded from the study.

Observer bias

Absence of a definitive test or the tarnished gold standard

This is probably the most common problem with studies of diagnostic tests. The gold standard must be reasonably defined. In most cases, no true gold standard exists, and a research study must make do with the best that is available. The authors ought to discuss the problem of lack of a gold standard as part of their results.

For example, patients with abdominal trauma may undergo a CT scan of the abdomen to look for internal organ damage. If the scan is positive, they are admitted to the hospital and may be operated upon. If it is negative, they are discharged and followed for a period of time to make sure a significant injury was not missed. However, if the follow-up time is too short or incomplete, there may be some patients with significant missed injuries who are not discovered and some may be lost to follow-up. The real gold standard, operating on everyone with abdominal trauma, would be ethically unacceptable.

Review or interpretation bias

Interpretation of a test can be affected by the knowledge of the results of other tests or clinical information. This can be prevented if the persons interpreting the test results are blinded to the nature of the patient's other test results or clinical presentation. If this bias is present, the test will appear to work better than it otherwise would in an uncontrolled clinical situation. There are two forms of review bias.

In **test review bias**, the person interpreting the tests has prior knowledge of the patient's outcome or their result on the gold-standard test. Therefore, they may be more likely to interpret the test so that it confirms the already known diagnosis. For example, a radiologist reading the myocardial perfusion scan mapping blood flow through the heart of a patient whom they know to have an AMI is more likely to read an equivocal area of the scan as showing no flow and therefore consistent with an MI. This is because he or she knows that there is a heart attack in that area that should show up with an area of diminished blood flow to some of the heart muscle. As a result the radiologist interprets the equivocal sign as definitely showing no flow, or a positive test for AMI.

In **diagnostic review bias**, the person interpreting the gold-standard test knows the result of the diagnostic test. This may change the interpretation of the gold standard, and make the diagnostic test look better since the reviewer will make it concur with the gold standard more often. This will not occur if the gold-standard test is completely objective by being totally automated with a dichotomous result or if the interpreter of the gold standard is blinded to the results of the diagnostic test. For example, a patient with a positive ultrasound of the leg veins is diagnosed with deep venous thrombosis or a blood clot in the veins. A radiologist reading the venogram, dye assisted x-ray of the veins, which is the gold standard in this case, is more likely to read an equivocal area as one showing blockage since he or she knows that the diagnostic test showed an area consistent with a clot.

Context bias

This is a common heuristic, or thought pattern. The person interpreting the test will base their reading of the test upon known clinical information. This can be a bias when determining raw test data or in a real-life situation. Radiologists are more likely to read pneumonia on a chest x-ray if they are told that the patient has classical findings of pneumonia such as cough, fever, and localized rales over one part of the lungs on examination. In daily clinical situations, this will make the correlation between clinical data and test results seem better than they may be in a situation in which the radiologist is given no clinical information, but asked only to interpret the x-ray findings.

Miscellaneous sources of bias

Indeterminate and uninterpretable results

Some tests have results that are not always clearly positive or negative, but may be unclear, indeterminate, or uninterpretable. If these are classified as positive or negative, the characteristics of the test will be changed. This makes calculation and manipulation of likelihood ratios or sensitivity and specificity much more complicated since categories are no longer dichotomous, but have other possible outcomes.

For example, some patients with pulmonary emboli have an indeterminate perfusion–ventilation lung scan showing the distribution of radioactive material in the lung. This means that the results are neither positive nor negative and the clinician is unsure about how to proceed. Similarly, the CT scan for appendicitis in some patients with the condition may not show the entire appendix. This is more likely to occur if the appendix lies in an unusual location such as in the pelvis or retrocecal area. In cases of patients who actually have the disease, if the result is classified as positive, the patient will be correctly classified. If however, the result is classified as negative, the patient will be incorrectly classified. Again the need for blinded reading and careful a-priori definitions of a positive and negative test can prevent the errors that go with this type of problem.

Reproducibility

The performance of a diagnostic test depends on the performance of the technician and the equipment used in performance of the test. Tests that are operator-dependent are most prone to error because of lack of reproducibility. They may perform very well when carried out in a research setting, but when extrapolated to the community setting, the persons performing them may never rise to the level of expertise required, either because they don't do enough of the tests to become really proficient or because they lack the enthusiasm or interest. For example, CT scans for appendicitis are harder to read than those taken for other GI problems. When tested in a center that was doing research on this use, they performed very well. When extrapolated to the community hospital setting, they did less well. Tests initially studied in one center should be studied in a wide variety of other settings before the results of their operating characteristics are accepted.

Post-hoc selection of test positivity criteria

This situation is often seen when a continuous variable is converted to a dichotomous one for purposes of defining the cutoff between normal and abnormal. In studying the test, it is discovered that most patients with the disease being sought have a test value above a certain threshold and most without the disease have a test value below that threshold. There is statistical significance for the difference in disease occurrence in these two groups ($P < 0.05$). That threshold is therefore selected as the cutoff point.

In some cases, the researchers looked at several cutoff points before deciding on a final one. Some of them produced differences that were not statistically significant. This is a form of data dredging and could be classified as a Type I error. A validation study should be done to verify this result and the results given as likelihood ratios rather than simple differences and P values. This problem can be evaluated by using likelihood ratios and sensitivity and specificity and plotting them on the Receiver Operating Characteristics curve for the data rather than using only statistical significance as the defining variables in test performance.

Temporal changes

Test characteristics measured at one point in time may change as the test is technically improved. The measures calculated from the studies of the newer technology will not apply to the older technology. This is especially true in radiology, where new generations of MRI machines, CT scanners, and other imaging modalities are regularly introduced. The results of a study done with the latest generation of CT scanners may not be seen if your hospital is still using the older scanners. Look for this problem in the use of newer biochemical or pathological tests, as well as in questionnaire tests if the questionnaire is constantly being improved. There may also be problems associated with the technological improvement in tests. Newer generations of CT scanners are more likely to deliver higher doses of radiation to the body.

Publication bias

Studies that are positive, that find a statistically significant difference between groups, are more likely to be published than those that find no difference. Consider the possibility that there may be several unpublished negative studies "out there" when deciding to accept the results of studies of a new test. Ideally, diagnostic tests should be studied in a variety of clinical settings and with different mixes of patients.

Words of caution: the manufacturers of a new test want as many physicians to use the test as often as possible and may sponsor studies that have various of the biases noted above. There is a lot of money to be made in the introduction of a new test, especially if it involves an expensive new technology. For example, a magnetic resonance imaging, MRI, machine costs several million dollars, which must be justified by the performance of lots of scans. These may not be justified based on good objective evidence obtained through well-conducted studies of the technology. As a conscientious physician, you must decide when these expensive technologies are truly useful to your patient. Working with well-done published guidelines and knowing the details of the studies of these new modalities can help to put their use into perspective.

Studies sponsored by the manufacturer of the test being studied are always open to extra scrutiny. Although this does not automatically make it a bad study, if the authors have a financial stake in the results of the study they often "spin" the results in the most favorable manner. Conversely, a company producing a diagnostic test will resist publication of a negative study, and this may lead to suppression of important medical information.

The ideal study of diagnostic tests

The following is a hypothetical example of an ideal research study of a diagnostic test. The study looked at the use of head CT in predicting the complications of stroke therapy with blood clot dissolving medication. Patients who are having a stroke get an immediate head CT. The scan is initially read by a community radiologist who is part of the treating physician group and not by a neuro-radiologist who specializes in reading head CTs. If in that radiologist's opinion the scan shows any sign of potential bleeding into the brain, that patient is excluded from the study.

This scan is then taken to two neuro-radiologists who are experts in reading head CTs. They read the scan without knowing the nature of the patient problem or each other's reading of the scan. If they disagree with each other's reading, a third radiologist is called in as a tiebreaker. All patients who are felt to be clinically eligible for the drug are randomized to be given either the drug or placebo. The rate of resolution of symptoms and the percentage of patients who make full recovery, do worse, and die are measured for each group.

The reference standard is the reading of the two blinded neuro-radiologists, or a majority of two in the case of disagreement. This is not perfect, but mirrors the best that could be done in any radiology setting. The outcome should then be judged by a clinician who would probably be a neurologist in this case and who is also blinded to the results of the CT and the group to which the patient was randomized. Although not perfect, and no study is, there are adequate safeguards to ensure the validity of the results. The inclusion criteria are specified and the filter for which patients are chosen is explicit. The biggest problem with this study is that patients who are excluded by the initial reading of the CT may in fact have been eligible for the treatment if a bleed was mistakenly read. However, in a real-life situation, this is what would occur, so the results are generalizable to the setting of a community hospital. This group with positive CT scans can be studied separately if all of their CT scans are taken and read by the same panel of neuro-radiologists who then record their final readings, the gold standard. This will tell us how accurate the reading of a bleed was on the CT scans by the community radiologists.

The gold standard is clearly defined and about as good as it gets. The test, CT read by community radiologists, and gold standard, CT read by neuro-radiology specialists, are independent of each other and read in a blinded manner since the two groups of radiologists are not communicating with each other. A more perfect gold standard could be another test such as magnetic resonance imaging, MRI, of the brain. All patients would need to have both the diagnostic test and the gold-standard test. The follow-up period must be made sufficiently long so that all possible outcome events are captured. That is not a significant problem here as all patients can be observed immediately for the outcome. The outcome is being measured by a clinician who is blinded to the results of the gold-standard test and the treatment given to the patient. The only potential problem is that the time factor to get the patient into a CT scan and then an MRI might make the time to getting the medication too long and lead to worse results for the patient.

How to evaluate research studies of diagnostic tests: putting it all together

All practicing physicians will be faced with the ability to order an ever-increasing number of diagnostic tests. Many of these will have only theoretical promise and may not have been tested very thoroughly in clinical practice. One must be able to critically evaluate the studies of diagnostic tests and determine for oneself whether the test is appropriate to use in your particular clinical setting. The criteria discussed in this chapter are taken with permission from the series called Users' Guides to the Medical Literature, published in *JAMA* (see Bibliography).

Are the results valid?

(1) Was there an independent, blind comparison with a reference (gold) standard of diagnosis?

Diagnostic test studies measure the degree of association between the predictor variable or test result and the outcome or disease. The presence or absence of the outcome or disease is determined by the result of a reference or gold-standard test. The diagnostic test under study cannot be used to determine the presence or absence of the disease. That would be an example of incorporation bias.

The term "normal" must be sensibly defined. How this term is arrived at must be specified. This could be done using a Gaussian distribution, percentile rank, risk factor presence or absence, culturally desirable outcome, diagnostic outcome, or therapeutic outcome and should be specified. If prolonged follow-up of apparently well patients is used to define the absence of disease, the period of follow-up must be reasonable so that almost all latent cases of the disease in question will develop to a stage where the disease can be readily identified.

Both the diagnostic test being studied and the gold standard must be applied to the study and control subjects in a standardized and blinded fashion. This should be done following a standardized protocol and using trained observers to improve reliability. Comparing the new test to the gold standard assesses accuracy and validity. Blinding reduces measurement bias. Ideally, the test should be automated and not operator-dependent, multiple measurements should be made, and at least two investigators involved. One will apply or interpret the new diagnostic test on the subjects while the second will apply or interpret the gold standard on the subjects.

(2) Was the study test described adequately?

The test results should be easily reproducible or reliable and easy to interpret with low inter-observer variation. Enough information should be present in the Methods section to perform the diagnostic test, including any special requirements, dosages, precautions, and timing sequences. An estimated cost of performing the test should be given, including reagents, physician or technician time, specialty care, and turn-around time. Long- and short-term side effects and complications associated with the test should be discussed. The test parameters may be very variable in different settings because test reliability varies. For "operator-dependent tests" the level of skill of the person performing the test should be noted and some discussion of how they are trained included in the description of the study so that this training program can be duplicated.

(3) Was the diagnostic test evaluated in an appropriate spectrum of patients?
In order to reduce sampling bias, the study patients should be adequately described and representative of the population likely to receive the test. The distribution of age, sex, and spectrum of other medical disorders unrelated to the outcome of interest should be representative of the population in whom the test will ultimately be used. The spectrum of disease should be wide enough to represent all the levels of patients for whom the test may be used and should include early disease, late disease, classical cases, and difficult-to-diagnose cases, those commonly confused with other disorders. If only very classical cases are studied, the diagnostic test may perform better than it would for less characteristic cases, an example of spectrum bias.

Frequently, research studies of diagnostic tests are done at referral centers that see many cases of severe, classical, or unmistakable disease. This may not correlate with the distribution of levels of disease seen in physicians' offices or community hospitals leading to referral or sampling bias. Investigators testing a new test will often choose a sample of subjects that have a higher-than-average prevalence of disease. This may not represent the prevalence of disease in the general population. If the study is a case–control study or retrospective study, typically 50% of the subjects will have disease and 50% will be normal, a ratio that is very unlikely to actually exist in the general population. Physicians tend to order testing in subjects who are less likely to have the disease than those usually studied when the test is developed.

There should be clear description of the way that people were selected for the test. This means that the reader should be able to clearly understand the selection filter that was used to preselect those people who are eligible for the test. They should be able to determine which patients are in the group most likely to have the disease as opposed to other patients who have a lower prevalence of the disease and yet might also be eligible for the test. In a case–control study, the control patients should be similar in every way to the diseased subjects except for the presence of disease. This cannot be done using only young healthy volunteers as the study subjects! The cases with the disease should be as much like the controls without the disease in every other way possible. The similarity of study and control subjects increases the possibility that the test is measuring differences due to disease and not age, sex, general health, or other factors or disease conditions.

(4) Was the reference standard applied regardless of the diagnostic test result?
The choice of a reference gold or diagnostic standard may be very difficult. The diagnostic standard test may be invasive, painful, costly, and possibly even dangerous to the patient, resulting in morbidity and even mortality. Obviously taking a surgical biopsy is a very good reference standard, but it may involve major

surgery for the patient. For that reason, many diseases will require prolonged follow-up of patients suspected as being free of the disease as an acceptable reference standard. How and for how long this follow-up is done will often determine the internal validity of the study. The study should be free of verification and other forms of review bias such as test review and context bias, which can occur during the process of observing patients who are suspected of having or not having the disease. Adequate blinding of observers is the best way to avoid these biases.

(5) Has the utility of the test been determined?

If the test is to be used or the investigators desire that it be used as part of a battery or sequence of tests, the contribution of this test to the overall validity of the battery or sequence must be determined. Is the patient better off for having the test done alone or as part of the battery of tests? Is the diagnosis made earlier, the treatment made more effective, the diagnosis made more cheaply, or more safely? These questions should all be answered especially before we use a new and very expensive or dangerous test. Some of these questions are answered by the magnitude of the results. But, there are always logistical questions that must be answered to determine the usefulness of a test in varied clinical situations.

What is the impact of the results?

The study results must be important. This means that the study must determine the likelihood ratios of the test. In most studies this will be done by calculation of the sensitivity and specificity. If these are reasonably good, the next step is deciding to which patients the results can be applied. Confidence intervals for the likelihood ratios should be given as part of the results. Where multiple test cutoff points are possible, an ROC curve should be provided and the best cutoff point determined. All of these points have associated confidence intervals. In any study of a diagnostic test, the initial study should be considered a derivation study and followed by one or more large validation studies. These will determine if the initial good results were actually true or if they were just that good by chance alone.

Can the results be applied to my patients?

Consider the population tested and the patient who is being evaluated. The answer to the question of generalizability or particularizability depends on how similar each individual patient is to the study population. You have to ask whether he or she would have been included in the sample being studied. Ideally the answer to that question ought always to be yes. But sometimes there are reasons for using a particular population. For example, studies done in the Veterans

Affairs Hospital System will be mostly of men. This does not automatically disqualify a female patient from having the test done for the target disorder. There ought to be a good physiological reason to exclude her from having the tests based on the results from a study of men. Perhaps there is a hormonal effect that will alter the results of the test. However, each physician must use their best clinical judgment to be able to determine whether the results of the study can be used in a given individual patient. Other factors which might affect the characteristics of the test in a single patient, include age and ethnic group.

(1) Is the diagnostic test available, affordable, accurate, and precise in my setting?

How do the capabilities of the lab or diagnostic center that one is working in compare with the one described in the study? This is a function of the type of equipment used and the operator-dependency of the test. Some very sophisticated and complex tests may only be available at referral or research centers and not readily available in the average community hospital setting. The estimated costs of false positive and false negative test results should be addressed, including the cost of repeat testing or further diagnostic procedures for false positive results and of a missed diagnosis due to false negative results. The cost of the test should be given, as well as the cost of following up on false positive tests and missing some patients with false negative tests. This could include the cost of malpractice insurance and payment of awards in cases of missed disease. This is very complex since the notion of negligence in missing a diagnosis depends more on one's pretest probability of disease and how one handles the occurrence of a false negative test.

(2) Can I come up with a reasonable pretest probability of disease for my patient?

This was addressed earlier, and although small deviations from the true pretest probability are not important, large variations are. One does not want to be very far off in estimating the prior probability. If the physician estimates that the patient has a 10% probability of disease and the true probability of disease is 90%, this will seriously and adversely decrease the ability to diagnose the problem. Data on pretest probability come from several sources including published studies of symptoms, one's personal experience, the study itself, if the sample is reasonably representative of the population of patients from which one's patient comes, and clinical judgment based on the information that is gathered in the history and physical exam process. If none of these gives a reasonable pretest probability, consider getting some help from an expert consultant. A colleague or consultant will probably be able to help here. Most reasonable and prudent physicians will agree on a ballpark figure, high, medium, or low, for the pretest probability in most patient presentations of illness.

Indication creep is a phenomenon that occurs when a diagnostic test is used in more and more patients who are less and less likely to have the disease being sought. This will happen after a test is studied in one group of patients, usually those with more severe or classical disease and then extended to patients with lower pretest probability of disease. As the test gets marketed and put into widespread clinical use, the type of patient who gets the test tends to be one with a lower and lower pretest probability of disease and eventually, the test is frequently done in patients who have almost zero pretest probability of disease. However, physicians are especially cautious to avoid missing anyone with a disease in the fear of being sued for malpractice. However, they must be equally cautious about over-testing those patients with such low probability of disease in whom almost all positive tests will be false positives.

(3) Will the post-test probability change my management of this patient?

This is probably the most important question to ask about the usefulness of a diagnostic test, and will determine whether the test should or should not be done. The first issue is a mathematical one. Will the resulting post-test probability move the probability across the testing or treatment threshold? If not, either do not do the test, or be prepared to do a second or even a third test to confirm the diagnosis.

Next, is the patient interested in having the test done and are they going to be "part of the team?" If the patient is not a willing partner in the process, it is not a good idea to begin doing the test or tests. Give the information to the patient in a manner they can understand and then ask them if they want to go through with the testing. They ought to understand the risks of disease, and of correct and incorrect results of testing, and the ramifications of a positive and negative test results. Incorporated in this is the question of the ultimate utility of the test. The prostate specific antigen (PSA) test to screen for prostate cancer is a good example since a positive test must be followed up with a prostate biopsy, which is invasive and potentially dangerous. In some men, a positive PSA test does not mean prostate cancer, but only an enlarged prostate, which could be diagnosed by other means. The decision making for this problem is very complex and should be done through careful consideration of all of the options and the patients' situation such as age, general health, and the presence of other medical conditions.

Finally, how will a positive or negative result help the patient reach his or her goals for treatment? If the patient has "heartburn" and you no longer suspect a cardiac problem, but suspect gastritis or peptic ulcers, will doing a test for *Helicobacter pylori* infection as a cause of ulcers and treatment with specific anti-microbial drugs if positive, or symptomatic treatment if negative, satisfy the patient that he or she does not have a gastric carcinoma? If not, then endoscopy, the gold standard in this case, ought to be considered without stopping for the intermediate test.

Studies of diagnostic tests should determine the sensitivity and specificity of the test under varying circumstances. The prevalence of disease in the population studied may be very different from that in most clinical practices. Therefore, predictive values reported in the literature should be reserved for validation studies and studies of the use of the test under well-defined clinical conditions. Remember that the predictive value of a test is dependent not only on the likelihood ratios, but also very directly on the pretest probability of disease.

Final thoughts about diagnostic test studies

It is critical to realize that studies of diagnostic tests done in the past were often done using different methodology than what is now recommended. Many of the studies done years ago only looked for the correlation between a diagnostic test and the final diagnosis. For example, a study of pneumonia might look at all physical examination findings for patients who were subjected to chest x-rays, and determine which correlated most closely with a positive chest x-ray, the gold standard.

There are two problems with these types of studies. First, the patients are selected by inclusion criteria that include getting the test done, here a chest x-ray, which already narrows down the probability that they have the illness. In other words, some selection filter was applied to the population. Second, correlation only tells us that you are more or less likely to find a certain clinical finding with an illness. It does not tell you what the probability of the illness is after application of that finding or test. The correlation does not give the same useful information that you get from likelihood ratios or sensitivity and specificity. Those will tell the clinician how certain diagnostic findings correlate with the presence of illness and how to use those clinical findings to determine the presence or absence of disease.

28

Screening tests

Detection is, or ought to be, an exact science, and should be treated in the same cold and unemotional manner. You have attempted to tinge it with romanticism, which produces much the same effect as if you worked a love-story or an elopement into the fifth proposition of Euclid.

Sir Arthur Conan Doyle (1859–1930): The Sign of Four, 1890

Learning objectives

In this chapter you will learn:
- the attributes of a good screening test
- the effects of lead-time and length-time biases and how to recognize them in evaluating a screening test
- how to evaluate the usefulness of a screening test
- how to evaluate studies of screening tests

Introduction

Screening tests are defined as diagnostic tests that are useful in detecting disease in asymptomatic or presymptomatic persons. The goal of all screening tests is to diagnose the disease at a stage when it is more easily curable (Fig. 28.1). This is usually earlier than the symptomatic stage and is one of the reasons for doing a diagnostic test to screen for disease.

Screening tests must rise to a higher level of utility since the majority of people being screened derive no benefit from having the test done. Because the vast majority of people who are screened do not have the disease, they get minimal reassurance from a negative test because their pretest probability of disease was low before the test was even done. However, for many people, the psychological relief of having a negative test, especially for something they are really scared of, is a worthwhile positive outcome.

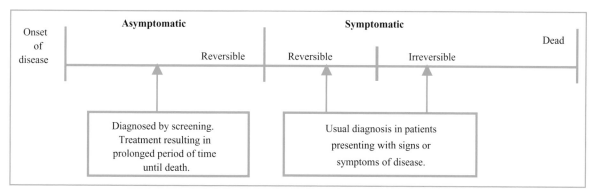

There are three rules for diagnostic tests that must be more carefully applied to screening tests. The first rule is that there is no free lunch. As the sensitivity of a test increases to detect a greater percentage of diseased persons, specificity falls and the number of false positives increases. The second rule is that the prevalence of the disease matters and as the prevalence decreases, the number of false positives increases and relative number of true positives to false positives decreases. The final rule is that the burden of proof regarding efficacy depends upon the clinical context, which can depend on multiple factors. If the intervention is innocuous and without side effects, screening should be done more often than if the intervention is dangerous, high-risk, or toxic. Similarly, if the test or treatment is very expensive, the level of proof of benefit of the screeing test must be greater.

During the 1950s the executive physical examination was used to screen for "all" diseases in corporate executives and other, mostly wealthy, people. It was a comprehensive set of diagnostic tests including multiple x-rays, blood tests, exercise stress tests, and others, usually administered while the patient spent a week in the hospital. It was justified by the thought that finding disease early was good and would lead to improved length and quality of life. The more diseases looked for, the more likely that disease would be found at an earlier phase in its course and treatment at this early stage would lead to better health outcomes. Subsequent analysis of the data from these extensive examination programs revealed no change in health outcomes as a result of these examinations. There were more people incorrectly labeled with diseases that they didn't have than there were diseases detected early enough to reduce mortality or morbidity. Ironically, most of the diseases that were identified in these programs could have been detected simply from a comprehensive history.

This is occurring again with the advent of full body CT scans to screen for hidden illness, mostly cancer. In this case most of the positive tests are false positives and the further testing that is required to determine wether the test is a false or true positive usually requires invasive testing such as operative biopsy. Finally,

Table 28.1. Criteria for a valid screening test

(1)	Burden of suffering	The disease must be relatively common. The burden of suffering must be sufficiently great.
(2)	Early detectability	The disease must be detectable at an early stage, preferably when totally curable.
(3)	Accuracy and validity	The test must be accurate and valid: it must reliably pick up disease (few misses) and not falsely label too many healthy people.
(4)	Acceptability	The test must be simple, inexpensive, not noxious, and easy to administer. It must be acceptable to the patient and to the health-care system.
(5)	Improved outcome	There must be treatment available, which if given at the time that early disease is detected, will result in improved outcome (lower mortality and morbidity) among those patients being screened.

it has recently been determined that the radiation exposure from the CT scans could actually cause more disease, specifically cancers, than would be picked up with the screening.

Criteria for screening

There are five criteria that must be fulfilled before a test should be used as a screening test. These are listed in Table 28.1. Following these rules will prevent the abuses of screening tests that occurred in the 1950s and 1960s and which continue today.

The disease must impose a significant burden of suffering on the population to be screened. This means either that the disease is common or that it results in serious or catastrophic disability. This disability may result in loss of productive employment, patient discomfort or dissatisfaction, as well as passing the disease on to others. It also means that it will cost someone a lot of money to care for persons with the disease. The hope is to reduce this cost both in human suffering and in dollars by treating at an earlier stage of disease and preventing complications or early death. This depends on well-designed studies of harm or risk to tell which diseases are likely to be encountered in a significant portion of the population in order to decide that screening for them is needed.

For example, it would be unreasonable to screen the population of all 20-year-old women for breast cancer with yearly mammography. The risk of disease is so low in this population that even a miniscule risk of increased cancer associated with the radiation from the examination may cause more cancers than the test would detect. Similarly, the prevalence of cancer in this population is so low that the likelihood a positive test would be cancer is very low and there will be many more false positives than true positives. Similarly screening for HIV in an extremely low-risk population would lead to incorrectly labeling many more people as being HIV-positive who were not affected and therefore, false positives. This could lead to a lot of psychological trauma and require lots of confirmatory testing in these positives, which would cost a huge amount of money to find one true case of HIV.

The screening test must be a good one and must accurately detect disease in the population of people who are in the presymptomatic phase of disease. This means that it must have high sensitivity. It should also reliably exclude disease in the population without disease or have high specificity. Of the two, we want the sensitivity to be perfect or almost perfect so that we can identify all patients with the disease. We'd like the specificity to be extremely high so that only a few people without disease are mislabeled leading to a high positive predictive value. This usually means that a reasonable confirmatory test must be available that will more accurately discriminate between those people with a positive screening test who do and don't have the disease. This confirmatory test ought to be very specific and acceptable to most people. It should be relatively comfortable, not very painful, should not cause serious side effects, and also be reasonably priced.

A screening test may be unacceptable if it produces too many false positives since those people will be falsely labeled as having the disease, a circumstance which could lead to psychological trauma, anxiety, insurance or employment discrimination, or social conflicts. False labeling has a deleterious effect on most people. Several studies have found significant increases in anxiety that interferes with life activities in persons who were falsely labeled as having disease on a screening test. This is an especially serious issue with genetic tests in which a positive test does not mean the disease will express itself, but only that a person has the gene for the disease.

There are practical qualities of a good screening test. The cost ought to be low so it can be economically done on large populations. It should be simple to perform with good accuracy and reliability. And finally, it must be acceptable to the patient. For screening tests, most people will tolerate only a low level of discomfort either from the test procedure itself or from the paperwork involved in getting the test done. People would much rather have their blood pressure taken to screen for hypertension than have a colonoscopy to look for early signs of colon cancer. Finally, people are more willing to have a test performed to detect disease when they are symptomatic than when they are well.

The mechanics of a screening program must be well planned if the plan is to give a huge number of people a diagnostic test. If the test is too complex such as screening colonoscopy for colon cancer, most people would not be willing to have it done. A test that is very uncomfortable such as a digital rectal exam for prostate or rectal cancer, may be refused by a large proportion of patients. Both examples also require more complex logistics such as individual examining rooms and sedation for the colonoscopy than a screening test such as blood pressure measurement. Screening tests must also be well advertised so that people will know why and how to have the test done.

Pitfalls in the screening process

Simply diagnosing the disease at an earlier stage is not helpful unless the prognosis is better if treatment is begun at that earlier stage of the illness. The treatment must be acceptable and more effective before people will be willing to accept treatment at an asymptomatic stage of illness. Why should someone take a drug for hypertension if they have no signs or symptoms of the disease when that drug can cause significant side effects and must be taken for a lifetime?

During the 1960s and 1970s, some lung cancers were detected at an earlier stage by routine screening chest x-rays. However, immediate treatment of these cancers did not result in increased survival and caused increased patient suffering due to serious side effects of the surgery and chemotherapeutic drugs. Therefore, even though cancers were detected at an earlier stage, mortality was the same.

The validity of a screening test can be determined from the evidence in the literature. Screening tests must balance the need to learn something about a patient, the diagnostic yield, with the ability to actively and effectively intervene in the disease process at an earlier stage.

There are three significant problems of studies of screening tests. These are **lead-time, length-time**, and **compliance biases**. Lead-time bias results in overoptimistic results of the screening test in the clinical study. The patients seem to live longer but this is only because their disease is detected earlier. In this case, the total time from onset of illness to death is the same in the group of patients who were screened and treated early compared with the unscreened group. The lead time is the time from diagnosis of disease by screening test to the appearance of symptoms. The time from appearance of symptoms to death is the same whether the disease was detected by the screening test or not. The total life span of the screened patient is no different from that of the unscreened patient. The time between early diagnosis with the screening test and appearance of symptoms, the lead time, will now be spent undergoing treatment (Fig. 28.2). This

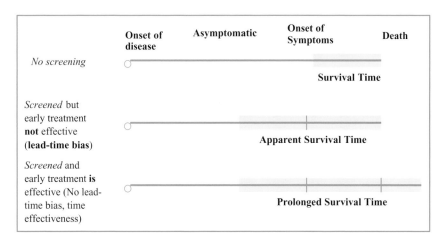

Fig. 28.2 Lead-time bias.

could be very uncomfortable due to the side effects of treatment or even dangerous if treatment can result in serious morbidity or death of the patient.

Length-time bias is much more likely to occur in observational studies. Patients are not randomized and the spectrum of disease may be very different in the screened group when compared to the unscreened group. A disease that is indolent and slowly progressive is more likely to be detected than one that is rapidly progressive and quickly fatal. Patients with aggressive cancers are more likely to die shortly after their cancer is detected. Those with slow-growing indolent tumors are more likely to be cured of their disease after screening and will live a long time until they die of other causes. There are some whose disease is too early to detect and who will be missed by screening. Without screening, his or her disease will be detected when it becomes symptomatic, which will be at a later stage. Length-time bias is illustrated in Fig. 28.3. This problem can be reduced in large population studies by effective randomization that ensures a similar spectrum of disease in screened and unscreened patients.

Compliance bias occurs because in general, patients who are compliant with therapy do better than those who are not regardless of the therapy. Compliant patients may have other characteristics such as being more health-conscious in their lifestyle choices, which lead to better outcomes. Studies of screening tests often compare a group of people who are in a screening program with people in the population who are not in the screening program. They are usually not randomized to be in either group. Therefore, the screened group is more likely to be composed of people who are more compliant or health-conscious, since they took advantage of the screening test in the first place. This will make it more likely that the screened group will do better since they may be the healthier patients in general. This bias can be avoided if patients in these studies are randomized before being put through the screening test. One way to test for this bias is to

Fig. 28.3 Length-time bias.

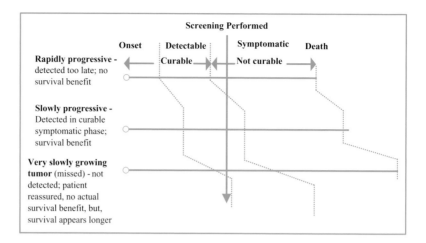

have two groups of patients, one that is randomized to receive the screening test or not and the other group that has a choice of whether to get screened or not. This was described in Chapter 15 on the randomized clinical trial (RCT).

Effectiveness of screening

Another problem with screening tests revolves around their overall effectiveness. For example, consider the use of mammograms for the early detection of breast cancer in young women. Women aged 50–70 in whom the cancer is detected at an early stage do appear to have better outcomes. The use of mammography for screening younger women (age 40–50) is still controversial. In studies of this group, it made very little difference in ultimate survival if the woman was screened. Early detection in this population resulted in a large number of false positive tests requiring biopsy and unnecessary worry for the women affected. It also resulted in an increased exposure to x-rays among these women and increased the cost of health care for everyone in the society.

A convenient concept to use in the calculation of benefit is the number needed to screen to get benefit (NNSB). Like the number needed to treat to get benefit (NNTB), it is simply 1/ARR, ARR being the absolute risk reduction or the difference in percentage response between the screened and unscreened groups. The ideal number to use here is the percentage of women who die from their cancer in the screened (EER) and unscreened (CER) groups. The NNSB can be used to balance the positive and negative effects of screening. For example, in the case of using mammograms to screen for breast cancer in women at age 40, we can make the spreadsheet as in Table 28.2.

Table 28.2. Screening 40- to 50-year-old women for breast cancer using mammography

	Screened	Not screened
Total population	1000	1000
Positive mammogram	300	–
Biopsies (invasive procedures)	150	–
New breast cancers	15	15
Deaths from breast cancer	5–8	7–8

Source: From: D. Eddy. *Clinical Decision Making.* Sudbury, MA: Jones & Bartlett, 1996.

On the benefit side, there is the prevention of at most three deaths per 1000 women screened. This leads to a large NNSB = 333. This means that 333 women must be screened to prevent one death from breast cancer.

$$CER = 8/1000 \; EER = 5/1000 \; ARR = (8/1000 - 5/1000) = 3/1000$$
$$NNSB = 1/ARR = 1/(3/1000) = 1/0.003 = 333$$

If the tests actually result in the same number of deaths from breast cancer, about 8% in both groups, the NNSB will be infinite and there will be no benefit of screening.

Typical acceptable NNSB for currently used screening modalities are in the 100–1000 range. If the test is relatively benign or treatment is very easy and the expected outcome is very good in the screened population a much larger NNSB is acceptable. More randomized clinical trials of screening tests are needed to determine acceptable levels of NNSB.

The United States Public Heath Service (USPHS) has published a set of criteria for an acceptable screening test. The test must be accurate and able to detect the target condition earlier than without screening and with sufficient accuracy to avoid producing large numbers of false positive and false negative results. Screening for and treating persons with early disease must be effective and should improve the likelihood of favorable health outcomes by reducing disease-specific mortality or morbidity compared to treating patients when they present with signs or symptoms of the disease. These criteria come from the USPHS *Guide to Clinical Preventive Services*, which also contains a compendium of recommendations for the use of the most important screening tests.[1] There are

[1] US Preventive Services Task Force. *Guide to Clinical Preventive Services.* 2nd edn. Washington, DC: USPHS, 1996. Available online through the National Library of Medicine's HSTAT service at hstat.nlm.nih.gov.

also very effective evidence-based guidelines for screening put out by the Agency for Healthcare Research and Quality.[2]

Critical appraisal of studies of screening tests[3]

(1) Are the recommendations valid?

    (a) Is there evidence from RCTs that earlier intervention works? Most screening strategies are based upon observational studies. Ideally, the intervention should be shown to be effective in a well-done RCT. The overall screening strategy should also be validated by an RCT. Only if the therapeutic intervention is extremely dramatic, which most aren't, is there likely to be no question about its efficacy. A good example of this would be in screening for hypothyroidism in the newborn. Early detection and treatment will prevent problems in this rare birth problem. Observational studies of screening tests are weaker than a well-done RCT. If there is an RCT of the screening modality, it should be first analyzed using the *Users' guide* for studies of therapy, which is also the guide that would be used to determine efficacy of prevention.

    (b) Were the data identified, selected, and combined in an unbiased fashion? Look for potential confounding factors during the process by which subjects are recruited or identified for inclusion in a study of screening. These may easily result in serious bias usually from confounding variables. Innate differences between the screened and not-screened groups should be aggressively sought. Frequently these differences are glossed over as being insignificant and they often are not and can lead to confounding bias.

(2) What are the recommendations and will they help me in caring for my patients? What are the benefits?

    (a) The benefits should be calculable using the NNSB (number needed to screen to benefit). The beneficial outcomes that the results refer to should be important for the patient. The confidence intervals should be narrow.

    (b) The harms or potential harms should be clearly identified. Persons who are labeled with the disease and who are really disease-free will at least be inconvenienced and may require additional testing that is not benign. At least they may have increased anxiety until the final diagnosis is made. Early treatment may result in such severe side effects that patients may

---

[2] Agency for Healthcare Research and Quality. www.ahrq.gov.
[3] Adapted with permission from the Users' Guides to the Medical Literature, published in *JAMA* (see Bibliography).

not want the treatment. You should be able to calculate the NNSH (number needed to screen to harm) of the intervention based upon the study data. This should be done with 95% confidence intervals to demonstrate the precision of that result.

(c) These should be compared in different people and with different screening strategies by looking at all possible screening strategies when evaluating a screening program. Different strategies may result in different outcomes either in final results or patient suffering, depending on the prevalence of disease in the population screened and the screening and verification strategy employed.

(d) Look for the impact of the screening test on people's values and preferences. There ought to be an evaluation of patient values as part of the study. These can be done using focus groups or qualitative studies of patient populations. If this is missing, be suspicious about the acceptability of the screening strategy. The study should be asking patients how they feel about the screening test itself as well as the possibility of being falsely labeled.

(e) The study should explore the impact of uncertainty by calculating a sensitivity analysis as described in Chapter 30. There is uncertainty associated with any study result and the 95% confidence intervals should be given.

(f) The cost-effectiveness should be evaluated considering all the possible costs associated with the screening, including but not limited to, setting up the program, advertising, following up positives, and excess testing and treatment of positives. A more complete guide to cost-effectiveness analysis is found in Chapter 31.

29

Practice guidelines and clinical prediction rules

Any fool can make a rule
And every fool will mind it.

Henry David Thoreau (1817–1862): Journal, 1860

Whoever controls guidelines controls medicine

D. Eddy, *JAMA*, 1990; 263: 877–880

Learning objectives

In this chapter you will learn:

- the reasons for and origins of practice guidelines
- the problems associated with practice guidelines and the process by which they are developed
- how to evaluate practice guidelines and how they are actually used in practice
- the process of clinical prediction rule development
- the significance of different levels of prediction rules

What are practice guidelines?

Practice guidelines have always been a part of medical practice. They are present in the "diagnosis" and "treatment" sections in medical textbooks. Unfortunately, published practice guidelines are not always evidence-based. As an example, for the treatment of frostbite on the fingers, a surgical textbook says that operation should wait until the frostbitten part falls off, yet there are no studies backing up this claim. Treatment guidelines for glaucoma state that treatment should be initiated if the intraocular pressure is over 30 mmHg or over a value in the middle 20 mmHg range if the patient has two or more risk factors. It then gives a list of over 100 risk factors but gives no probability estimates of the increased rate of glaucoma attributable to any single risk factor. Clearly these are not evidence-based or particularly helpful to the individual practitioner.

Practice guidelines are simply an explicit set of steps that when followed will result in the best outcome. In the past, they have been used for good reasons such as hand washing before vaginal delivery to prevent childbed fever or puerperal sepsis and for bad ones such as frontal lobotomies to treat schizophrenia. In some cases they are promulgated as a result of political pressure. One recent example is breast-cancer screening with mammograms in women between 40 and 50 years old. This has been instituted in spite of lack of good evidence of improved outcomes. This particular program can cost a billion dollars a year without saving very many lives and can irrationally shape physician and patient behavior for years.

A physician in 1916 said "once a Caesarian section, always a Caesarian section," meaning that if a woman required a Caesarian section for delivery, all subsequent deliveries should be by Caesarian section. As a result of this one statement, the practice became institutionalized. This particular "guideline" was based on a bad outcome in just a few patients. It may have been valuable 85 years ago, but with modern obstetrical techniques it is less useful now. Many recent studies have cast doubts on the validity of this guideline, but a new study suggests that there is a slightly increased risk of uterine rupture and poor outcome for mother and baby if vaginal delivery is attempted in these women. Clearly the jury is still out on this one and it is up to the individual patient with her doctor's input to make the best decision for her and her baby.

Practice guidelines are used for a variety of purposes. Primarily they ought to be used as a template for optimal patient care. This should be the best reason for their implementation and use in clinical practice. When evidence-based practice guidelines are written, reviewed, and based upon solid high-quality evidence, they should be implemented by all physicians. A good example of an evidence-based clinical guideline in current use is weight-based dosing of the anticoagulant heparin for the treatment of deep venous thrombosis (DVT). When the guideline is used, there are fewer adverse effects of treatment, treatment failure, or excess bleeding and better outcomes leading to more rapid resolution of the DVT.

However, there are "darker" consequences that accompany the use of practice guidelines. They can be used as means of accreditation or certification. Currently several specialty boards use chart-review processes as part of their specialty recertification process. Managed care organizations (MCOs) can develop accreditation rules that depend on physician adherence to practice guidelines in the majority of their patients with a given problem. Performance criteria can be used as incentives in the determination of merit pay or bonuses, a process called Pay for Performance (P4P).

In the last 30 years there has been an increase in the use of practice guidelines in determining the proper utilization of hospital beds. Utilization review has resulted in the reduction of hospital stays, which occurred in most cases

Table 29.1. Desirable attributes of a clinical guideline

(1)	Accurate	the methods used must be based on good-quality evidence
(2)	Accountable	the readers (users) must be able to evaluate the guideline for themselves
(3)	Evaluable	the readers must be able to evaluate the health and fiscal consequences of applying the guideline
(4)	Facilitate resolution of conflict	the sources of disagreement should be able to be identified, addressed, and corrected
(5)	Facilitate application	the guidelines must be able to be applied to the individual patient situation

without any increase in mortality or morbidity. The process of utilization review is strongly supported by managed care organizations and third-party payors. The guidelines upon which these rules are based ought to be evidence-based (Table 29.1).

Development of practice guidelines

How should practice guidelines be developed? The process of guideline development should be evidence-based. Ideally a panel of interested physicians is assembled and collects the evidence for and against the use of a particular set of diagnostic or therapeutic maneuvers. Some guidelines are simply consensus- or expert-based and the results may not be consistent with the best available evidence.

When evaluating a guideline it ought to be possible to determine the process by which the guideline was developed. These are summarized using the AGREE criteria.[1] This working group of evidence-based practitioners have developed six domains for the evaluation of the quality of the process of making a practice guideline. These domains are: scope and purpose of the guideline, stakeholder involvement, rigor of development, clarity and presentation, applicability and editorial independence. This process only indirectly assesses the quality of the studies that make up the evidence used to create the guideline.

There are several general issues that should be evaluated when appraising the validity of a practice guideline. First, the appropriate and important health outcomes must be specified. They should be those outcomes that will matter to patients and all relevant outcomes should be included in the guideline. These include pain, anxiety, death, disfigurement, and disability. They should not be chemical or surrogate markers of disease. Next, the evidence must be analyzed

[1] AGREE criteria: Found at website of the AGREE Collaboration: http://www.agreecollaboration.org

for validity and the effect of these interventions on the outcomes of interest. This must include explicit descriptions of the manner in which the evidence was collected, evaluated, and combined. The quality of the evidence used should be explicitly given.

The magnitudes of benefits and risks should be estimated and benefits compared to harms. This must include the interests of all parties involved in providing care for the patient. These are the patient, health-care providers, third-party payors, and society at large. The preferences assigned to the outcomes should reflect those of the people or patients who will receive those outcomes.

The costs both economic and non-economic should be estimated and the net health benefits compared to the costs of providing that benefit. Alternative procedures should be compared to the standard therapies in order to determine the best therapy. Finally, the analysis of the guideline must incorporate reasonable variations in care provided by reasonable clinicians. A sensitivity analysis accounting for this reasonable variation must be part of the guideline.

Once a guideline is developed, physicians who will use this guideline in practice must evaluate its use. If the guideline is not acceptable for the practitioner, it will not be used. For example, in 1992 a clinical guideline was developed for the management of children aged 3 to 36 months with fever but no resources to detect and treat occult bacteremia. This guideline was published simultaneously in the professional journals *Annals of Emergency Medicine* and *Pediatrics*. After a few years, the guideline was only selectively used by pediatricians, but almost universally used by emergency physicians. Why? The patients seen in pediatricians' offices are significantly different than those seen in emergency departments (ED). Sicker kids are sent to the ED by their pediatricians for further evaluation. The pediatricians are able to closely follow their febrile kids while emergency physicians are unable to do this. Therefore, emergency physicians felt better doing more testing and treating of febrile children in the belief that they would prevent serious sequelae. Finally, testing was easier to do in an ED than in a pediatrician's office. This guideline has been removed since most of the children in this age group are now immunized against the worst bacteria causing occult bacteremia, hemophilus and pneumococcus.

Even if a practice guideline is validated and generally accepted by most physicians, there may still be a delay in the general acceptance of this guideline. This is mostly because of inertia. Physicians' behavior has been studied and certain interventions have been found to change behavior. These include direct intervention such as reminders on a computer or ordering forms for drugs or diagnostic tests, follow-up by allied health-care personnel, and education from opinion leaders in their field. One of the most effective interventions involved using prompts on a computer when ordering tests or drugs. These resulted in improved drug-ordering practices and long-term changes in physician behavior. Less effective were audits of patient care charts and distributed educational materials. Least effective were formal continuing medical education (CME) presentations especially if they were of brief duration (less than 1 day). In some cases, these very short presentations actually produced negative results leading to lower use of high quality evidence in physician practices. The construct called Pathman's Pipeline demonstrating the barriers to uptake of validated evidence was discussed in Chapter 17.

Practice guidelines should be developed using a preset process called the evidence- and outcomes-based approach. Separate the main steps of the policy-making process, the outcome and desirability. First estimate the specific outcomes and probability of each one of the proposed interventions. Then, make judgments about the desirability of each of the outcomes. Explicitly estimate the effect of the intervention on all outcomes that are important to patients. Estimate how the outcomes will likely vary with different patient characteristics and based on estimates of outcomes from the highest-quality experimental evidence available. Use formal methods such as systematic reviews or formal critical appraisal of the component studies to analyze the evidence and estimate the outcomes. To accurately understand patient preferences, use actual assessments of patients' preferences to determine the desirability of the outcomes.

Critical appraisal of clinical practice guidelines[2]

(1) Are the recommendations valid?
   (a) Were all important options and outcomes considered? These must be considered from the perspective of the patient as well as the physician. All reasonable physician options should be considered including comments on those options not evidence-based but in common practice.
   (b) Was a reasonable, explicit, and sensible process used to identify, select, and combine evidence? This must be reproducible by anyone reading the paper outlining how the guideline was developed. Explicit rationale for choice of studies should be done. Evidence should be presented and graded by quality indicators.
   (c) Was a reasonable, explicit, and sensible process used to consider the relative value of different outcomes? The different outcomes should be described explicitly and the reasons why each outcome was chosen should be given. Patient values should be used where available.
   (d) Is the guideline likely to account for recent developments of importance? The bibliography should include the most recent evidence regarding the topic.
   (e) Has a peer-review and testing process been applied to the guideline? Ideally, clinicians who are expert in the area of the guideline should develop

---

[2] Adapted with permission from the Users' Guides to the Medical Literature, published in *JAMA* (see Bibliography).

and review the guideline. The guideline developers must balance the need to have experts create a guideline with the potential conflicts of interest of those experts. It should be tested in various settings to determine if physicians are willing to use it and to ensure that it accomplishes its stated goals.

(2) What are the recommendations?

    (a) Are practical and clinically important recommendations made? The guidelines should be simple enough and make enough sense for most clinicians to use them.

    (b) How strong are the recommendations? The evidence for the guideline should be explicitly listed and graded using a commonly used grading scheme. Currently the GRADE criteria or the levels of evidence from the Centre for Evidence-Based Medicine at Oxford University are probably the grading schemes most often used. The results of the studies should be compelling with large effect sizes to back up the use of the evidence.

    (c) How much uncertainty is associated with the evidence and values used in creating the guideline? It should be clear from the presentation of the evidence how uncertainty in the evidence has been handled. Some sort of sensitivity analysis should be included. What happens when basic assumptions are changed within the limits of the 95% CI of the different outcomes?

(3) Will the recommendations help me in caring for my patients?

    (a) Is the primary objective of the guideline important clinically? The guidelines ought to meet your needs for improving the care of the patient you are seeing. They should be consistent with your patient's health objectives.

    (b) How are the recommendations applicable to your patients? The patient must meet the criteria for inclusion into the guideline. Patient preferences must be considered after a thorough discussion of all the options. It must be reasonable for any physician to provide the needed follow-up and support for patients who require the recommended health care.

Clinical prediction rules

Physicians are constantly looking for sets of rules to assist them in the diagnostic process. Prediction rules are more specific than clinical guidelines for certain diagnoses. The definition of clinical prediction rules is that they are a decision-making support tool that can help physicians to make a diagnosis. They are derived from original research and incorporate three or more variables into the decision process.

The Ottawa ankle rules

The Ottawa ankle rules were first developed in the early 1990s and are now in universal use in most ED and primary-care practices. Their development is an excellent model for how prediction rules should be created. The main reason for developing this rule was to attempt to decrease the number of ankle x-rays ordered for relatively minor trauma. The rule has been successfully applied in various settings and resulted in decreased use of ankle x-rays. This has become the prototype for the development of clinical prediction rules.

The first step in the development of these rules was to determine the underlying processes in making a particular diagnosis and initiating treatment modalities. In the case of the Ottawa ankle rules, this involved defining the components of the ankle examination, determining whether physicians could accurately assess them, and attempting to duplicate the results in a variety of settings. In the case of the ankle rules, it was found that only a few physical examination findings could be reliably and reproducibly assessed. Surprisingly, not all physicians reliably documented findings as apparently obvious as the presence of ecchymosis. For some of the physical-examination findings the kappa values were less than 0.6. This level was considered to be the minimum acceptable level of agreement.

The next step was to take all these physical-examination variables and apply them to a group of patients with the complaint of traumatic ankle pain. The authors determined which of these multiple variables were the most predictive of an ankle fracture. These variables were then applied to a group of patients and a statistical model was used to determine the final variables in the rule. When combined, these gave the rule the best operating characteristics. This means that when these variables are correctly applied to a patient they have the best sensitivity and specificity for diagnosing ankle fractures. In this case the rule creators decided that they wanted 100% sensitivity and were willing to sacrifice some specificity in the attempt. The process of determining which variables will be part of the rules is pure and simple data dredging. The results of this study become the derivation set for the prediction rule. This is defined as a Level-4 prediction rule. It is developed in a derivation set and ready for testing prospectively in the medical community as a validation set in different settings. For the Ottawa ankle rules, the clinical prediction rule was positive and required that an x-ray be taken if the patient could not walk four steps immediately and in the Emergency Department and if they had tenderness over the lateral or medial malleoli of the ankle.

Following this the rules were applied to another group of patients, the validation set. The same rules were applied to a new population in a prospective manner. In this case the rule functioned perfectly. This raised the rule to a Level-2 rule, since it had been validated in a different study population. If the rule were only valid in a small subpopulation, it would be a Level-3 rule. In this

Table 29.2. Levels of clinical decision rules

Level 1	Rule that can be used in a wide variety of settings with confidence that it can change clinician behavior and improve patient outcomes. At least one prospective validation in a different population and one impact analysis demonstrating change in clinician behavior with beneficial consequences.
Level 2	Rule that can be used in various settings with confidence in its accuracy. Demonstrated accuracy in at least one prospective study including a broad spectrum of patients and clinicians or validated in several smaller settings that differ from one another.
Level 3	Rule that clinicians may consider using with caution and only if patients in the study are similar to those in the clinician's clinical setting. Validated in only one narrow prospective sample.
Level 4	Rule that is derived but not validated or validated only in split samples, large retrospective databases, or by statistical techniques.

Source: From T. G. McGinn, G. H. Guyatt, P. C. Wyer, C. D. Naylor, I. G. Stiell & W. S. Richardson. Users' guides to the medical literature. XXII. How to use articles about clinical decision rules. Evidence-based medicine working group. *JAMA* 2000; 284: 79–84. Used with permission.

case, the rule was tried in a cross-section of the population that included men and women of all ages. There was not a large ethnic mix in the population, but this is a relatively minor point in this disease since there is no a-priori reason to think that African-Americans or other non-Caucasian ethnic groups will react differently in an ankle examination than Caucasians.

Finally, a Level-1 rule is one that is ready for general use and has been shown to work effectively in many clinical settings. It should also show that the savings predicted from the initial study were maintained when the rule was applied in other clinical settings. This is now true of the Ottawa ankle rules.

There are some published standards for clinical prediction rules. Wasson and others developed these in 1985, and a modified version was published in *JAMA* in 2000 (Table 29.2).

Methodological standards for developing clinical decision rules

The clinical problem addressed should be a fairly commonly encountered condition. It will be very difficult if not impossible to determine the accuracy of the examination or laboratory tests for uncommon or rare illnesses. The clinical predicament should have led to variable practices by physicians in order to support the need for a clinical prediction rule. This means that physicians act in very different ways when faced with several patients who have the same set of symptoms. There should also be general agreement that the current diagnostic practice is not fully effective, and a desire on the part of many physicians for this to change.

There must be an explicit definition of findings used to predict the outcome. Ideally the inter-observer agreement should be able to be determined. Only those with a high enough inter-observer reliability as demonstrated by a high kappa value should then be used as part of the final rule. There are several versions of the kappa test. For most dichotomous data the simple kappa is used. Other statistical methods are used for more complex data such as the weighted kappa for ordinal data and intra-class correlation coefficient for continuous interval data. Once tested, only those signs also called predictor variables with good agreement across various levels of provider experience should be used in the final rule.

All the important predictor variables must be included in the derivation process. These predictors are the components of the history and physical exam that will be in the rule to be developed. If significant components are left out of the prediction rule, providers are less likely to use the rule, as it will not have face validity for them. The predictor variables all must be present in a significant proportion of the study population or they are not likely to be useful in making the diagnosis.

Next, there should be an explicit definition of the outcomes. They must be easily understandable by all providers and be clinically important to the patient. Finding people with a genetic defect that is not clinically important may be interesting for physicians and researchers, but may not directly benefit patients. Therefore, most providers will not be interested in this outcome and will not seek to accomplish it using that particular guideline.

The outcome event should be assessed in a blinded manner to prevent bias. The persons observing the outcome should be different from those recording and assessing the predictor variables. In cases where the person assessing the predictor variable is also the one determining the outcome, observation bias can occur. This occurs when the people doing the study are aware of the assessment and the outcome and may change their definitions of the outcome or the assessment of the patient. This may occur in subtle ways yet still produce dramatic alterations in the results.

The subjects should be carefully selected. There should be a range of ages, ethnic groups, and genders of patients. The selection of a sample should include the process of selection, inclusion and exclusion criteria, and the clinical and demographic characteristics of the sample. Patient selection should be free of bias and there should be a wide spectrum of patient and disease characteristics. The study should determine the population of patients to which this rule will be applied. This gives the clinician the parameters for application of the rule. In the Ottawa ankle rules, there were no children under age 18 and therefore initially the rule could not be applied to them. Subsequent studies found that the rule applied equally well in children as young as 12.

The setting should also be described. Studies that are done only in a specialized setting will result in referral bias. In these cases, the rules developed may not apply in settings where physicians are not as academic or where the patient base has a broader spectrum of the target disorder. A rule that is validated in a specialized setting must be further validated in more diverse community settings. The original Ottawa ankle rule was derived and validated in both a university-teaching-hospital emergency department and a community hospital. The results were the same in both settings.

The sample size and number of outcome events should be large enough to prevent a Type II error. If there are too few outcome events, the rule will not be particularly accurate or precise and have wide confidence intervals for sensitivity or specificity. As a rule of thumb, there should be at least 10–20 desired outcome events for each independent variable. For example, if we want to study a prediction rule for cervical spine fracture in injured patients and have five predictor variables, we should have at least 50 and preferably 100 significant cervical spine fractures. A Type I error can also occur if there are too many predictor variables compared to the number of outcome events. If the rule worked perfectly, it would have a sensitivity of 100%, the definition of a perfect screening rule. This rule will rule out disease if it is completely negative. It will not rule in disease if positive. However since a sample size of 50 patients without cervical spine fractures is pretty small, the confidence intervals on this would go from 94% to 100%. If the outcome is not too bad, this is a reasonable rule. However if the outcome were possible paralysis, missing up to 6% of the patients with a potential for this outcome would be disastrous. This would prevent that rule from being universally used.

The mathematical model used to create the rule should be adequately described. The most common methods are recursive partitioning and classification and regression trees (CART) analysis. In each of these, the various predictor variables are modeled to see how well they can predict the ultimate outcome. In the recursive-partitioning method, the most powerful predictor variable is tested to see which of the positive patients are identified. Those patients are then removed from the analysis and the rest are tested with the next most powerful predictor variable. This is continued until all patients with the desired outcome are identified. The CART methodology, a form of logistic regression analysis, is much more complex and beyond the scope of this text.

There must be complete follow-up, ideally 100% of all patients enrolled in the study. If fewer patients are followed to completion of the study, the effect of patient loss should be assessed. This can be done with a best case/worst case analysis, which will give a range of values of sensitivity and specificity within which the rule can be expected to operate.

The rule should be sensible. This means it must be clinically reasonable, easy to use, and with a clear-cut course of action if the rule is positive or negative. A nine-point checklist for determining which heart-attack patient should go to the intensive care unit and which can be admitted to a lower level of care is not likely to be useful to most clinicians. There are just too many variables for anyone to remember. One way of making it useful is to incorporate it into the order form for admitting patients to these units, or creating a clinical pathway with a written checklist that incorporates the rule and must be used prior to admission to the cardiac unit.

For most physicians, rules that give probability of the outcome are less useful than those that tell the physician there are specific things that must be done when a certain outcome is achieved. However, future physicians, who will be better versed in the techniques of Bayesian medical decision making, will have an easier time using rules that give probability of disease rather than specific outcome actions. They will also be better able to explain the rationale for a particular decision to their patients. The Wells criteria for risk-stratifying patients in whom you suspect deep vein thrombosis (DVT) are an example of probabilities as the outcome of the rule.[3] The final outcome classifies patients into high, moderate, and low levels of risk for having a DVT. Each of these has a probability that is pretty well defined through the use of experimental studies of diagnostic tests.

The rule should be tested in a prospective manner. Ideally this should be done with a population and setting different than that used in the derivation set. This is a test for misclassification when the rule is put into effect prospectively. If the rule still functions in the same manner that it did in the derivation set, it has passed the test of applicability. This is where provider training in the use of the rule can be studied. How long does it take to learn to use the rule? If it takes too long, most providers in community settings will be reluctant to take the time to learn it. They will feel that the rule is something that will be only marginally useful in a few instances. Providers who have a stake in development of the rule are more likely to use it better and more effectively than those who are grudgingly goaded into using it by an outside agency.

---

[3] P. S. Wells, D. R. Anderson, J. Bormanis, F. Guy, M. Mitchell, L. Gray, C. Clement, K. S. Robinson & B. Lewandowski. Value of assessment of pretest probability of deep-vein thrombosis in clinical management. *Lancet* 1997; 350: 1795–1798.

It must still be tested in other sites and with other practitioners in order to determine the effect of clinical use in other sites. This testing should be done in a prospective manner. As part of this testing, the use of the rule should be able to reduce unnecessary medical care. This should result in automatic cost-effectiveness of the rule. A rule designed to reduce the number of x-rays taken of the neck, if correctly applied, will result in less x-rays ordered. There is no question that there will be an overall cost saving. Of course, if there is a complex and lengthy training process involved some of the cost savings will be transferred to the training program, making the rule less effective. Of course, if the rule doesn't work well, it may lead to malpractice suits because of errors in patient care making it even more expensive.

Critical appraisal of prediction rules

(1) Is the study valid?
   (a) Were all important predictors included in the derivation process? The model should include all those factors that physicians might take into account when making the diagnosis.
   (b) Were all important predictors present in a significant proportion of the study population? The predictor variables should be those that are common. No specific percentage is required, but clinical judgment should decide this.
   (c) Were all the outcome events and predictors clearly defined? The description of the outcomes and predictors should be easily reproducible by anyone in clinical practice.
   (d) Were those assessing the outcome event blinded to the presence of the predictors and those assessing the presence of predictors blinded to the outcome event?
   (e) Was the sample size adequate and did it include adequate outcome events? There should be at least 10–20 cases of the desired outcome, patients with a positive diagnosis, for each of the predictor variables being tested.
   (f) Does the rule make clinical sense? The rule should not fly in the face of current clinical practice otherwise it will not be used.
(2) What are the results?
   (a) How well do clinicians agree on the presence or absence of the findings incorporated into the rule? Inter- and intra-rater agreement and kappa values with confidence intervals should be given.
   (b) What is the sensitivity and specificity of the prediction rule? The rule should lead to a high LR+, ideally > 10, and a low LR−, ideally < 0.1.

    (c) How well does the rule predict the outcome? Depending on the severity of the outcome, the rule should find patients with the desired outcome almost all of the time. Is the post-test probability for the rule high in all clinical scenarios?

(3) How can I apply the results to my patients?

    (a) Are the patients in the study similar enough to my patient?

    (b) Can I efficiently and effectively use the rule with my patients?

30

Decision analysis and quantifying patient values

Chance favors only the prepared mind.

Louis Pasteur (1822–1895)

Learning objectives

In this chapter you will learn:
- the function of each part of a decision tree
- how to use a decision tree in conjunction with the uncertainties of a diagnostic test to assist in decision making for patients
- different ways of quantifying patient values using linear rating scales, time trade-off, and standard gamble
- how to define and use QALYs

Introduction

How do physicians choose between various treatment options? For the individual physician treating a single patient, it is a matter of obtaining the relevant clinical information to make a diagnosis. This is followed by treatment as set down in some sort of clinical practice guideline or from the results of a well-done RCT. However, these results may have a high degree of uncertainty with large 95% CI and may not consider the patient's preferences or values. To help deal with these issues there are some statistical techniques that we can apply to quantify the process.

To put the concept of risk into perspective, we must briefly go back a few hundred years. Girolamo Cardano (1545) and Blaise Pascal (1660) noted that in making a decision that involved any risk there were two elements that were completely unique and yet both were required to make the decision. These were the objective facts about the likelihood of the risk and the subjective views on the part of the risk taker about the utility of the outcomes involved in the risk. This second factor leads to the usefulness or expected value of the outcomes expected from the risk. This involved weighing the gains and losses involved in taking each of the potential risks and attaching a value to each outcome. Pascal created the first recorded decision tree when deciding whether or not to believe in God.

The Port Royal text on logic (1662) noted that people who are "pathologically risk-averse" make all their choices based only upon the consequences and will refuse to make a choice if there is even the remotest possibility of an adverse consequence. They do not consider the statistical likelihood of that particular consequence in making a decision. Later, in the early eighteenth century, Daniel Bernoulli noted that those who make choices based only upon the probability of an outcome without any regard for the quality of the risk involved with that particular outcome would be considered foolhardy. Most of us are somewhere in between, which takes us to the modern era in medical decision making.

There is a systematic way in which the components of decision making can be incorporated to make a clinical decision and determine the best course of therapy. This statistical method for determining the best path to diagnosis and treatment is called expected-values decision making. Given the probability of each of the risks and benefits of treatment, which strategy will produce the greatest overall benefit for the patient? The theory of expected-values decision making is based on the assumption that there is a risk associated with every treatment option and uncertainty associated with each risk.

By using the technique known as instrumental rationality the clinician can calculate the treatment strategy which will produce the most benefit for the average or typical patient. The clinician quantifies each treatment strategy by assigning a numerical value to each outcome called the **utility** and multiplying that value by the **probability** of the occurrence of that outcome. The utilities and probabilities can be varied to account for variation in patient values and likelihood of outcomes.

The vocabulary of expected-values decision making: expected value = utility × probability

The probability is a number from 0 to 1 that represents the likelihood of a particular outcome of interest. You must know as much about each outcome of the various treatment options as possible. The probability of each outcome (P) comes from clinical research studies of patient populations. Ideally, they will have the same or similar characteristics as the patient or population that is being treated. These can also come from systematic reviews of many clinical studies or meta-analyses. They are usually not exact, but are only a best approximation, and ought to come with 95% confidence intervals attached.

There must then be an assignment of a value or utility (U) to each outcome that quantifies the desirability or undesirability of that outcome. A utility of 1 is assigned to a perfect outcome, usually meaning a complete cure or perfect health. A utility of 0 is usually thought of as a totally unacceptable outcome, usually reserved for death. Intermediate utility values are assigned to other outcomes. The quality of life resulting from each intermediate outcome will be less than expected with a total cure but more than death. This outcome state may be wholly or partially unbearable due to treatment side effects or adverse effects of the illness. A numerical value for utility between 1 and 0 is then assigned to this outcome. Recent studies of patient values for outcomes of cardiopulmonary resuscitation (CPR) revealed that some patients will give negative scores to outcomes such as surviving in a persistent vegetative state and being maintained on a ventilator. This means that they consider these outcomes to be worse than death. As research into the development of patient values has continued, it is clear that there are many outcomes that are valued as less than zero. A recent example was a study that requested patients to determine their values in stroke care. Being alive but with a severe disability was rated as less than zero.

A decision tree illustrating treatment options can then be constructed, as seen from the following clinical example. Thrombolytic therapy, the use of clot-dissolving medication called t-PA, can be used to treat acute embolic or thrombotic cerebrovascular accident, a CVA, or stroke due to a blood clot in the brain. Consider a patient who is a 60-year-old man with sudden onset of weakness of the right arm and leg associated with inability to speak. A stroke is suspected and the physician wants to try this new form of treatment to dissolve the suspected clot in the artery supplying the left parietal area of the brain. A CT scan shows no apparent bleeding in the brain. There are two options for the patient at this point. Thrombolytic therapy (t-PA) can be given to dissolve the clot or the patient can be treated using traditional methods of anticoagulation and intensive physical rehabilitation therapy.

The first step is to list the possible outcomes for each therapy. For purposes of the exercise we will greatly simplify this process and assume that there are only three possible outcomes. Thrombolytic therapy can result in one of two outcomes, either a cure with complete resolution of the symptoms or death from intracranial hemorrhage, bleeding into the substance of the brain. Traditional medical therapy will result in some improvement in the clinical symptoms in all patients but leave all of them with some residual deficit.

Next, find the probabilities of each of the outcomes. Outcome probabilities are obtained from studies of populations of patients with similarities for both the stroke and risk factors for bleeding. The probability of death from thrombolyic therapy is P_d, for complete cure it is P_c, which is equal to $1 - P_d$, and for partial improvement with medical therapy in this example only, the probability is 1.

The next step is to assign a utility to each of the outcomes. The utility of complete cure is 1, death is 0, and the unknown residual chronic disability is U_x. These values are obtained from studies of patient attitudes toward each of the outcomes in question and will be discussed in more detail shortly.

Mechanics of constructing a decision tree

There are three components to any decision tree. Nodes are junctures where something happens. There are three types of nodes: decision, probability or chance, and stationary. A decision node is the point where the clinician or patient must choose between two or more possible options. A probability node is the point where one of two or more possible outcomes can occur by chance. A stationary node is the point where the patient starts, their initial presentation, or finishes, their ultimate outcome. The symbols for the nodes are shown in Fig. 30.1.

Fig. 30.1 Symbols used in a decision tree.

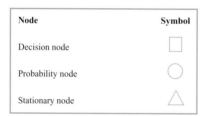

Node	Symbol
Decision node	□
Probability node	○
Stationary node	△

Arms connect the nodes. Each arm represents one treatment or management strategy. Figure 30.2 shows a simple decision tree for our problem. In this simplified decision tree for stroke, one arm represents thrombolytic therapy and the other represents standard medical therapy. The thrombolytic therapy arm has a probability node and then two other arms come from that. These are cure or death.

In the simplified stroke-therapy example calculate the expected values in each arm of the tree by multiplying the utility and probability and summing their values around each node. Therefore, for thrombolytic therapy the expected value E will equal $1(1 - P_d) + 0(P_d)$. For standard medical therapy, since the utility of chronic residual disability is U_x and since all patients have this intermediate outcome, the expected value E is U_x. The patient should always prefer the strategy that leads to the highest expected value. In this example, the patient would always choose standard medical treatment for stroke if the expected value for this arm is 100%, which will occur if $U_x = 1$ and if there is a measurable death rate for treating with thrombolytic therapy, making the expected value of the thrombolytic arm $100\% - P_d$.

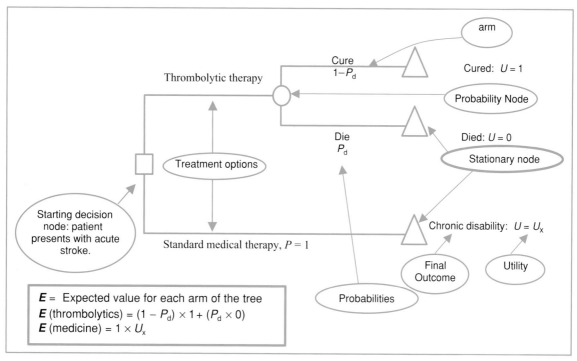

Fig. 30.2 Decision tree for thrombolytic therapy.

However, the value of a lifetime of chronic neurological disability is not 100%, and lets assume for this example that it is 0.9. This means that living with chronic neurological disability is somehow equated with living 90% of a normal life. Recalculating the expected value of each arm will determine what probability of death from thrombolytics would result in wanting to choose thrombolytics over medical therapy. We must solve the equation $1 - P_d = 0.9$. Since the value of E for the medicine arm is now 0.9, thrombolytic therapy should be the chosen modality as long as $P_d < 0.10$.

Disagreeable events such as side effects may reduce the value of a given arm. For example, if the experience of getting thrombolytics were unpleasant, that may lead to a utility reduction of 0.01, changing the expected value of that arm to $1 - 0.01 - P_d$. In the example, and if U_x were still 0.9, thrombolytics would be favored as long as $P_d < 0.09$.

In reality, there are more outcomes than shown in this example. For the thrombolytic-therapy arm, the clot can be dissolved successfully, there can be residual deficit, or the patient may have an intracranial bleed resulting in death, or have partial improvement but be left with a residual deficit. The degree of deficit can also be divided into different categories, for example using the Modified Rankin Scale to create six criteria for outcomes. The thrombolytic arm of the decision tree would then look as shown in Fig. 30.3, where P_c is the probability of

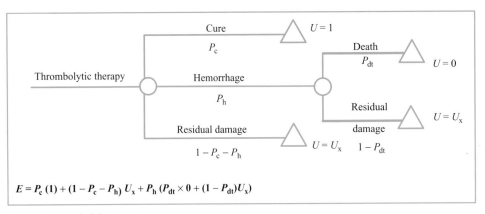

$$E = P_c\,(1) + (1 - P_c - P_h)\,U_x + P_h\,(P_{dt} \times 0 + (1 - P_{dt})U_x)$$

Fig. 30.3 Expanded decision tree for thrombolytic therapy.

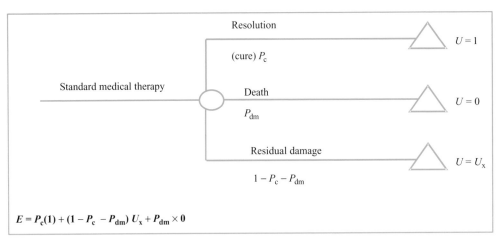

$$E = P_c(1) + (1 - P_c - P_{dm})\,U_x + P_{dm} \times 0$$

Fig. 30.4 Expanded decision tree for standard medical therapy.

cure and P_h the probability of hemorrhage. The probability of death due to hemorrhage is P_{dt} and for residual damage due to hemorrhage is $1 - P_{dt}$. For residual damage we will use the same utility, $U_x = 0.9$ as in the previous example for the standard-therapy arm.

Similarly, standard medical treatment can result in spontaneous cure or death. This will result in that side of the decision tree looking like Fig. 30.4. Here P_c is the probability of complete resolution and P_{dm} the probability of death.

The reason that a decision tree is needed at all is because while there is an increase in complete cures with thrombolytic therapy there is also an increase in intracranial hemorrhage leading to residual damage or death. Simply balancing the two, using NNTB for cure and NNTH for death due to hemorrhage, ignores the patient's values for each of these outcomes. This is especially true when one or both of the alternative outcomes can lead to a lifetime of disability.

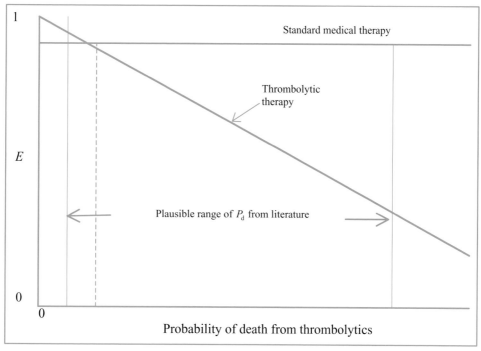

Fig. 30.5 One-way sensitivity analysis of a simplified hypothetical stroke therapy model.

Sensitivity analysis

Sensitivity analysis is a way to deal with imprecision in the data used to create the decision tree. We have discussed that this is true of almost all data obtained from the medical literature and insist that the results of any kind of study have appropriate confidence intervals to give the uncertainty of the result. A sensitivity analysis tests the "robustness" of the conclusions over a range of different values of probabilities for each branch of the decision tree. Sensitivity analysis asks what would happen to the expected value of thrombolytics against standard medical management if we varied the probability or utility of any of the outcomes. One simple way of doing this it to take the 95% confidence intervals of the probabilities and use them as the extreme used in the sensitivity analysis. In other words, recalculate the expected values of each arm of the tree using first the upper and then the lower 95% CI value as the new probability for one arm.

If there is very little difference between the expected values of the two treatments being compared, then a slight change in the probabilities assigned to each arm could easily alter the direction of the decision. In that case, if the values of the probabilities are off by just a little bit, the entire result will change and the patient and physician will have little useful information regarding the relative merits of the two treatments, or which one is superior.

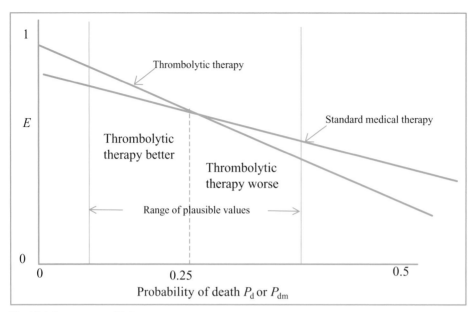

Fig. 30.6 One-way sensitivity
analysis of a more complex
hypothetical model for stroke
therapy.

Sensitivity analysis determines how much variation in the final outcome will result from plausible variations in each of the input variables. One-way sensitivity analysis changes only one parameter at a time (Figs. 30.5, 30.6). Multi-way sensitivity analysis looks for the variable that causes the biggest change in the value of the overall model. Then the analysis changes all those assumptions that are "very sensitive" to see what happens to the model. Finally, a curve is drawn to show what happens to the expected values when the two most "sensitive" variables are changed (Fig. 30.7).

The results of a sensitivity analysis can be graphed, showing the effect on the final outcomes with a change in each of these values. Expected values are usually calculated for each branch of the decision tree as quality-adjusted life years (QALYs). A QALY equals $E \times$ life expectancy, where E is the expected value calculated from the decision tree.

In the decision tree on thrombolytic therapy and stroke, adding the uncertainty associated with the results of a CT scan which checks for early signs of intracranial bleeding as the cause of the stroke, complicates the previous example of thrombolytic therapy in stroke. This is because the presence of a small amount of bleeding is difficult to diagnose on the CT scan, and if thrombolytic therapy is given in the presence of even a very small bleed the likelihood of a serious and possibly fatal intracranial hemorrhagic stroke increases. Since the presence of a bleed is not always detected, the CT is not always a valid test and the construction of the decision tree must incorporate the possibilities of incorrect interpretations of the CT. The sensitivity and specificity of the CT in stroke

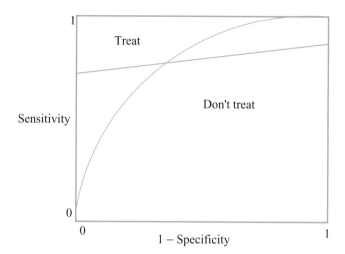

Fig. 30.7 Two-way sensitivity analysis of a complex model of treatment for stroke based on the results of the CT scan. (Yes, the graph of sensitivity vs. 1 – specificity is the ROC curve.)

patients would help to calcluate the probabilities associated with these additions to the tree.

It is now possible to determine the probability of giving thrombolytic therapy when there actually is a bleed and the CT scan is read incorrectly causing a false negative CT, and of not giving the therapy when there is truly no bleed and yet one is read on the CT scan, a false positive CT. The ultimate decision should still be based on whichever strategy gives the highest final expected utility. Figure 30.8 shows this more complex but also more realistic decision tree of thrombolytic therapy in stroke.

Reality check! (disclaimer)

This is not a model of what doctors actually do now at the bedside but a mathematical modeling technique that can help doctors and patients find the best possible way of making complex medical decisions. It can be used to create health policy or to determine the best strategy for a practice guideline. In actuality, physicians have trouble applying decision analysis to individual patients even when there is a clearly superior treatment. Also, the model requires that the outcomes be put into a few discrete categories when in fact there are many outcomes that are not as clear-cut as in the model.

In this example, thrombolytic therapy complications can vary from serious to mild in severity. Chronic disability can also vary from a mild to a constant disabling deficit, which can be very severe and last for only a brief period of time and then spontaneously resolve. Standard medical treatment may actually result in more patients having only a small amount of residual deficit. On the other

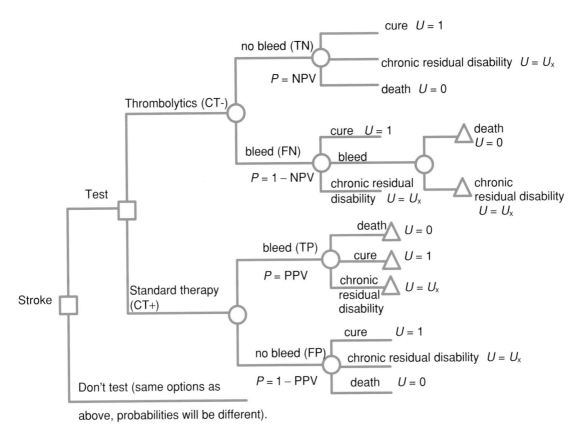

Fig. 30.8 Complex decision tree incorporating the use of CT scans in decision making for stroke. The probabilities have been omitted for clarity.

hand, thrombolytic treatment may result in more cases with increased residual deficit or death, both unsatisfactory outcomes. This can occur even if a "cure" is obtained in a few more patients in the thrombolytic group. You must include all of these outcomes to make this a more realistic model of the situation. Finally, any decision analysis must include a reasonable "time horizon" over which the outcomes should be assessed.

Computers can be used to show patients how their personal values for each outcome will change the expected value of each treatment. There are computer programs that have been developed to assist patients in making difficult decisions about whether or not to have prostate cancer screening and what options to take if the screening test is positive, but they are not yet commercially available and are currently used only in research programs. This is clearly a direction for future research in decision-making theory. The development of user-friendly computerized interfaces will help improve the quality of patient decisions. This will never make the doctor obsolete. The doctor must continue to be able to educate his or her patient about the consequences of each action and describe the objective reality of each disease state and treatment options for them so that the patient can make appropriate decisions on the utility they want to assign to each outcome. In short, the role of the health-care provider is to give their patients the facts and probability of the outcomes and help the patient decide on their utility for each outcome.

Threshold approach to decision making

Earlier, in Chapter 26, we talked about the treatment and testing thresholds. The threshold approach to testing and treatment can use decision trees to determine when diagnostic testing should be done. Consider the situation of a patient complaining of shortness of breath in whom you suspect a pulmonary embolism or blood clot in the lungs. Should you order a pulmonary angiogram test in which dye is injected into the pulmonary arteries? The test itself is very uncomfortable, causes some complications, and can rarely cause death. There are basically three options:

(1) Treat based on clinical examination and give the patient an anticoagulant without doing the test. Do this if the probability of disease is above the Treatment Threshold.
(2) Test first and treat only if the test is positive.
(3) Neither test nor treat if one is very certain that the disease is not present. Do this if the probability of disease is below the Testing Threshold.

The treatment threshold is the probability of disease above which a physician should initiate treatment for the disease without first doing the test for the disease. This is the level above which, testing will produce an unacceptable number of false negatives and the patient would then be denied the benefits of treatment. "The pretest probability of disease is so great that I will treat regardless of the results of the test."

The testing threshold is the probability of a disease above which a physician should test before initiating treatment for that disease. This is the probability below which, there are an unacceptable number of false positives and patients would then be unnecessarily exposed to the side effects of treatment. "The pretest probability of disease is so small that I will not treat even if the test is positive."

If the post-test probability of disease after a positive test, the positive predictive value, is still below the treatment threshold, don't start treatment. It may take another test to decide if the patient has the disease or not. If the post-test probability after a negative test, the false reassurance rate, falls below the testing threshold, it was a worthwhile test and the patient does not need treatment. It took the probability of disease from a value of probability at which testing should precede treating, to one at which neither treatment nor further testing is beneficial. In essence this means that disease has been ruled out. Decision trees are another way to determine the cutoffs for testing and treating.

In order to complete the decision tree for our example of thrombolytic therapy and stroke, the posterior probability that an intracranial bleed has occurred when the CT scan has been read as negative must be known. This requires knowing the sensitivity and specificity of the CT scan and the prevalence of intracranial bleeding. If the post-test probability of a bleed is low, thrombolytic treatment will be better and a worsening bleed is very unlikely with t-PA, making thrombolytic therapy more beneficial and conversely standard medical therapy less beneficial. If the post-test probability of a bleed is high, standard treatment is likely to be better, since thrombolytic therapy is more likely to lead to increased bleeding in the brain.

Both of the thresholds are dependent on prevalence or pretest probability! At a low pretest probability, even a positive CT ought not make a difference since there would be many false positives and you shouldn't do the test at all since you are more likely to have a false positive and unnecessarily give thrombolytic therapy to someone who won't benefit. At a high pretest probability, even a negative CT ought not make a difference since there would be many false negatives and you shouldn't do the test at all since you are more likely to have a false negative and withhold thrombolytic therapy from someone who would benefit. An example would be a person with known atrial fibrillation, not on anticoagulants, who had a sudden onset of severe left hemiparesis without a headache. Changing one fact of this pattern would change the probability of a bleed and the final decision. The consequence of giving thrombolytic therapy to someone with a bleed makes the CT worthwhile, since treating anyone with a positive scan will result in a real tragedy.

At a high pretest probability the clinical picture is so strong that the test shouldn't be done at all since a false negative is much more likely than a true negative leading to treatment of someone with a potential bleed. An example would be someone with a sudden onset of the worst headache of their life with their only deficit being slight weakness of their non-dominant hand. Here the potential of giving thrombolytic therapy to someone with a bleed is too high and the projected benefit not great enough.

Mathematical expression of threshold approach to testing

There are formulas for calculating these thresholds, but please don't memorize them.

Test threshold =

$$\frac{(\text{FP rate})\,(\text{risk of inappropriate Rx}) + (\text{risk of test})}{(\text{FP rate})(\text{risk of inappropriate Rx}) + (\text{TP rate})(\text{benefit of appropriate Rx})}$$

Treatment threshold =

$$\frac{(\text{TN rate})\,(\text{risk of inappropriate Rx}) - (\text{risk of test})}{(\text{TN rate})(\text{risk of inappropriate Rx}) + (\text{FN rate})(\text{benefit of appropriate Rx})}$$

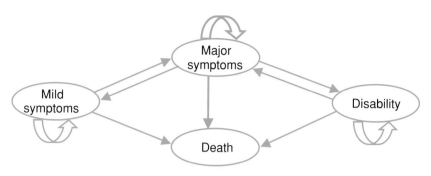

Fig. 30.9 Markov model schematic. From F. A. Sonnenberg & J. R. Beck. Markov models in medical decision making: a practical guide. *Med. Decis. Making* 1993; 13: 322–338.

Determining the risks and benefits of incorrect diagnosis will set these thresholds. A false positive test resulting in unnecessary use of risky tests or treatments such as cardiac catheterization or cardiac drugs or a false negative test resulting in unnecessarily withholding beneficial tests or treatments are both adverse outcomes of testing. You can substitute different values of test characteristics, different positive and negative predictive values, and different values of the benefit and risk of treatment in a sensitivity analysis of the decision tree and determine what the effect of these changes will be on the utility of each treatment arm.

Markov models

Another method of making a decision analysis is through the use of Markov models. These consider the simultaneous interaction of all possible health states. A patient can be in only one health state at a time. The difficulty with these is that there must be some data on the average time a given individual patient spends in each health state. This is then weighted by considering the quality of life for each state.

Ovals are states of health associated with quality measures such as death ($U = 0$), complete health or cure ($U = 1$), and other outcomes (U varies from 0 to 1). Arrows are transitions between states or within a state and are attached to probabilities or the likelihood of changing states or remaining in the same state. This type of model is ideal for putting into a computer to get the final expected values. A Markov model of health decision making is diagrammed in Fig. 30.9.

Ethical issues

Finally, there are significant ethical issues raised by the use of decision trees and expected-values decision making. After performing a decision tree, one must place ethical values on the decisions. Issues of morality and fairness must be considered. When there are limited resources, is it more just to spend a large amount of resources for a small gain? Is a small gain defined as one affecting only a few people or one having only a small health benefit? Some of these questions can be answered using cost-effectiveness analyses and will be covered in the next chapter.

The use of a decision tree in making medical decisions can help the patient, provider, and society decide which treatment modality will be most just. Look for treatments that benefit the most people or have the largest overall improvement in health outcome. Ethical problems arise when a choice has to be made on whether to consider the best outcome from the perspective of a large population or the individual patient. If we take the perspective of the individual patient, how are we to know that the treatment will benefit that particular patient, the next patient, or the next 20 patients? Should we use the perspective of statistical significance ($P < 0.05$) or is it fairer to use NNTB? Is the decision up to each individual or should the decision be legislated by society?

Decision trees allow the provider, society, and the patient to decide which therapy is going to be the most beneficial for the most people. Whether decision trees are a mathematical expression of utilitarianism is a hotly debated issue among bioethicists.

Siegler's schema (Table 30.1) is useful for using these models in medical and ethical decision making. The basic perspectives of medical care within the traditional patient–physician relationship include medical indications, which are physician-directed, and patient preferences, which are patient-driven. Both of these are input variables in the decision tree. Current or added perspectives modify the decision and include quality of life, which considers the impact on the individual of high-technology interventions and contextual features, which are cultural, societal, family, religious or spiritual, community, and economic factors. These are all part of the discussion between the provider and the patient and form the basis of the provider–patient relationship.

Assessing patient values

Patient values must be incorporated into medical decision making and healthcare policies by providers, government, managed care organizations, and other decision makers. The output of decision trees is variable and ultimately is based on the patient preferences. We can measure and quantify patient values and use them in decision trees to help patients make difficult decisions.

Using unadjusted life expectancy or life years cannot compare various states of health in cases with the same number of years of life because they do not quantify the quality of those years. Quality-of-life scales or measures of status rated by others or by the patient themself include health status, functional status, well-being, or patient satisfaction. Common scales are the Activities of Daily Living or ADL and the Arthritis Activity Scale used in rheumatoid arthritis. These

Table 30.1. Seigler's schema for ethical decision making in medicine

Ethical concern	Ethical principle
MEDICAL INDICATION What is the best treatment? What are the alternatives?	BENEFICENCE The duty to promote the good of the patient
PATIENT PREFERENCES What does the patient want? What outcome does the patient prefer?	AUTONOMY Respect for the patient's right to self-determination
QUALITY OF LIFE What impact will the proposed treatment or lack of it have on the patient's life?	NON-MALEFICENCE The duty not to inflict harm or injury
SOCIECONOMIC ISSUES (CONTEXTUAL FEATURES) What does the patient want within their own socioeconomic milieu? What are the needs of the patient's society?	JUSTICE The patient is given what is their "due"

Source: From A. R. Jonsen, M. Siegler & W. J. Winslade. *Clinical Ethics.* 3rd edn. New York: McGraw-Hill, 1992. pp. 1–10.

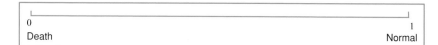

Fig. 30.10 Linear rating scale. Simply measure the patient's mark on the scale as a percentage of the entire length of the scale.

are difficult to use in a quantitative manner. This discussion will present several standardized quantitative measures of patient preference that can be used to measure the relative preference that a patient has for one or another outcome.

The linear-rating-scale method utilizes a 10-cm visual analog scale (VAS) with one end being zero or death and the other end one or a completely healthy life (Fig. 30.10.) The patient is asked "where on this scale would you rate your life if you had to live with chronic disease?" In the t-PA in stroke example that would be the residual neurological deficit from the stroke syndrome. The resultant value of U is the percentage of the total length of the line.

The time trade-off method for this example asks "suppose you have 10 years left to live with chronic residual neurological disability from the stroke. If you could trade those 10 years for x years without any residual neurological deficit, what is the smallest number of years you would trade to be deficit-free?" Since it is a direct question, there is a lot of variability attached to the answer between patients.

Fig. 30.11 Standard gamble.

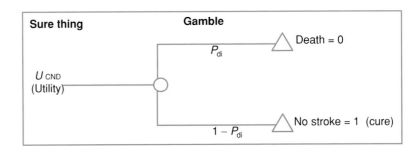

The standard-gamble or utility method attempts to find out how much risk the patient is willing to take. The patient is told to consider an imaginary situation in which you will give them a pill that will instantly cure their stroke. However, there is a risk in that it occasionally causes instant but painless death. If there were 100% cure and 0% death, every patient would always take the pill. On the other hand, if there were 0% cure and 100% death no one would ever take the pill unless the patient is extremely depressed and considers their life totally worthless. Continue to change the cure-to-death ratio until the person cannot decide which course of action to take. This is the point of indifference. "At what level of risk would you be indifferent to the outcome?" In our stroke example, the sure thing is chronic residual neurological deficit and the gamble is no deficit or death. Set up a "mini decision tree" and solve for the utility of living with chronic neurological deficit. This is diagrammed in Fig. 30.11, where:

   P_{di} is the probability of death at the point of indifference, the information learned when using the standard gamble.

   $U_{CND} = (0 \times P_{di}) + (1 - P_{di}) 1$ or

   $U_{CND} = 1 - P_{di}$. This is the value of living with a chronic stroke syndrome that the patient assigns as an outcome through a standard gamble.

QALYs are the units of the standardized measure that combines the quality of life and life expectancy. It is the output measure that is commonly used in decision analyses. It combines total life expectancy with a quantitative measure of patient value. A decision analysis can determine how many QALYs result from each strategy. The QALY is determined by taking the normal life expectancy and multiplying it by the patient value or utility of 1 year of life.

Different values will be obtained from each method used to measure patient values. The linear rating scale measures the quality of functionality of life, the time trade-off introduces a choice between two certainties, and the standard gamble introduces probability and willingness to take risks into the equation.

Attitudes toward risk and framing effects

Attitudes toward risk vary with individuals and at different periods of time during their lives. Patient values can be related to special events such as the birth of a child or marriage, habits such as smoking or drinking, or age. The length of time involved in the trade-off will be different if asked of a younger or older person since a younger person may be less likely to be willing to trade off years. Also personal preferences related to the amount of risk a person is generally willing to take in other activities, such as sky-diving, play a role in determining patient values. Since values tend to be very personal, providers should not be the ones to assign these values. Values based on the provider's own risk-taking behavior will not accurately measure the values of their patient.

How the questions are worded or framed will influence the answer to the question. Asking what probability of death a patient is willing to accept will likely give a lower number than asking what probability of survival they are willing to accept. The framing of the questions may reflect the risk-taking attitude of the provider. A patient is more likely to prefer a treatment if told that 90% of those treated are alive 5 years later than if told that 10% are dead after the same time period, even though the outcome is exactly the same. The feelings aroused by the idea of death are more likely to lead to the rejection of an option framed from the perspective of death when this same option would be endorsed in the opposite framing of the choice, the perspective of survival. Although apparently inconsistent and irrational, this effect is a recurring phenomenon. This irrationality is not due to lack of knowledge since physicians respond no differently than non-physician patients.

Probability means different things to different people. This is related to how individuals relate to numbers and how well people understand probabilities. In general, people (including physicians and other health-care providers) do not understand probabilities very well. Physicians tend to give qualitative rather than quantitative expressions of risk in many different and ambiguous ways. For example, what does a "rare risk" of death mean? Does it mean 1% of the time or one in a million? From the patient perspective, a rare event happens 100% of the time if it happens to them.

Finally, patient values change when they have the disease in question as opposed to when they do not. Patients who are having a stroke are much more willing to accept moderate disability than well persons who are asked about the abstract notion of disability if they were to get a stroke. This means that stroke patients assign a higher value to the utility (U) of residual deficit than well people asked in the abstract. Most clinical studies of these issues that are now being done have quality-of-life and patient-preference measures attached to possible outcomes. They should help clarify the effects of variations in patient values on the outcomes of decision trees.

31

Cost-effectiveness analysis

When gold argues the cause, eloquence is important.

Publilius Syrus (first century BC): Moral Sayings

Learning objectives

In this chapter you will learn:

- the process of evaluating an article on cost-effectiveness
- the concepts of marginal cost and marginal benefit
- how to use these tools to help make medical decisions for a population
- how to calculate a simple cost-effectiveness problem and evaluate the cost-effectiveness of a specific therapy

The cost of medical care is constantly rising. The health-care provider of the future will seek to use the most cost-efficient methods to care for her or his patients. Cost-effectiveness analysis can be used to help choose between treatment options for an individual patient or for large populations. Governments and managed care organizations use cost-effectiveness techniques to justify their coverage for various health-care "products." Drug companies often produce cost-effectiveness studies to show that their more expensive drugs are actually cheaper in the long run by being cheaper to administer or by saving future health-care costs. Health-care providers, policy makers, and insurance-plan administrators must be able to evaluate the validity of these claims through the critical analysis of cost-effectiveness studies.

How do we decide if a test or treatment is worth it?

If one treatment costs less and is clearly more effective than the alternative option, there is no question about which treatment to use. Similarly, if the treatment costs more and is clearly less effective, there will also be no question about which to use. Treatment with the most effective treatment modality would proceed for the patient and that would also save money in the process. More often than not, however, the situation arises for which one therapy costs much more and is marginally more effective than a much less expensive therapy or the converse, where one therapy is clearly less effective but is also less expensive. Cost-effectiveness analysis gives us the data to answer the question "how much more will this extra effectiveness cost or how much more will use of the less effective therapy ultimately cost?"

This is a serious ethical issue for society and relates to a concept called **opportunity costs**. If one very expensive treatment is beneficial for a few people and we decide to pay for that treatment, we may be unable to afford other equally or more effective treatments that may help many more people. There is only so much money to go around and you can't spend the same dollar twice! If we fund bone marrow transplants for questionably beneficial indications, we may not be able to pay for hypertension screening leading to treatment that could prevent the need for certain other high cost therapies like kidney or heart organ transplants in the future. A bone marrow transplant may prolong one life by 6 years, yet result in loss of funds for hypertension screening and treatment programs which could prevent six new deaths from uncontrolled hypertension in that same period. Cost-effectiveness analysis should be able to tell if the cost of a new therapy is "worth it" or if we should be paying for some other, cheaper, and possibly more effective therapy.

Cost rationing has always been a contentious issue in medicine. The wealthy can get any medical procedure done regardless of efficacy or cost while the poor must wait for available services. This is known as de-facto rationing and is manifested by long waiting times in a municipal hospital emergency department or for an appointment to be examined by a specialist or get diagnostic studies done. In the United States, there may be reduced availability of certain drugs to patients in some managed care organizations, on Medicaid and certainly to uninsured working people who cannot afford to pay for that drug out of their own pockets. The State of Oregon used a type of cost-effectiveness analysis to decide what services the State Medicaid program should cover. We are constantly making value judgments over how we as a society will spend our money. The ethical issues will be left to the politicians and ethicists to discuss. This chapter will present the tools needed to evaluate studies of cost-effectiveness.

Cost-effectiveness studies can be very complex to evaluate. On the most basic level, they simply add up all the costs of a particular procedure, subtract from them the cost of the comparison procedure that is in current use, and divide by the benefit, usually the number of additional QALYs obtained by using the new procedure. These are the same QALYs that were calculated in the previous chapter on Expected Values Decision Making. However, the manner in which the analysis is set up will have an enormous impact on what kind of result will be obtained. It is difficult to do a good and fair cost analysis and relatively simple to do a bad and often biased one. Therefore it is up to the reader to apply a few simple rules when reading a cost analysis. If these rules are followed, you can be fairly sure the analysis is relatively fair and usually valid.

Guidelines for assessing an economic analysis of clinical care

Was a broad enough viewpoint adopted?

Is there a specified point of view, either a hospital, health insurance entity, ministry of health, or preferably society as a whole, from which the costs and effects are being viewed?[1] The viewpoint should be given from the perspective of who is paying for the treatment and who is affected by the decision outcome of what to treat and not treat. Often these studies compare usual fee for service or third-party insurance against managed-care costs. However, the comparison may simply be for the costs of the treatments only without a specific viewpoint on who is paying for them or how much is being reimbursed.

There is a disconnect between costs and charges in health-care finances because of the large amount of uncompensated and negotiated care that is delivered. This must be considered in any economic analysis. Costs are the amount of money that is required to initiate and run a particular intervention. Charges are the amount of money that is going to be requested from the payors. It is disingenuous to use charges since they always overestimate the costs. However, when using simple costs only, the cost of treating non-insured patients must be factored into the accounting.

The different programs being compared must be adequately described. It should be possible from reading the article's methods to set up the same program in any comparable setting. This requires a full description of the process of setting up the program, the costs and effects of the program, and how these were measured.

Were all the relevant clinical strategies compared?

Does the analysis compare well-defined alternative courses of action? The comparison between treatment options must be specified. Typically two treatment options or treatment as opposed to non-treatment are considered in a cost-effectiveness analysis. The treatment options ought to be those that are in

---

1 Adapted with permission from the User's Guide to the Medical Literature, published by *JAMA* (see Bibliography).

common use by the bulk of physicians in a particular field and not just fringe practitioners. Using treatments that are no longer in common use will give a biased result to the analysis.

Was clinical effectiveness established?

The program's effectiveness should have been validated. There should be hard evidence from well-done randomized clinical trials to show that the intervention is effective, and this should be explicitly stated. Where not previously done, a systematic review or meta-analysis should be performed as part of the analysis. A cost-effectiveness analysis should not be done based on the assumption that because we can do something it is good. If no RCT is available that looks at the relevant clinical question, observational studies can be used, but with the caveat that they are more prone to bias especially from confounding variables.

Were the costs measured accurately?

Does the analysis identify all the important and relevant costs and effects that could be important? Were credible measures selected for the costs and effects that were incorporated into the analysis? On the cost side this includes the actual costs of organization and setting up a program and continuing operations, additional costs to patient and family, costs outside the health-care system like time lost from work and decreased productivity, and intangible costs such as loss of pleasure or loss of companionship. These costs must be compared for both doing the intervention program and not doing the program but doing the alternatives.

On the effect side, the analysis should include "hard" clinical outcomes: mortality, morbidity, residual functional ability, quality of life and utility of life, and the effect on future resources. These include the availability of services and future costs of health care and other services incurred by extending life. For example, it may be fiscally better to allow people to continue to smoke since this will reduce their life span and save money on end-of-life care for those people who die prematurely. This doesn't mean we should encourage smoking.

The error made most often in performing cost-effectiveness analyses is the omission of consideration of opportunity costs that were referred to at the start of this chapter. If you pay for one therapeutic intervention you may not be able to pay for some other one. Cost-effectiveness analyses must include an analysis of these opportunity costs so that the reader can see what equivalent types of programs might need to be cut from the health-care budget in order to finance the new and presumably better intervention. Analyses that do not consider this issue are giving a biased view of the usefulness of the new program and keeping it out of the context of the most good for the greater society.

Table 31.1. Comparing inpatient vein stripping (IP Stripping) to outpatient injection (OP Injections) of varicose veins

Treatment	Outcomes			
	Cost to hospital per patient (indexed)	No further treatement needed	Support stockings needed	Further treatment needed
OP injections	9.77	78%	9%	13%
IP stripping	44.22	86%	11%	3%

What is the resulting cost or cost per unit health gained and is this gain impressive?

The marginal or incremental gain for both the costs and effects should be calculated. First, the degree of risk reduction is determined. On a superficial basis, a very simple way to do a quick cost-effectiveness analysis is with the number needed to treat to benefit (NNTB). This is the number of patients you must treat in order to achieve the desired effect in one additional patient. It is the inverse of the attributable risk reduction (ARR) between the two therapies. This is compared to the marginal cost of the better treatment to get a cost-effectiveness estimate.

For example, in the GUSTO trial of thrombolytic therapy for myocardial infarction, a difference in outcomes was found when t-PA was used instead of streptokinase: t-PA at $2000/dose resulted in 6.5% mortality while streptokinase at $200/dose resulted in 7.5% mortality. The ARR is the difference between the two, or 1%. The NNTB for t-PA is 100 (1/ARR) which is how many patients must be treated with t-PA instead of streptokinase to prevent one additional death. The marginal or incremental cost per life saved is then $180 000 [($2000 − $200) × 100 lives].

The prices used to calculate costs should be appropriate to the time and place. The use of US dollars in studies on Canadian health-care resources will not translate into a credible cost analysis. Also, the effects measured should include lives or years of life saved, improvement in level of function, or utility of the outcome for the patient.

There are several different ways to analyze costs and effects. In a cost-minimization analysis only costs are compared. This works if the effects of the two interventions are equal or minimally different. For example, when comparing inpatient vein stripping to outpatient injection of varicose veins, the results shown in Table 31.1 were obtained. Here the cost is so different that even if 13% of outpatients require additional hospitalization (and therefore we must pay for

Table 31.2. Comparing doxycycline to azithromycin for *Chlamydia* infections

Treatment	Outcomes			
	Cost to hospital per patient	No further treatement needed	Adverse effects	Compliance rate
Doxycycline	3	77%	29%	70%
Azithromycin	30	81%	23%	100%

Source: Data extracted from A. C. Haddix, S. D. Hillis & W. J. Kassler. The cost effectiveness of azithromycin for *Chlamydia trachomatis* infections in women. *Sex. Transm. Dis.* 1995; 22: 274–280.

both procedures) you will still save money by performing outpatient injections. We are assuming that the end results are similar in both groups.

Another analysis compared doxycycline 100 mg twice a day for 7 days to azithromycin 1 g given as a one-time dose for the treatment of *Chlamydia* infections in women. It found that some patients do not complete the full 7-day course for doxycycline and then need to be retreated, and can infect other people during that period of time (Table 31.2). The cost of azithromycin that would make the use of this drug cost-effective for all patients can then be calculated. In this case, the drug company making azithromycin actually lowered their price for the drug by over 50% based on that analysis, to a level that would make azithromycin more cost-effective.

In a cost-effectiveness analysis the researcher seeks to determine how much more has to be paid in order to achieve a benefit of preventing death or disability time. Here, the effects are unequal and all outcomes must be compared. These include costs, well years, total years, and utility or benefits. The outcome is expressed as incremental or marginal cost over benefit. Commonly used units are additional dollars per QALY or life saved.

The first step in a cost-effectiveness analysis is to determine the difference in the benefits or effects of the two treatment strategies or policies being compared. This gives the incremental or marginal gain expressed in QALYs or other units of utility. This is done using an Expected Values Decision Analysis as described in Chapter 30. It is possible that one of the tested strategies may have a relatively small benefit and yet be overall more cost-effective than others therapies, which although only slightly less effective are very much more expensive.

Next the difference in cost of the two treatment strategies or policies must be determined, to get the incremental or marginal cost. The cost-effectiveness is the ratio of the incremental cost to the incremental gain. Consider the example of two strategies, A and B. In the first (A), the quality-adjusted life expectancy is 15 QALYs and the cost per case is $10 000. In the second (B), the life expectancy is 20 QALYs, a definite improvement, but at a cost of $110 000 per case. The cost-effectiveness of B as compared to A is the difference in cost divided by the difference in effects. This is $(110\,000 - 10\,000)/(20 - 15) = \$20\,000/\text{QALY}$ gained. Note that if the more effective treatment had also cost less, you should obviously use the more effective one unless it has other serious drawbacks such as serious known side effects. Calculate this only when the more effective treatment strategy or policy is also more costly.

Are the conclusions unlikely to change with sensible changes in costs and outcomes?

Since most research on a given therapy is done at different times, changes over time must be accounted for. This process is called discounting and considers inflation and depreciation. It takes into account that inflation occurs and that, instead of paying for a program now, those costs can be invested now and other funds used to pay for solving the problem later. For example, you can pay $200 a year for 10 years or $2000 in 10 years. The future costs are usually expressed in current dollars since $200 in the future is equivalent to less than $200 today. Actuarial and accounting methods used should be specified in the methods section of the analysis.

Setting up a program is usually a greater cost than running it and initial costs are usually amortized over several decades. Discounting the value side of the equation considers that the value of a year of life saved now may be greater than a year saved later. Adding a year of life to someone at age 40 may mean more to them than adding a year of life to a 40-year-old but only after they reach the age of 60. This was considered in the discussion on patient preferences and values in Chapter 30.

As with any other clinical research study, the numbers used to perform the analysis are only approximations and have 95% confidence levels attached. Therefore, a sensitivity analysis should always be done to check on the assumptions made in the analysis. This is a process by which the results of the analysis are changed based on reasonable changes in costs or effects that are statistically expected based upon the 95% CI values. Suitable graphs can demonstrate the change in the overall cost-effectiveness based on changes in one or more parameters. If the cost curve is relatively flat, a large change in a baseline characteristic does not result in much change in the cost-effectiveness of the intervention.

Are the estimates of the costs and outcomes appropriately related to the baseline risk in the population?

There may be various levels of risk within the population. What is cost-effective for one subgroup may not be cost-effective for another. The study should attempt to identify these subgroups and assign individual cost-effectiveness analyses to each of them. For example, if looking at the cost-effectiveness of positive inotropic agents in the treatment of heart failure, it may be that for severe heart failure their use is cost-effective, while for less severe cases it is not. The use of beta-blocker drugs in heart failure has been studied, and the cost-effectiveness is much greater when the drug is used in high-risk patients than in low-risk patients. However, it is above the usual definition of the threshold for saving a life in both circumstances.

Final comments: ethical issues

How much are we willing to spend to save a life? What is an acceptable cost per QALY gained? A commonly accepted figure in the decision-analysis literature is $40 000 to $60 000 per QALY, approximately the cost to maintain a person on dialysis for 1 year. This number has increased only slightly over the past 40 years since renal dialysis is more common although more expensive. In the United Kingdom, the National Institute for Health and Clinical Excellence (NICE) considers a threshold of cost-effectiveness to be between £20 000 and £30 000 per QALY.

There are multiple ethical issues involved in the use of cost-effectiveness analyses. The provider is being asked to take sides with the option that will cost the least, or at least be the most cost-effective. This may not be the best option for each patient. Cost-effectiveness analyses are really more useful as political tools for making decisions on coverage by insurance schemes rather than for daily use in bedside clinical decision making.

There are some cases when cost-effectiveness is the best thing to do for the individual patient. Universally these situations occur when the best practice is the cheapest. One example is the use of antibiotics for treating urethral *Chlamydia* infections that was mentioned earlier. More importantly, since most physicians cannot understand the issues involved in cost-effectiveness analyses when these come up in health policy areas, they should turn to agencies that are doing these on a regular basis. These are the AHRQ in the United States and NICE in the United Kingdom. Pharmaceutical and medical instrument and device manufacturers and some specialty physicians are often trying to assert that their service, product, or procedure is the best and most cost-effective because, although more expensive now, it will lead to savings later. This can occur because of the "spin" that is put on their cost-effectiveness analysis. To be able to pick up the inconsistencies and omissions from a cost-effectiveness analysis is very difficult. However, most physicians ought to be able at least to understand the analysis and subsequent comments made by people who are more highly trained in evaluating this type of study. Recognizing the presence or absence of conflict of interest in these commentaries is of utmost importance.

One current debate is over the use of chest pain evaluation units (CPEU) in Emergency Departments (ED) of acute care hospitals. These are for patients who are at low risk of having a myocardial infarction and for whom a stay of 48 hours in an intensive care unit is very expensive and probably unnecessary. In this discussion, it is assumed that discharge home from the ED is not safe as up to 4% of acute MIs are missed by emergency physicians. Proponents of these CPEUs point out that a lot of money will be saved if these low-risk patients are put into the CPEU rather than the acute-care hospital bed. They have done cost-effectiveness analyses that show only a slight overall increase in costs under the assumptions of the current admission rate of these patients to the hospital. However, if now all the extremely low-risk patients, including those who have virtually no risk, are admitted to the CPEU, the overall admission rate may actually increase, resulting in markedly increased costs. Clearly there must be a search for some other method of dealing with these patients, which will be cost-effective and result in decreased hospital-bed utilization. The methods of cost-effectiveness analysis must look at all eventualities.

32

Survival analysis and studies of prognosis

He ended; and thus Adam last replied:
How soon hath thy prediction, seer blest,
Measured this transient world, the race of time,
Till time stand fixed! Beyond is all abyss,
Eternity, whose end no eye can reach.

John Milton (1608–1674): Paradise Lost

Learning objectives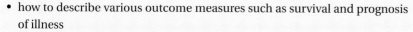

In this chapter you will learn:

- how to describe various outcome measures such as survival and prognosis of illness
- the ways outcomes may be compared
- the steps in reviewing an article which measures survival or prognosis

One of the most important pieces of information that patients want is to know what is going to happen to them during their illness. The clinician must be able to provide information about prognosis to the patient in all medical encounters. Patients want to know the details of the outcomes they can expect from their disease and treatment. Evaluation of the clinical research literature on prognosis is a required skill for the health-care provider of the future. Outcome analysis looks at the interplay of three factors: the patient, the intervention, and the outcome. We want to know how long a patient with the given illness will survive if given one of two possible treatments. These treatments can be two active therapies or therapy and placebo. Studies of outcomes or prognosis should clearly define these three elements.

The patient: the inception cohort

To start an outcome study, an appropriate inception cohort must be assembled. This means a group of patients for whom the disease is identified at a uniform point in the course of the disease, called the inception. This can occur at the appearance of the first unambiguous sign or symptom of a disease or at the first application of testing or therapy. Ideally this should be as early in the disease as possible. However, it should be at a stage where most reasonably prudent providers can make the diagnosis and not sooner as most providers won't be able to make the diagnosis and initiate therapy at that earlier stage of disease. Collection of the cohort after the occurrence of the outcome event and looking backward will distort the results either in a positive or negative way if some patients with the disease die before diagnosis or commonly have spontaneous remissions soon after diagnosis. A study of survival of patients with acute myocardial infarction who are studied from the time they arrive in the coronary care unit will miss those who die suddenly either before seeking care or in the emergency department.

Incidence/prevalence bias can be a fatal flaw in the study if the inception cohort is assembled at different stages of illness. This confuses new from ongoing cases of the illness. There may be very different prognoses for patients at these various stages of the illness. Lead-time and length-time bias occurring as the result of screening programs should be avoided by proper randomization. These were discussed in detail in Chapter 28 on screening tests.

Diagnostic criteria, disease severity, referral pattern, comorbidity, and demographic details for inclusion of patients into the study must be specified. Patients referred from a primary-care center may be different than those referred from a specialty or tertiary-care center. Termed referral filter bias, this is due to an over-representation of patients with later stages of disease or more complex illness who are more likely to have poor results. Centripetal bias is another name for cases referred to tertiary-care centers because of the need for special expertise. Popularity bias occurs when the more challenging and interesting cases only are referred to the experts in the tertiary care center. The results of these biases limit external validity in other settings where most patients will present with earlier or milder disease.

All members of the inception cohort should be accounted for at the end of the study and their outcomes known. This is much more important in these types of studies as we really want to know all of the possible outcomes of the illness. There are non-trivial reasons why patients drop out of a study. These include recovery, death, refusal of therapy due to the disease, side effects of therapy, loss of interest, or moving away. One study showed that patients in a study who were harder to track and more likely to drop out had a higher mortality rate.

There are several rules of thumb to use in determining the effect of incomplete follow-up. First, identify the outcome of most interest to you and determine the fraction of patients who had this outcome. Then add the patients "lost to follow-up" to both the numerator and the denominator, which gives the result if all patients lost had the outcome of interest. Now add the patients lost to follow-up

Table 32.1. A study of 71 patients 6 of whom were lost to follow-up

	Original study	"Highest" case	"Lowest" case
Relapse rate	$39/65 = 60\%$	$45/71 = 63\%$	$39/71 = 55\%$
Mortality rate	$1/65 = 1.5\%$	$7/71 = 10\%$	$1/71 = 1.4\%$

to only the denominator, giving the lowest result if no patient lost had the outcome of interest. Compare these two results. If they are very close to each other, the result is still useful. If not the result of the study may be useless. In the example in Table 32.1, the difference in relapse rates is minor while the difference in mortality is quite large. As a general rule, the lower the rate of an outcome, the more likely it is to be affected by patients lost to follow-up.

The intervention

There should be a clear and easily reproducible description of the intervention being tested. All details of a therapeutic program should be described in the study. The reader should be able to duplicate the process of the study at another institution. All the interventions tested or compared should be those that make a difference. It is of paramount importance that the intervention proposed in the study be one that can be performed in settings other than at the most advanced tertiary care setting only. Similarly, testing a drug against placebo may not be as important or useful as testing it against the drug that is currently the most favorite for that indication. Most of these issues have been discussed in the chapter on randomized clinical trials in Chapter 15.

The outcome

The outcome criteria should be objective, reproducible, and accurate. The outcome assessment should also be done in a blinded manner to avoid diagnostic suspicion and expectation bias in the assessment of patient outcomes. There can be significant bias introduced into the study if the outcomes are not measured in a consistent manner. Ideally, the outcome measures should be unmistakably objective. Death or life are clear and easily measured outcome variables although the cause of death as measured on a death certificate is not always a reliable, clear, or objective outcome measure of the actual cause of death. Admission to the hospital appears to be clear and objective, but the reasons or threshold for admission to the hospital may be very subjective and subject to significant inter-rater variability. Outcomes such as "full recovery at home" or "feeling better" have a higher degree of subjectivity associated with them.

There should be adjustment for extraneous prognostic factors. The researcher should determine whether the prognostic factor is merely a marker or actually a factor that is responsible for the causation. This determines whether or not there are alternative explanations for the outcomes due to some confounding variable. Count on the article being reviewed by a statistician who can determine if the authors used the correct statistical analysis, but be aware that the correct adjustment for extraneous factors may not have been done correctly if at all. If the authors suggest that a group of signs, symptoms, or diagnostic tests accurately predict an outcome, look for a validation sample in a second study which attempts to verify that indeed these results occurred because of a causal relationship and not just by chance. Look for at least 10 and preferably 20 patients who actually had the outcome of interest for each prognostic factor that is evaluated to give clinically and statistically significant results. Chapter 14 has a more detailed discussion of multivariate analysis.

Most often outcomes are expressed as a dichotomous nominal variable (e.g., dead or alive, disease or no disease, a patent or occluded bypass, improved or worse, it works or it doesn't, etc.). One is interested in the association of an independent variable such as drug use, therapy, risk factor, diagnostic test result, tumor stage, age of patient, or blood pressure with the dependent or outcome variable.

Diagnostic-suspicion bias occurs when the physician caring for the patient knows the nature and purpose of the outcomes being measured and as a result, changes the interpretation of a diagnostic test, the actual care or observation of the patient. Expectation bias occurs when the person measuring the outcome knows the clinical features of the case or the results of a diagnostic test and alters their interpretation of the outcome event. This is less likely when the intervention and outcome measures are clearly objective. Ideally blind diagnosis, treatment, and assessment of all the patients going through the study will prevent these biases.

Another problem in the outcomes selected occurs when multiple outcomes are lumped together. Many more studies of therapy are comparing two groups for several outcomes at once and these so-called composite outcomes have been discussed in Chapter 11 in greater detail. Commonly used measures of heart therapies might include death, an important outcome, non-fatal myocardial infarction, important but less than death and need for revascularization procedure much less important than death. The use of these measures can lead to over-optimistic conclusions regarding the therapy being tested. If each outcome were measured alone, none would have statistical significance, which could be due to a possible Type II error. When combined, multiple or composite outcomes may then show statistical significance.

One example is the recent CAPRIE trial comparing clopidogrel, an antiplatelet agent, against aspirin. The primary outcome measures were overall number of deaths, and of deaths due to stroke, myocardial infarction, or vascular causes. The definition of vascular causes was not made clear. The end result was that there were no decreases in death from stroke or myocardial infarction, but a 20% reduction in deaths in the patients with peripheral arterial disease. The absolute reduction was 1.09% (from 4.80% to 3.71%, giving an NNTB of 91). If these patient outcomes were considered as separate groups, the differences would not have been statistically significant. Another danger is that some patients may be counted several times because they have several of the outcomes. Finally, the clinical significance of the combined outcome is unknown.

There are basically three types of data that are used to indicate risk of an outcome. Interval data such as blood pressure is usually considered to be normally distributed and measured on a continuous scale. Nominal data like tumor type or treatment options is categorical and often dichotomous like alive and dead or positive and negative test results. Ordinal data such as tumor stage is also categorical but with some relation between the categories. There are three types of analyses applied to this type of problem: frequency tables, logistic analysis, and survival analysis. Decision theory uses probability distributions to estimate the probability of an outcome. A loss function measures the relative benefit or utility of that outcome.

Frequency tables

Frequency tables use a chi-square analysis to compare the association of the outcome with risk factors that are nominal or ordinal. For the chi-square analysis, data are usually presented in a table where columns are outcomes, rows are risk factors, and the frequencies appear as table entries. The observed data are compared with the data that would be expected if there were no association. The analysis results in a P value which indicates the probability that the observed outcome could have been obtained by chance when it was really no different from the expected value. Fisher's exact test is used when the observed value of any cell is less than 5.

Logistic analysis

This is a more general approach to measuring outcomes than using frequency tables. Logistic regression estimates the probability of an outcome based on one or more risk factors. The risk factors may be interval, ordinal, or nominal variables. Results of logistic regression analysis are often reported as the odds ratio, relative risk, or hazard ratio. For one independent variable of interval-type data and relative risk, this method calculates how much of an increase in the risk of the outcome occurs for each incremental increase in the exposure to the risk factor. An example of this would answer the question "how much additional risk of stroke will occur for each increase of 10 mm Hg in systolic blood pressure?" For ordinal data the analysis calculates the probability of an outcome based on the stage of disease for example, the recurrence of a stage 4 compared to a stage 2 tumor.

For multiple variables, is there some combination of risk factors that will better predict an outcome than one risk factor alone? Which of these risk factors will be the best predictor of that outcome? The identification of significant risk factors can be done using multiple regressions or stepwise regression analyses as we discussed in Chapter 29 on clinical prediction rules.

Survival analysis

In the real world the ultimate outcome is often not known and could be dead as opposed to "so far, so good" or not dead yet. It would be difficult to justify waiting until all patients in a study die so that survival in two treatment or risk groups can be compared. Besides, another common problem with comparing survival between groups occurs in trying to determine what to do with patients who are doing fine but die of an incident unrelated to their medical problem such as death in a motor-vehicle accident of a patent who had a bypass graft 15 years earlier. This will alter the information used in the analysis of time to occlusion with two different types of bypasses. Finally, how should the study handle the patient who simply moves away and is lost to follow-up?

The situations described above are examples of **censored** data. The data consist of a time interval and a dichotomous variable indicating status, either failure (dead, graft occluded, etc.) or censored (i.e., not dead yet, success so far, etc.). In the latter case, the patient may still be alive, have died but not from the disease of interest, or been alive when last seen but could not be located again.

A potential problem in these analyses is the definition of the start time. Early diagnosis may automatically confer longer survival if the time of diagnosis is the start time. This is also called lead-time bias, as discussed in Chapter 28, and is a common problem with screening tests. **Censoring bias** occurs when one of the treatment groups is more likely to be censored than the other. If certain patients are lost as a result of treatment (e.g., harmful side effects) their chances of being censored are not independent of their survival times. A survival analysis initially assumes that any patient censoring is independent of the outcome. Figure 32.1 shows an example of the effects of censoring on a hypothetical study.

Survival curves

The distribution of survival times is most often displayed as a survivor function, also called a survival curve. This is a plot of the proportion of subjects surviving versus time. It is important to note that "surviving" may indicate things other

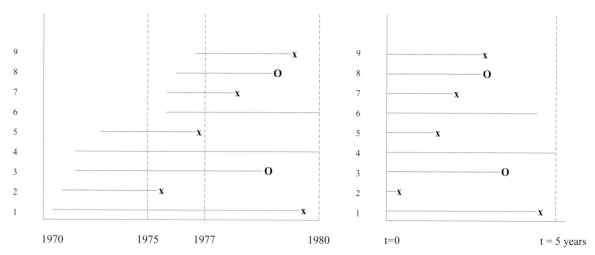

Fig. 32.1 Censoring. Patients are enrolled in a study over a 2-year period (1975–1977). All are followed until 1980 and patients who die are marked with an x. Some patients (2 and 5) are enrolled at a late stage of their disease. Their inclusion will bias the cohort toward poorer survival. Two patients (4 and 6) are still alive at the end of the observation period. Patient 1 lived longer than everyone except patient 4, although it appears that patient 1 didn't live so long, since their previous survival (pre-1975) does not count in the analysis. We don't know how long patient 4 will live since he or she is still alive at the end of the observation period and their data are censored at t = 5 years. Two other patients (3 and 8) are lost to follow-up, and their data are censored early (o).

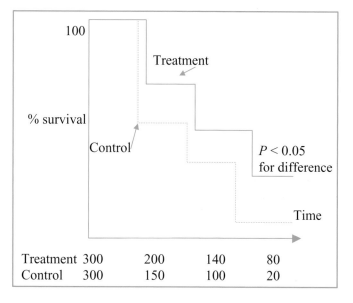

Fig. 32.2 Kaplan–Meier survival curve.

than actual survival (i.e., life vs. death), such as success of therapy (i.e., patent vs. non-patent coronary bypass grafts). These curves can be deceptive since the number of individuals represented by the curve decreases as time increases. It is key that a statistical analysis is applied at several times to the results of the curves. The number of patients at each stage of the curve should also be given. The Kaplan-Meier curve is the one most commonly used.

There is one primary method for plotting and analyzing survival curves. The actuarial-life-table method measures the length of time from the moment the patient is entered into the study until failure occurs. The product-limit method is a graphic representation of the actuarial-life-table method and is also known as the Kaplan–Meier method. It is the plot of survival that is most commonly used in medicine. The analysis looks at the period of time, the month or year since the subject entered the study, in which the outcome of interest occurred. A typical Kaplan–Meier curve is shown in Fig. 32.2.

There are several tests of equality of these survivor functions or curves that are commonly performed. One of the most popular is the Mantel–Cox also known as log-rank test. The Cox proportional-hazard model uses interval data as the independent variable determining how much the odds of survival are altered by each unit of change in the independent variable. This answers the question of how much the risk of stroke is increased with each increase of 10 mm Hg in mean arterial blood pressure. Further discussion of survival curves and outcome analysis is beyond the scope of this book. Two of the Users' Guides to the Medical Literature articles provide more detail.[1,2]

[1] A. Laupacis, G. Wells, W. S. Richardson & P. Tugwell. Users' guides to the medical literature. V. How to use an article about prognosis. Evidence-Based Medicine Working Group. *JAMA* 1994; 272: 234–237.
[2] C. D. Naylor & G. H. Guyatt. Users' guides to the medical literature. X. How to use an article reporting variations in the outcomes of health services. Evidence-Based Medicine Working Group. *JAMA* 1996; 275: 554–558.

33

Meta-analysis and systematic reviews

Common sense is the collection of prejudices acquired by age eighteen.

Albert Einstein (1879–1955)

Learning objectives

In this chapter you will learn:

- the principles of evaluating meta-analyses and systematic reviews
- the concepts of heterogeneity and homogeneity
- the use of L'Abbé, forest, and funnel plots
- measures commonly used in systematic reviews: odds ratios and effect size
- how to review a published meta-analysis and use the results to solve a clinical problem

Background and rationale for performing meta-analysis

Over the past 50 years there has been an explosion of research in the medical literature. In the worldwide English-language medical literature alone, there were 1,300 biomedical journals in 1940, while in 2000 there were over 14,000. It has become almost impossible for the individual practitioner to keep up with the literature. This is more frustrating when contradictory studies are published about a given topic. Meta-analyses and systematic reviews are relatively new techniques used to synthesize and summarize the results of multiple research studies on the same topic.

A primary analysis refers to the original analysis of research data as presented in an observational study or randomized clinical trial (RCT). Secondary analysis is a re-analysis of the original data either using another statistical technique or answering new questions with previously obtained data.

The traditional review article is a qualitative review. It is a summary of all primary research on a given topic and it may provide good background information that is more up to date than a textbook. But review articles have the disadvantage of being somewhat subjective and reflecting the biases of the author, who may be very selective of the articles chosen for review. One must be knowledgeable of the literature being reviewed in order to evaluate this type of article critically.

Meta-analysis is more comprehensive or "transcends" traditional analysis of data. Typically, a meta-analysis looks at data from multiple studies of the same clinical question and uses a variety of statistical techniques to integrate their findings. It may be called a quantitative systematic review and represents the rigorous application of research techniques and statistical analysis to present an overview of a given topic.

A meta-analysis is usually done to reconcile studies with different results. It can look at multiple negative studies to uncover Type II errors or at clinical problems where there are some negative and some positive studies to uncover Type I or Type II errors. It can help uncover a single study which has totally different results because of systematic error or bias in the research process. Large confidence intervals in some studies may be narrowed by combining them. For example, multiple small trials done before 1971 showed both positive and negative effects of light or phototherapy on hyperbilirubinemia in newborns. A meta-analysis in 1985 showed an overall positive effect.

Occasionally a large trial shows an opposite effect from that found in multiple small trials. This is often due to procedural or methodologic study design differences in the trials. However, as a general rule, correctly done large cooperative trials are more reliable than meta-analysis of many smaller trials. For example a meta-analysis of multiple small trials of magnesium in acute myocardial infarction (AMI) showed a positive effect on decreasing mortality. The ISIS-4 trial, a large multicenter RCT where magnesium was given in one arm of the study, showed no benefit, although it was given later in the course of the AMI than it had been in the smaller studies. The disparity of study methodologies in this case required that the researchers set up a new multicenter study of the use of magnesium in AMI. Called MAGIC, it is now in progress. The use of meta-analysis does not reduce the need for large well-done studies of primary clinical modalities.

Guidelines for evaluation of systematic reviews

Were the question and methods clearly stated and were comprehensive search methods used to locate relevant studies?

In meta-analysis, the process of article selection and analysis should proceed by a preset protocol. By not changing the process in mid-analysis the author's bias and retrospective bias are minimized. This means that the definitions of outcome and predictor or therapy variables of the analysis are not changed in mid-stream. The research question must be clearly defined, including a defined patient population and clear and consistent definitions of the disease, interventions, and outcomes.

A carefully defined search strategy must be used to detect and prevent publication bias. This bias occurs because trials with positive results and those with large sample sizes are more likely to be published. Sources should include conference proceedings, dissertation abstracts, and other databases, as well as the usual search of MEDLINE. A manual search of relevant journals may uncover some additional studies. The bibliographies of all relevant articles found should be hand searched to find any misclassified articles that were missed in the original search.

The authors must cite where they looked and should be exhaustive in looking for unpublished studies. Not using foreign studies may introduce bias since some foreign studies are published in English-language journals while others may be missed. The authors should also contact the authors of all the studies found and ask them about other researchers working in the area who may have unpublished studies available. The Cochrane Collaboration maintains a register of controlled trials called CENTRAL, which attempts to document all current trials regardless of result. Also, the National Library of Medicine and the National Institutes of Health in the United States have an online repository of clinical trials called www.clinicaltrials.gov, which can be accessed to determine if a clinical trial is ongoing and proceeding according to its original plan.

Were explicit methods used to determine which articles to include in the review and were the selection and assessment of the methodologic quality of the primary studies reproducible and free from bias?

Objective selection of articles for the meta-analysis should be clearly laid out and include inclusion and exclusion criteria. The objectives and procedures must be defined ahead of time. This includes a clearly defined research and abstraction method and a scoring system for assessing the quality of the included studies. For each study several factors ought to be assessed. The publication status may suggest stronger studies in that those that were never published or only published in abstract form may be significantly deficient in methodological areas.

The strength of the study design will determine the ability to prove causation. Randomized clinical trials are the strongest study design. A well-designed observational study with appropriate safeguards to prevent or minimize bias and confounding, will also give very strong results. The methods of meta-analysis include ranking or grading the quality of the evidence. The Cochrane Collaboration is using the new GRADE recommendations to rank the quality of studies in their systematic reviews. Appendix 1 gives two commonly used criteria for grading various levels of evidence, the one used by the Centre for Evidence-Based Medicine at Oxford and the GRADE criteria. The full set of GRADE criteria can be downloaded from the Cochrane Collaboration's website, www.cochrane.org.

The study sites and patient populations of the individual studies may limit generalizability of the meta-analysis. The interventions or exposures should be similar between studies. Finally, the studies should be measuring the same or very similar outcomes. We will discuss issues of how to judge homogeneity and combine heterogeneous studies.

Independent review of the methods section looks at inclusion and exclusion criteria, coding, and replication issues. There must be accurate and objective abstraction of the data, ideally done by blinded abstracters. Two abstracters should gather the data independently and the author should check for inter-rater agreement. The methods and results sections should be disguised to prevent reviewers from discovering the source of the research. Inter-rater reliability of coders should be maximized with a minimal level of 0.9 on the kappa statistic. Once this has been established, a single coder can code all the remaining study results.

Were the differences in individual study results adequately explained and were the results of the primary studies combined appropriately?

Studies may be homogeneous or heterogeneous. There are both qualitative and quantitative measures of heterogeneity. Testing for heterogeneity of the studies is done to determine if the studies are qualitatively similar enough to combine. The tests for heterogeneity include the Mantel–Haentszel chi-squared test, the Breslow–Day test, and the Q statistic by the DerSimonian and Laird method. They all suffer from low power so are likely to have a Type II error. If the test statistic is statistically significant ($P < 0.05$), the studies are likely to be heterogeneous. However, the absence of statistical significance does not mean homogeneity and may only be present due to low power of the statistical test for heterogeneity.

The presence of heterogeneity among the studies analyzed will result in erroneous interpretation of the statistical results. If the studies are very heterogeneous, one strategy for analyzing them is to remove the study with most extreme or outlier results and recalculate the statistic. If the statistic is no longer statistically significant, it can be assumed that the outlier study was responsible for all or most of the heterogeneity. That study should then be examined more closely to determine what about the study design might have caused the observed extreme result. This could be due to differences in the population studied or systematic bias in the conduct of the study.

Analysis and aggregation of the data can be done in several ways, but should consider sample sizes and magnitude of effects. A simple vote count in which the number of studies with positive results is directly compared with the number of studies with negative results is not an acceptable method since neither effect size nor sample size are considered. Pooled analysis or lumped data add numerators and denominators of each study together to produce a new result. This is better than a vote count, but still not acceptable since that process ignores the confidence intervals for each study and allows errors to multiply in the process of adding the results. Simple combination of *P* values is not acceptable because this does not consider the direction of the effect or magnitude of the effect size.

Weighted outcomes compare small and large studies, analyze them as equals, and then weight the results by the sample size. This involves adjusting each outcome by a value that accounts for the sample size and degree of variation. Confidence intervals should be applied to the mean results of each study evaluated. Aggregate study and control-group means and confidence intervals can then be calculated. Subgroups should be analyzed where appropriate, recognizing the potential for making a Type I error. There are two standard measures for evaluating the results of a meta-analysis: the odds ratio and the effect size.

The odds ratio (OR) is the most common way of combining results in meta-analysis. The odds ratio can be calculated for each study showing whether the intervention increases or decreases the odds of a favorable outcome. These can then be combined statistically and the 95% confidence intervals calculated for all the odds ratios. If we are looking at a positive outcome such as % still alive, an OR > 1 favors the experimental treatment. If looking at a negative outcome such as mortality rates, an OR < 1 favors the experimental treatment. The OR is used rather than the relative risk (RR) even though the studies are usually RCTs. This is done because of the mathematical problems when using the RR. Newer calculation techniques are making it possible to calculate an aggregate RR, and this is becoming more common in meta-analyses.

The effect size (*d* or δ) is a standard metric compared across studies. It is a relative and not an absolute value. The equation for effect size is $d = (m_1 - m_2)/\text{SD}$, where m_1 and m_2 are the means of the two groups being studied and SD is the standard deviation of either sample population. A difference (δ) in SD units of 0.2 SD is a small effect, 0.5 SD a moderate effect, and >0.8 SD, a large effect. If the data are skewed, it is better to use median rather than mean of the data to calculate the effect size, but this requires the use of other, more complex statistical methods to accomplish the analysis.

The statistical analytic procedures usually employed in systematic reviews are far too complex to discuss here. However, there are important distinctions between the methods used in the presence and in the absence of heterogeneity of the results of the studies, which the reader should be aware of. If the data are relatively homogeneous, a statistical process called the fixed-effects model can be used. This assumes that all the studies can be statistically analyzed as equals. However, if the data are very heterogeneous, a statistical process called the random-effects model should be used. This is more complex and takes into account that the various studies are part of a population of studies of the events.

Fig. 33.1 Hypothetical meta-analysis. Initial studies (except one) lacked power to find a difference. A difference was found when all studies were combined.

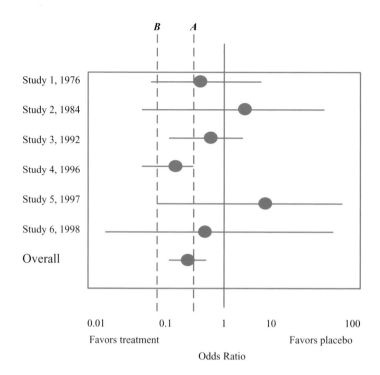

The result is the presence of wider confidence intervals. Unfortunately, the methods used for the random-effects model give more weight to the smaller studies, which is a potential source of bias if there are more small studies with positive results, a result of publication bias. Frequently, a single meta-analysis will use both methods to determine statistical significance. If the two methods give the same result, the statistical significance is more "powerful" than if one method finds statistical significance and the other does not.

There are three graphic techniques that can be used to look at the overall data. These all demonstrate the effect of the problem of publication bias but in different ways. Large studies or those showing positive effects are more likely to be published. It is very likely that if one small study showed a positive effect it would be published. Conversely if a small study showed a negative effect or no difference between the groups, it is less likely to be published. It is important to be able to estimate the effect of this phenomenon on the results of the meta analysis.

Graphic displays are a powerful tool to show the difference in study results. The most common way of graphing meta-analysis results is called the Forest Plot. This shows the results of each study as a point estimate for the rate, risk difference, or ratio (odds ratio, relative risk, or effect size) and a line for the 95% confidence intervals on this point estimate. A log scale is commonly used so that the reciprocal values are an equal distance from 1 (Fig. 33.1). Always be careful

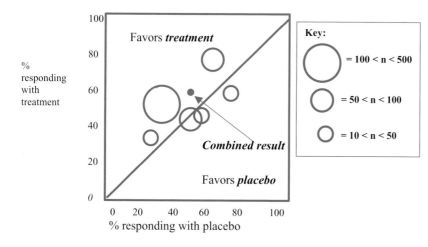

Fig. 33.2 L'Abbé plot of a hypothetical meta-analysis. The largest studies showed the most effect of the treatment, suggesting that the smaller studies lacked power.

to check the scales. It is easy to see if the confidence interval crosses the point of no significance, 0 for differences or 1 for ratios.

There is a visual guide that can suggest heterogeneity in this type of plot.[1] Simply draw a perpendicular from the higher end of the 95% CI for the study with the lowest point value. In Fig. 33.1 this is line A drawn through the higher end of the 95% CI of study 4. Draw a similar line through the lower end of the 95% CI of the study with the highest point value. Here it is line B, through the lower point of study 5. If the confidence intervals of all of the studies appear in the space between these two lines, the studies are probably not heterogeneous. Any study outside this area may be the cause of significant heterogeneity in the aggregate analysis of the study results.

The L'Abbé plot in Fig. 33.2, is used to show how much each individual study contributes to the outcome. The two possible outcome rates, for the control and intervention groups are plotted on the x- and y-axis, respectively. A circle, the diameter of which is proportional to the sample size, represents each study. A key to the sample size is given with the plot. The L'Abbé plot is a better visual aid to see the differences between study results and how much those depend on the sample size.

Finally, the funnel plot shown in Fig. 33.3 is another way to show the effect of sample size on the effect size. This is a plot of the effect size (δ) on the x-axis and sample size on the y-axis. If there are many positive small studies with large effect sizes, the resulting plot will look like an asymmetric triangle or half of an upside-down funnel. This suggests that the overall result of the meta-analysis is being unduly influenced by these many, very positive, small studies, which could

---

[1] Shown to me by Rose Hatala, M.D., from the Department of Medicine of the University of British Columbia, Vancouver, BC, Canada.

Fig. 33.3 Funnel plot of six studies. Notice that the largest effect sizes were found in the smallest studies. A plot with this configuration suggests publication bias.

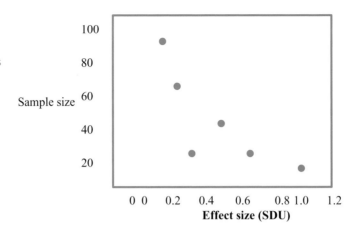

be due to publication bias or that all of these studies may have similar systematic biases and perhaps fatal flaws in their execution.

Were the reviewers' conclusions supported by the data cited?

A sensitivity analysis should be done to address the possibility of publication bias also called the "file-drawer effect." Negative and unpublished studies are frequently small and usually won't be able to drastically change the results of the meta-analysis. Using the funnel or the L'Abbé plots and other methods will help alert the reader to the potential presence of publication bias.

There is a way of calculating the potential effect of publication bias. Fail-safe N is an estimate of the number of negative studies you would need in order to eliminate the difference between treatment and outcome or cause and effect that was found. This can mean to reverse the δ value or increase the overall probability of finding a difference when one doesn't exist to a value higher than the δ level (i.e., $P > 0.05$). If a large part of the positive effect found is due to a few small and very positive studies, it is possible that there are also a few small and clearly negative studies that because of publication bias have never been published. If the fail-safe N is small it means that only a few small negative studies would be needed to reverse the finding. This is a plausible occurrence. But if fail-safe N is very large, it is unlikely that there are that many negative studies "out there" that have never been published and you would accept the results as being positive.

Some common problems with meta-analyses are that they may be comparing diverse studies with different designs or over different time periods. There may be excessive inter-observer variability in deciding on which trials to evaluate, and how much weight to give to each trial. These issues ought to be addressed by the authors and difference in the results explained. In many cases, the methodologies will contribute biases that can be uncovered in the meta-analysis process.

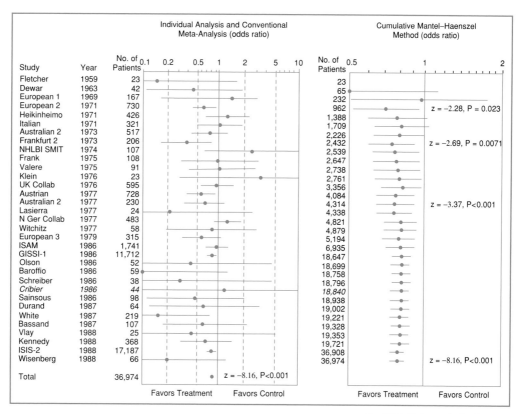

Study	Year	No. of Patients	Individual Analysis and Conventional Meta-Analysis (odds ratio)	No. of Patients	Cumulative Mantel–Haenszel Method (odds ratio)
Fletcher	1959	23		23	
Dewar	1963	42		65	
European 1	1969	167		232	
European 2	1971	730		962	z = −2.28, P = 0.023
Heikinheimo	1971	426		1,388	
Italian	1971	321		1,709	
Australian 2	1973	517		2,226	
Frankfurt 2	1973	206		2,432	z = −2.69, P = 0.0071
NHLBI SMIT	1974	107		2,539	
Frank	1975	108		2,647	
Valere	1975	91		2,738	
Klein	1976	23		2,761	
UK Collab	1976	595		3,356	
Austrian	1977	728		4,084	
Australian 2	1977	230		4,314	z = −3.37, P<0.001
Lasierra	1977	24		4,338	
N Ger Collab	1977	483		4,821	
Witchitz	1977	58		4,879	
European 3	1979	315		5,194	
ISAM	1986	1,741		6,935	
GISSI-1	1986	11,712		18,647	
Olson	1986	52		18,699	
Baroffio	1986	59		18,758	
Schreiber	1986	38		18,796	
Cribier	*1986*	*44*		*18,840*	
Sainsous	1986	98		18,938	
Durand	1987	64		19,002	
White	1987	219		19,221	
Bassand	1987	107		19,328	
Vlay	1988	25		19,353	
Kennedy	1988	368		19,721	
ISIS-2	1988	17,187		36,908	
Wisenberg	1988	66		36,974	z = −8.16, P<0.001
Total		36,974	z = −8.16, P<0.001		

Favors Treatment   Favors Control   Favors Treatment   Favors Control

Fig. 33.4 Meta-analysis of therapeutic trials for myocardial infarction. From J. Lau, E. M. Antman, J. Jimenez-Silva, B. Kupelnick, F. Mosteller, T. C. Chalmers. Cumulative meta-analysis of therapeutic trials for myocardial infarction. *N. Engl. J. Med.* 1992; 327: 248–254. Used with permission.

Cumulative meta-analysis is a meta-analytic approach that doesn't look at each study individually, but looks at them cumulatively. There are two ways of doing this. In one, the studies are looked at chronologically. Each study's results are combined with the ones done before to give a new estimate of the effect size. You can look and see where in the progression of these studies the results became statistically significant.

Another way of doing this is by beginning with the study with smallest sample size and then successively adding larger ones. This is a good way to uncover Type II errors. You can see where in the progression of studies the results become statistically significant. If they only become statistically significant after the vast majority of the studies had been done, the results are not as strong as if they had become statistically significant after only a few studies. This implies that there is a difference between the two groups, but that difference is relatively small clinically, even though eventually it becomes statistically significant. The chronological cumulative meta-analysis by Lau and colleagues of therapeutic trials of streptokinase in myocardial infarction showed statistical significance after the sixth trial was completed, of a total of 33 studies (Fig. 33.4).

A recent addition to the quantitative systematic review literature comes from the Cochrane Collaboration, which was described in Chapter 5. The Cochrane Collaboration is now a worldwide network of interested clinicians, epidemiologists, and scientists who perform systematic reviews and meta-analyses of clinical questions. Their reviews are standardized, of the highest quality, and updated regularly as more information becomes available. They are available online in the Cochrane Library.

Additional guidelines for meta-analysis

There are some additional guidelines for creating and reviewing meta-analyses that were published in 1985 by Green and Hall and are still very useful to follow.[2]

The inclusion and exclusion criteria for the relevant studies should be defined and reported. This may lead to substantive and conceptual issues such as how to handle a study with missing or incomplete data. The coding categories should be developed in a manner that will accommodate the largest proportion of the identified literature. Over-coding of characteristics of studies is better than under-coding. The following characteristics should be coded: type and length of the intervention, sample characteristics, research design characteristics and quality, source of the study (e.g., published, dissertation, internal report, and the like), date of study, and so on. The reliability of the coders should be checked with the kappa statistic.

Multiple independent and dependent variables should be separately evaluated using a sensitivity analysis. Interactions between variables outside the principal relationship being reviewed should be looked for. The distribution of results should be examined and graphed. Look at outliers more closely. Perform statistical tests for the heterogeneity of results. If the studies are found to be heterogeneous, a sensitivity analysis should be performed to identify the outlier study. The effect size should be specified and level of significance or confidence intervals given. Effect sizes should be recalculated to give both unadjusted and adjusted results. Where necessary, nonparametric and parametric effect size estimates should be calculated.

In the conclusions, the authors should examine other approaches to the same problem. Quantitative evaluation of all studies should be combined with qualitative reviews of the topic. This should look at the comparability of treatment and control groups from study to study. They should also look at other potentially interesting and worthwhile studies that are not part of the quantitative review. Finally, the limitations of the review and ideas for future research should be

---

[2] B. F. Green & J. A. Hall. Quantitative methods for literature review. *Annu. Rev. Psychol.* 1984; 35: 37–54.

discussed. For the reader, it is well to remember that "data analysis is an aid to thought, not a substitute."[3]

The same is true of evidence-based medicine in general. It should be an aid to thought, and an encouragement to integrate the science of medical research into clinical practice. But, it is not a substitute for critical thinking and the art of medicine. There is a great tendency to accept meta-analyses as the ultimate word in evidence. The results of such an analysis are only as good as the evidence upon which it is based. Then again, this statement can apply to all evidence in medicine. We will always be faced with making difficult decisions in the face of uncertainty. In that setting, it takes our clinical experience, intuition, common sense, and good communications with our patients to decide upon the best way to use the best evidence.

[3] B. F. Green & J. H. Hall. *Ibid.*

Appendix 1   Levels of evidence and grades of recommendations

Adapted and used with permission from the Oxford Centre for Evidence-Based Medicine *Levels of Evidence* (May 2001), available at www.cebm.net/levels_of_evidence.asp.

Adapted and used with permission from the GRADE working group of the Cochrane Collaboration.

Levels of evidence

Level	Therapy/Prevention, Etiology/Harm	Prognosis	Diagnosis	Differential diagnosis/Symptom prevalence study	Economic and decision analyses
1a	SR (with homogeneity) of RCTs[a]	SR (with homogeneity) of inception cohort studies; CDR validated in different populations[d]	SR (with homogeneity) of Level 1 diagnostic studies; CDR with 1b studies from different clinical centers	SR (with homogeneity) of prospective cohort studies	SR (with homogeneity) of Level 1 economic studies
1b	Individual RCT (with narrow confidence interval)	Individual inception cohort study with ≥80% follow-up; CDR validated in a single population	Validating cohort study with good reference standards; or CDR tested within one clinical center[gh]	Prospective cohort study with good follow-up[j]	Analysis based on clinically sensible costs or alternatives; systematic review(s) of the evidence; and including multi-way sensitivity analyses
1c	All or none[b]	All-or-none case series	Absolute SpIns and SnOuts[i]	All-or-none case series	Absolute better-value or worse-value analyses[k]
2a	SR (with homogeneity) of cohort studies	SR (with homogeneity) of either retrospective cohort studies or untreated control groups in RCTs	SR (with homogeneity) of Level >2 diagnostic studies	SR (with homogeneity) of 2b and better studies	SR (with homogeneity) of Level >2 economic studies
2b	Individual cohort study (including low-quality RCT; e.g., <80% follow-up)	Retrospective cohort study or follow-up of untreated control patients in an RCT; Derivation of CDR or validated on split-sample only[e]	Exploratory cohort study with good reference standards; CDR after derivation, or validated only on split-sample or databases	Retrospective cohort study, or poor follow-up	Analysis based on clinically sensible costs or alternatives; limited review(s) of the evidence, or single studies; and including multi-way sensitivity analyses
2c	"Outcomes" research; ecological studies	"Outcomes" research		Ecological studies	Audit or outcomes research

(cont.)

Levels of evidence (cont.)

Level	Therapy/Prevention, Etiology/Harm	Prognosis	Diagnosis	Differential diagnosis/Symptom prevalence study	Economic and decision analyses
3a	SR (with homogeneity) of case–control studies		SR (with homogeneity) of 3b and better studies	SR (with homogeneity) of 3b and better studies	SR (with homogeneity) of 3b and better studies
3b	Individual case–control study		Non-consecutive study; or without consistently applied reference standards	Non-consecutive cohort study, or very limited population	Analysis based on limited alternatives or costs, poor quality estimates of data, but including sensitivity analyses incorporating clinically sensible variations.
4	Case series (and poor-quality cohort and case–control studies)^c	Case series (and poor-quality prognostic cohort studies)^f	Case–control study, poor or non-independent reference standard	Case series or superseded reference standards	Analysis with no sensitivity analysis
5	Expert opinion without explicit critical appraisal or based on physiology, bench research, economic theory or "first principles".				

SR = Systematic review

CDR = Clinical Decision Rule

Users can add a minus sign to denote the level of evidence that fails to provide a conclusive answer because of:

- EITHER a single result with a wide confidence interval (such that, for example, an ARR in an RCT is not statistically significant but whose confidence intervals fail to exclude clinically important benefit or harm)
- OR a systematic review with troublesome (and statistically significant) heterogeneity.

Such evidence is inconclusive, and therefore can only generate Grade D recommendations.

^{a} By homogeneity we mean a systematic review that is free of worrisome variations (heterogeneity) in the directions and degrees of results between individual studies. Not all systematic reviews with statistically significant heterogeneity need be worrisome, and not all worrisome heterogeneity need be statistically significant. As noted above, studies displaying worrisome heterogeneity should be tagged with a "–" (minus sign) at the end of their designated level.

^{b} All or none: met when *all* patients died before the therapy became available, but some now survive on it; or when some patients died before the therapy became available, but *none* now die on it.

[c] By poor-quality *cohort* study we mean one that failed to clearly define comparison groups and/or failed to measure exposures and outcomes in the same (preferably blinded) objective way in both exposed and non-exposed individuals and/or failed to identify or appropriately control known confounders and/or failed to carry out a sufficiently long and complete follow-up of patients. By poor-quality *case-control* study we mean one that failed to clearly define comparison groups and/or failed to measure exposures and outcomes in the same (preferably blinded) objective way in both cases and controls and/or failed to identify or appropriately control known confounders.

[d] Clinical Decision Rules are algorithms or scoring systems which lead to a prognostic estimation or a diagnostic category.

[e] Split-sample validation is achieved by collecting all the information in a single group, then artificially dividing this into "derivation" and "validation" samples.

[f] By poor-quality prognostic cohort study we mean one in which sampling was biased in favour of patients who already had the target outcome, or the measurement of outcomes was accomplished in <80% of study patients, or outcomes were determined in an unblinded, non-objective way, or there was no correction for confounding factors.

[g] Validating studies test the quality of a specific diagnostic test, based on prior evidence. An exploratory study collects information and trawls the data (e.g., using a regression analysis) to find which factors are "significant."

[h] *Good* reference standards are independent of the test, and applied blindly or objectively to all patients. *Poor* reference standards are haphazardly applied, but still independent of the test. Use of a non-independent reference standard (where the "test" is included in the "reference," or where the "testing" affects the "reference") implies a level 4 study.

[i] An "Absolute SpPin" is a diagnostic finding whose Specificity is so high that a Positive result rules in the diagnosis. An "Absolute SnNout" is a diagnostic finding whose Sensitivity is so high that a Negative result rules out the diagnosis.

[j] Good follow-up in a differential diagnosis study is >80%, with adequate time for alternative diagnoses to emerge (e.g., 1–6 months acute, 1–5 years chronic).

[k] Better-value treatments are clearly as good but cheaper, or better at the same or reduced cost. Worse-value treatments are as good and more expensive, or worse and equally or more expensive.

Grades of recommendation

A consistent level 1 studies

B consistent level 2 or 3 studies *or* extrapolations from level 1 studies

C level 4 studies *or* extrapolations from level 2 or 3 studies

D level 5 evidence *or* troublingly inconsistent or inconclusive studies of any level

"Extrapolations" are where data are used in a situation which has potentially clinically important differences from the original study situation.

GRADE quality assessment criteria

Quality of evidence	Study design	Lower if *	Higher if *
High	Randomized trial	**Study quality:** −1 Serious limitations −2 Very serious limitations	**Strong association:** + 1 Strong, no plausible confounders, consistent and direct evidence**
Moderate			
Low	Observational study	−1 Important **inconsistency**	+ 2 Very strong, no major threats to validity and direct evidence***
Very low		**Directness:** −1 Some uncertainty −2 Major uncertainty	
		−1 **Sparse data**	+ 1 Evidence of a **Dose response** gradient
		−1 High probability of **Reporting bias**	+ 1 All **plausible confounders** would have reduced the effect

* 1 = move up or down one grade (for example from high to moderate); 2 = move up or down two grades (for example from high to low).

** A statistically significant relative risk of >2 (<0.5), based on consistent evidence from two or more observational studies, with no plausible confounders.

*** A statistically significant relative risk of >5 (<0.2), based on direct evidence with no major threats to validity.

Moving from strong to weak recommendations

Factors that can weaken the strength of a recommendation	Decision explanation
Absence of high quality evidence	• Yes • No
Imprecise estimates	• Yes • No
Uncertainty or variation in how different individuals value the outcomes	• Yes • No
Small net benefits	• Yes • No
Uncertainty about whether the net benefits are worth the costs (including the costs of implementing the recommendation)	• Yes • No

Frequent "yes" answers will increase the likelihood of a weak recommendation

- **Strong recommendation:** the panel is confident that the desirable effects of adherence to a recommendation outweigh the undesirable effects.
- **Weak recommendation:** the panel concludes that the desirable effects of adherence to a recommendation probably outweigh the undesirable effects, but is not confident.

Appendix 2   Overview of critical appraisal

Adapted from G. Guyatt & D. Rennie (eds.) *Users' Guides to the Medical Literature: a Manual for Evidence-Based Clinical Practice.* Chicago: AMA, 2002. Used with permission.

(1) Randomized clinical trials (commonly studies of therapy or prevention)
- (a) Are the results valid?
    - (i) Were the patients randomly assigned to treatment and was allocation effectively concealed?
    - (ii) Were the baseline characteristics of all groups similar at the start of the study?
    - (iii) Were the patients who entered the study fully accounted for at its conclusion?
    - (iv) Were participating patients, family members, treating clinicians, and other people (observers or managers) involved in the study "blind" to the treatment received?
    - (v) Were all measurements made in an objective and reproducible manner?
    - (vi) With the exception of the experimental intervention, were all patients treated equally?
    - (vii) Were the patients analyzed in the groups to which they were randomized?
    - (viii) Was follow-up complete?
- (b) What are the results?
    - (i) What is the treatment effect? (Absolute Rate Reduction, Relative Rate Reduction, Number Needed to Treat)
    - (ii) What is the variability of this effect? (Confidence Intervals)
- (c) Will the results help me in my patient care?
    - (i) Were all clinically important outcomes considered in the study?
    - (ii) Will the benefits of the experimental treatment counterbalance any harms and additional costs?
    - (iii) Can the results of this study be applied to most of my patients with this or similar problems?

(2) Cohort studies (commonly studies of risk or harm or etiology)
- (a) Are the results valid?
    - (i) With the exception of the risk factor under study, were all groups similar to each other at the start of the study?
    - (ii) Were all measurements (outcome and exposure) made in an objective and reproducible manner and carried out in the same ways in all groups?

      (iii) Were all patients that were entered into the study accounted for at the end of the study and was the follow-up for a sufficiently long time?

  (b) What are the results?

      (i) Is the temporal relationship between the cause and effect correct?

      (ii) Is there a dose–response gradient between the cause and effect?

      (iii) How strong is the association between cause and effect? (Relative Risk Reduction, Relative Risk, Absolute Risk Reduction, Number Needed to Harm)

      (iv) What is the variability of this effect? (Confidence Intervals)

  (c) Will the results help me in my patient care?

      (i) What is the relative magnitude of the risk in my patient population?

      (ii) Can the results of this study be applied to most of my patients with this or similar problems?

      (iii) Should I encourage the patient to stop the exposure? If yes, how soon?

(3) Case–control studies (commonly studies of etiology or risk or harm)

  (a) Are the results valid?

      (i) With the exception of the presence of the disease under study, were all groups similar to each other at the start of the study?

      (ii) Were all measurements (disease and exposure) made in an objective and reproducible manner and carried out in the same ways in all groups? Was an explicit chart review method used for all patients?

      (iii) Was the risk factor information obtained for all patients who were entered into the study?

  (b) What are the results?

      (i) Is there a dose–response gradient between the cause and effect?

      (ii) How strong is the association between cause and effect? (Odds Ratio)

      (iii) What is the variability of this effect? (Confidence Intervals)

  (c) Will the results help me in my patient care?

      (i) What is the relative magnitude of the risk in my patient population?

      (ii) Can the results of this study be applied to most of my patients with this or similar problems?

      (iii) Should I encourage the patient to stop the exposure? If yes, how soon?

Hierarchy of relative study strength

RCT > Cohort > Case–control > Case series

(4) Studies of diagnosis (commonly cohort or case–control studies)

  (a) Are the results valid?

      (i) Were all the patients in the study similar to those patients for whom the test would be used in general medical practice?

      (ii) Was there a reasonable spectrum of disease in the patients in the study?

      (iii) Were the details of the diagnostic test described adequately?

      (iv) Were all diagnostic and outcome measurements made in an objective and reproducible manner and carried out in the same ways in all patients?

      (v) Was both the test under study and a reasonable reference standard used to test all patients?

(vi) Was the comparison of the test under study to the reference standard done in a blinded manner?

(vii) Did the results of the test being studied influence the decision to perform the reference standard test?

(b) What are the results?

(i) How strong is the diagnostic test? (Likelihood Ratios, Sensitivity and Specificity)

(ii) What is the variability of this result? (Confidence Intervals)

(c) Will the results help me in my patient care?

(i) Can the test be used in my patient population when considering factors of availability, performance, and cost?

(ii) Can I determine a reasonable pretest probability of disease in my patients?

(iii) Will the performance of the test result in significant change in management for my patients?

(iv) Will my patient be better off as a result of having obtained the test?

Appendix 3 Commonly used statistical tests

The following is a very simplistic summary of the usual tests used in statistical inference.

Descriptive statistics

Type of variable	What is being described	Statistic	Graph
Single variable			
Ratio or interval	Central tendency	Mean	Histogram Stem–leaf plot Frequency polygon Box plot
	Dispersion	Standard deviation	
	Deviation from normality	Skew or Kurtosis	
Ranks	Central tendency	Median	Box plot (ordinal) Bar chart
	Dispersion	Range	Interquartile range
Named	Central tendency	Mode	Bar chart (nominal) Dot plot
	Dispersion	Number of categories	
Two variables			
Ratio or interval	Association	Pearson's r	Scatter plot
Nominal or ordinal	Comparison	Kappa, phi, rho Weighted kappa	Paired bar chart Scatter plot

Inferential statistics

Type of dependent variables	Number and type of independent variables	Test
Ratio or interval data		
One or two means	None	t-test or z-test ($n > 100$)
	Continuous	F-test or t-test
	Nominal	t-test
(Multiple regression)	Multiple continuous	F-test
(ANOVA)	Multiple nominal	F-test or Student Newman–Keuls test
(ANCOVA)	Multiple continuous and nominal	F-test
	Association	Pearson's r
	Predicting variable values	Regression
Ordinal data	None	Wilcoxon signed rank test
	Ordinal	Spearman's test
	Nominal	Mann–Whitney test
	Multiple ordinal	χ^2-test
	Multiple nominal	Kruskal–Wallis test
	Association	Spearman's ρ
Nominal data	None (affected by time)	Normal approximation to Poisson
	Nominal (paired)	McNemar's test
	Nominal (unpaired)	χ^2-test, normal approximation, or Mantel–Haenszel test
	Continuous	χ^2-test for trend
	Multiple continuous or nominal	χ^2-test
	Multiple nominal	Mantel–Haenszel test

Multivariate analysis

Multiple linear regression is used when the outcome variable is continuous

Multiple logistic regression is used when the outcome variable is binary event (e.g., alive or dead, disease-free or recurrent disease, etc.)

Discriminant function analysis is used when the outcome variable is categorical (better, worse, or about the same)

Proportional hazards regression (Cox regression) is used when the outcome variable is the time to the occurrence of a binary event (e.g., time to death or tumor recurrence)

Appendix 4   Formulas

Descriptive statistics

Mean: $\mu = (\Sigma x_i)/n$
   where x_i-the numerical value of the i th data point, and n-the total number of data
   points.
Variance (s^2 or σ^2): $s^2 = (\Sigma(x_i - \mu)^2)/(n - 1)$.
Standard deviation (SD, s, or σ): $s = \sqrt{s^2}$

Confidence intervals using the standard error of the mean

95% CI $= \mu \pm Z_{95\%}(\sigma/\sqrt{n})$
$Z_{95\%} = 1.96$ (number of standard deviations defining 95% of the data)
SEM $= \sigma/\sqrt{n}$
95% CI $= \mu \pm 1.96$ (SEM)

Basic probability

Probability that event a or event b will occur: P (a or b) $= P$ (a) $+ P$ (b)
Probability that event a and event b will occur: P (a and b) $= P$ (a) $\times P$ (b)
Probability that at least one of several mutually exclusive events will occur $= 1 - P$ (none of
the events will occur)
   where P (none of the events will occur) $= P$ (not a) $\times P$ (not b) $\times P$ (not c) $\times$ ...

Event rates (Fig A.4.1)

Control event rate $=$ CER $=$ control patients with outcome of interest/all control
patients $=$ A/CE
Experimental event rate $=$ EER $=$ experimental patients with outcome of interest/all exper-
imental patients $=$ C/EE
Absolute rate reduction $=$ ARR $=$ |EER $-$ CER|
Relative rate reduction $=$ RRR $=$ (CER $-$ EER)/CER
Number needed to treat to benefit $=$ NNTB $= 1$/ARR

Relative risk and odds ratio (Fig A.4.2)

Absolute risk of disease in risk group $=$ A/(A $+$ B)
Absolute risk of disease in no risk group $=$ C/(C $+$ D)

Fig. A.4.1 Event-rate
calculations: 2 × 2 table.

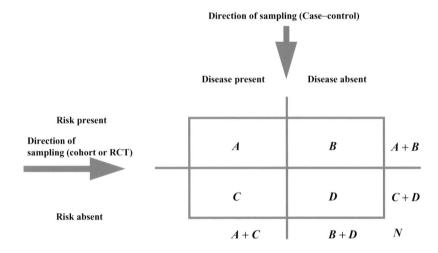

	Events of interest	Other events		
Control or placebo group	A	B	CE	Control group events
Experimental group	C	D	EE	Experimental group events

Fig. A.4.2 Relative-risk and
odds-ratio calculations: 2 × 2
table.

Direction of sampling (Case–control)

Disease present   **Disease absent**

Risk present

**Direction of
sampling (cohort or RCT)**

A	B	$A + B$
C	D	$C + D$

Risk absent

$A + C$ $B + D$ N

population

Relative risk of disease $= RR = [A/(A + B)]/[C/(C + D)]$
Absolute attributable risk $= AAR = [A/(A + B)] - [C/(C + D)]$
Attributable risk percent relative to no-risk group $= [A/(A + B) - C/(C + D)]/[C/(C + D)]$
   Also called relative attributable risk. Dependent on which variable you want to measure this relative to, it can also be written as;
Attributable risk percent relative to risk group $= [A/(A + B) - C/(C + D)]/[A/(A + B)]$
Number needed to treat to harm $= NNTH = 1/AAR$
Odds of risk factor if diseased $= A/C$
Odds of risk factor if not diseased $= B/D$
Odds ratio $= OR = [A/C]/[B/D] = AD/BC$

Confidence intervals (Fig. A.4.3)

For odds ration: Confidence Interval $= CI = \text{expln}(OR) \pm 1.96\sqrt{(1/A + 1/B + 1/C + 1/D)}$
For relative risk: Confidence Interval $= CI = \text{expln}(RR) \pm 1.96\sqrt{([(1 - (A/(A + B)))/A])}$
   $+ [(1 - (C/(C + D))/D])$
Let the computer do the calculations!

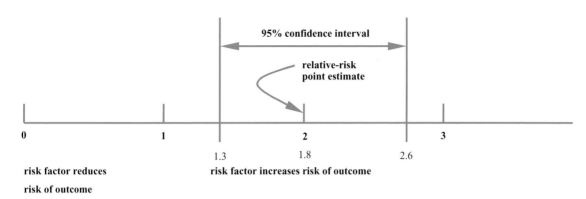

Fig. A.4.3 Confidence interval for relative risk.

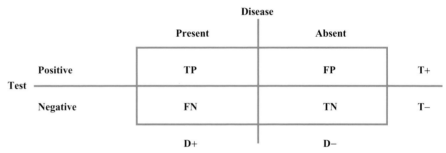

Fig. A.4.4 Diagnostic tests: 2 × 2 table.

Diagnostic tests (Fig. A.4.4)

True positive rate = TPR = TP/D+ = sensitivity
False positive rate = FPR = FP/D− = 1 − specificity
False negative rate = FNR = FN/D+ = 1 − sensitivity
True negative rate = TNR = TN/D− = specificity
Likelihood ratio of a positive test = LR+ = sensitivity/(1 − specificity)
Likelihood ratio of a negative test = LR− = (1 − sensitivity)/specificity
Positive predictive value = PPV = TP/T+
Negative predictive value = NPV = TN/T−
False alarm rate = FAR = 1 − PPV
False reassurance rate = FRR = 1 − NPV

Bayes' theorem

Odds = probability/(1 − probability)
Post-test odds = pretest odds × likelihood ratio (this is PPV if LR+ is used and FRR if LR−
is used)
Probability = odds/(1 + odds)

Appendix 5 Proof of Bayes' theorem

For a given test with the following parameters:

Sensitivity = N Specificity = S Pretest probability (prevalence of disease) = P, the 2×2 table will be as shown in Fig. A.5.1.

Using the sensitivity and specificity:

$$PPV = \frac{NP}{T+} = \frac{NP}{NP + ((1 - S)(1 - P))}$$

Using Bayes' theorem:

$O(pre) = P/(1 - P)$ and

$O(post) = O(pre) \times LR+$

$LR+ = N/(1 - S)$

$O(post) = [P/(1 - P)] \times [(N)/(1 - S)] = NP/((1 - S)(1 - P))$

$$P(post) = O/(1 + O) = \frac{NP/((1 - S)(1 - P))}{1 + (NP/((1 - S)(1 - P)))}$$

Now multiply top and bottom by $(1 - S)(1 - P)$:

$$= \frac{NP}{((1 - S)(1 - P)) + NP} \text{ or } \frac{NP}{NP + ((1 - S)(1 - P))}$$

The same as the PPV.

Similarly:

$$FRR = 1 - NPV = \frac{(1 - N)P}{T-} = \frac{P(1 - N)}{S(1 - P) + P(1 - N)}$$

$LR- = (1 - N)/S$

$O(post) = (P/(1 - P)) \times ((1 - N)/S) = P(1 - N)/S(1 - P)$

$$P(post) = \frac{P(1 - N)/S(1 - P)}{1 + (P(1 - N)/S(1 - P))}$$

Now multiply top and bottom by $S(1 - P)$:

$$P(post) = \frac{P(1 - N)}{S(1 - P) + P(1 - N)}$$

The same as the FRR (Fig. A.5.1).

	D+	D−	
T+	NP	(1−S)(1−P)	NP + (1−S)(1−P)
T−	(1−N)P	S(1−P)	(1−N)P + S(1−P)
	P	1−P	

Fig. A.5.1 Bayes' theorem: 2 × 2 table.

Appendix 6   Using balance sheets to calculate thresholds

Strep throat

Suppose you are examining a 36-year-old white male with a sore throat and want to know whether treatment for strep throat is a good idea. Exam is equivocal with large tonsils with exudate, but no cervical nodes or scarlatiniform rash, and only slight coryza.[1]

Disease   Strep throat

Prevalence in the literature   About 20% for large tonsils with exudate. If no exudate this drops to about 10%, and if also tender cervical nodes it increases to 40%.

Estimate the treatment threshold.

Potential harm from antibiotic treatment   4–5% of patients will get a rash or diarrhea, both of which are uncomfortable but not life-threatening. Anaphylaxis (life-threatening allergy) is very rare ($< 1 : 200\,000$) and will not be counted in the analysis. Harm $= 0.05$.

Impact of this harm   Discomfort for about 2–3 days, gets about 0.1 on a 0–1 scale. It could be greater if the patient modeled swimwear and a rash would put him or her out of work for those days. Impact $= 0.1$.

Impact of improvement   Since treatment results in relief of symptoms about 1 day sooner, this should be similar to the harm impact, 0.1 on the 0–1 scale. Impact $= 0.1$. Improvement $= 1$ (100% get better by this 1 day).

Action or treatment threshold   (Harm $\times$ harm impact) / (improvement $\times$ improvement impact) $= (0.1 \times 0.05) / (0.1 \times 1) = 0.05$.

This is the threshold for treatment without testing.

Will a test change your mind if the pretest probability is 20%?

The sensitivity and specificity of throat culture is 0.9 and 0.85 respectively. If you apply these to a pretest probability of 20%, a negative test will result in NPV $= 0.03$ (3%). This is below the action (treatment) threshold (5%) and so treatment would not be initiated if the test were negative. Therefore it pays to do the test.

Tuberculosis

Now let's consider a different problem in an Asian man with lung lesions, fever, and cough, and let's use a slightly different methodology. The differential is between

---

[1] From R. Gross. *Making Medical Decisions: an Approach to Clinical Decision Making for Practicing Physicians*. Philadelphia, PA: American College of Physicians, 1999.

tuberculosis (highly contagious and treated with antibiotics) and sarcoidosis (not contagious and treated with steroids). The initial testing is negative for both. How should the patient be treated while waiting for the results of the culture for TB (gold standard)? Clinical probability of TB estimated at 70% before initial testing, 40% after initial testing (normal angiotensin-converting-enzyme level, negative TB skin test, noncaseating granulomas on biopsy).

> Normal angiotensin-converting-enzyme level: against sarcoidosis but poor sensitivity
> Negative TB skin test: against TB, but can be present in overwhelming TB infection (poor sensitivity)
> Noncaseating granulomas on biopsy: against TB and for sarcoidosis
> Benefit (B) = untreated TB mortality − treated TB mortality = 50% − 20% = 30%
> Risk (R) = death from hepatitis due to treatment = prevalence of hepatitis in Asian men treated with TB medications (2%) × risk for death from hepatitis (7.6%) = 0.15%

> Treatment threshold = $1/(B : R + 1)$

> $B : R = 30 : 0.15 = 200$

Treatment threshold = $1/201 = 0.005$

> Therefore treat with TB medications since the estimated probability of disease in this patient is 40%, greater than the treatment threshold. If B is very high and R is very low, you will almost always treat regardless of the test result. If the converse (R high and B low) you will be much less likely to treat without fairly high degree of evidence of the target disorder.

Acute myocardial infarction

In this case, you must consider how sure you are of the diagnosis to use the more expensive thrombolytic therapy (t-PA) rather than the cheaper streptokinase (SK).

> $B = 0.01 − 1\%$ (difference between the mortality of AMI with t-PA compared to SK)
> $R = 0.008 − 0.8\%$ (difference between the occurrence of acute cerebral bleed from t-PA over SK)

> Therefore $B : R = 1.2$

B:R + 1 = 2.2 and T = 1/2.2 = 0.45 and you would not initiate thrombolytic therapy unless the probability of thrombotic MI was greater than 45%.

Glossary

2AFC (two-alternative-forced-choice) problem The probability that one can identify an abnormal patient from a normal patient using this test alone.

Absolute risk The percentage of subjects in a group that experiences a discrete outcome.

Absolute risk (rate) reduction (ARR) The difference in rates of outcomes between the control group and the experimental or exposed group. An efficacious therapy serves to reduce that risk. For example, if 15% of the placebo group died and 10% of the treatment group died, ARR or the absolute reduction in the risk of death is 5%.

Accuracy Closeness of a given observation to the true value of that state.

Adjustment Changing the probability of disease as a result of performing a diagnostic maneuver (additional history, physical exam, or diagnostic test of some kind).

Algorithm A preset path which takes the clinician from the patient's presenting complaints to a final management decision through a series of predetermined branching decision points.

All-or-none case series In previous studies all the patients who were not given the intervention died and now some survive, or many of the patients previously died and now none die.

Alternative hypothesis There is a difference between groups or an association between predictor and outcome variables. Example: the patients being treated with a newer antihypertensive drug will have a lower blood pressure than those treated with the older drug.

Anchoring The initial assignment of pretest probability of disease based upon elements of the history and physical.

Applicability The degree to which the results of a study are likely to hold true in your practice setting. Also called **external validity, generalizability, particularizability, relevance**.

Arm (of decision tree) A particular diagnostic modality, risk factor, or treatment method.

Assessment Clinician's inferences on the nature of the patient's problem. Synonymous with differential diagnosis or hypotheses of cause of the underlying problems.

AUC (area under the ROC curve) Probability that one can identify a diseased patient from a healthy one using this test alone.

Availability heuristic The ability to think of something depends upon how recently you studied that fact.

Bayes' theorem What we know after doing a test equals what we knew before doing the test times a modifier (based on the test results). Post-test odds = pretest odds × likelihood ratio.

Bias Any factor other than the experimental therapy that could change the study results in a non-random way. The direction of bias offset may be unpredictable. The validity of a study is integrally related to the degree to which the results could have been affected by biased factors.

Blinding Masking or concealment from study subjects, caregivers, observers, or others involved in the study of some or all details of the study. Process by which neither the subject nor the research team members who have contact with the subject know to which treatment condition the subject is assigned. Single-blind means that one person (patient or physician) does not know what is going on. Double-blind means that at least two people (usually patient and treating physician) don't know what's going on. Triple-blind means that patient, treating physician, and person measuring outcome don't know to which group patient is assigned. It can also mean that the paper is written before the results are tabulated. The whole point of blinding is to prevent bias.

Case–control study Subjects are grouped by outcome, cases having the disease or outcome of interest and controls. The presence of the risk factor of interest is then compared in the two groups. These studies are usually retrospective.

Case report or case series One or a group of cases of a particular disease or outcome of interest with no control group.

Clinical guideline An algorithm used in making clinical decisions. Also called a *Practice guideline*.

Clinical significance Results that make enough difference to you and your patient to justify changing your way of doing things. For example, a drug which is found in a megatrial of 50 000 adults with acute asthma to increase FEV1 by only 0.5% ($P < 0.0001$)

would fail this test of significance. The findings must have practical importance as well as statistical importance.

Cochrane collaboration   An internationally organized effort to catalog and systematically evaluate all existing clinical studies into systematic reviews easily accessible to practicing clinicians so as to facilitate the process of using the best clinical evidence in patient care.

Cohort study   Subjects are grouped by the risk factor, and those with and without the risk factor are followed to see who develops the disease and who doesn't. The occurrence of the outcome of interest is compared in the two groups. These studies can be prospective or retrospective (non-concurrent).

Cointervention   A treatment that is not under investigation given to a study patient. Can be a source of bias in the study.

Competing-hypotheses heuristic   A way of thinking in which all possible hypotheses are evaluated for their likelihood and final decision is based on the most likely hypothesis modified by secondary evaluations.

Confidence intervals   An interval around an observed parameter guaranteed to include the true value to some level of confidence (usually 95%). The true value can be expected to be within that interval with 95% confidence.

Continuous test results   A test resulting in an infinite number of possible outcome values.

Control group   The subjects in an experiment who do not receive the treatment procedure being studied. They may get nothing, a placebo, or a standard or previously validated therapy.

Controlled clinical trial   Any study that compares two groups for exposure to different therapies or risk factors. A true experiment in which one group is given the experimental intervention and the other group is a control group.

Cost-effectiveness   Marginal cost divided by marginal benefit. (Cost of treatment A – cost of treatment B)/(benefit of treatment A – benefit of treatment B).

Cost-effectiveness (or cost–benefit) analysis   Research study which determines how much more has to be paid in order to achieve a given benefit of preventing death, disability days, or another outcome.

Cost-minimization analysis   Analysis in which only costs are compared.

Criterion-based validity   How well a measurement agrees with other approaches for measuring the same characteristic.

Critical appraisal   The process of assessing and interpreting evidence systematically, considering its validity, results, and relevance.

Critical value   Value of a test statistic to which the observed value is compared to determine statistical significance. The observed test statistic indicates significant differences or associations exist if its value is greater than the critical value.

Critically appraised topic (CAT)   A summary of a search and critical appraisal of the literature related to a focused clinical question. Catalogue of these kept in an easily accessible place (e.g., online) can be used to help make real-time clinical decisions.

Decision analysis   Systematic way in which the components of decision making can be incorporated to make the best possible clinical decision using a mathematical model. Also known as *Expected values decision making*.

Decision node   A point on a branching decision tree at which the clinician must make a decision to either perform a clinical maneuver (diagnosis or management) or not.

Degrees of freedom (df)   A number used to select the appropriate critical value of a statistic from a table of critical values.

Dependent variable   The outcome variable that is influenced by changes in the independent variable of a study.

Descriptive research   Study which summarizes, tabulates, or organizes a set of measures (i.e., answers the questions who, what, when, where, and how).

Descriptive statistics   The branch of statistics that summarizes, tabulates, and organizes data for the purpose of describing observations or measurements.

Diagnostic test characteristics   Those qualities of a diagnostic test that are important to understand how valuable it would be in a clinical setting. These include sensitivity, specificity, accuracy, precision, and reliability.

Diagnostic tests   Modalities which can be used to increase the accuracy of a clinical assessment by helping to narrow the list of possible diseases that a patient can have.

Dichotomous outcome   Any outcome measure for which there are only two possibilities, like dead/alive, admitted/discharged, graduated/sent to glue factory. Beware of potentially fake dichotomous outcome reports such as "improved/not improved", particularly when derived from continuous outcome measures. For example, if I define a 10-point or greater increase in a continuous variable as "improved," I may show what looks like a tremendous benefit when that result is clinically insignificant. This is lesson 2a in "How to lie with statistics."

Dichotomous test results　　Only two possible outcome values, yes or no, positive or negative, alive or dead, etc.

Differential diagnosis　　A list of possible diseases that your patient can have in descending order of clinical probability.

Effect size　　The amount of change measured in a given variable as a result of the experiment. In meta-analyses when different studies have measured somewhat different things, a statistically derived generic size of the combined result.

Effectiveness　　How well the proposed intervention works in a clinical trial to produce a desired and measurable effect in a well-done clinical trial. These results may not be duplicated in "real life."

Efficacy　　How well the proposed intervention actually works in practice to produce a desired outcome in other more generalized clinical situations. This is usually the desired outcome for the patient and society.

Event rate　　The percentage of events of interest in one or the other of the groups in an experiment. These rates are compared to calculate number needed to treat. This is also a term for absolute risk.

Expected values (E)　　Probability × Utility ($P \times U$). The value of each arm of the decision tree or the entire decision tree (sum of $P \times U$).

Expected-values decision making　　See *Decision analysis.*

Experimental group(s)　　The subjects in an experiment who receive the treatment procedure or manipulation that is being proposed to improve health or treat illness.

Explanatory research – experimental　　Study in which the independent variable (usually a treatment) is changed by the researcher who then observes the effect of this change on the dependent variable (usually an outcome). The key here is the willful manipulation of the two variables.

Explanatory research – observational　　Study looking for possible causes of disease (dependent variable) based upon exposure to one or more risk factors (independent variable) in the population.

Exposure　　Any type of contact with a substance that causes an outcome. A drug, a surgical procedure, risk factor, even a diagnostic test can be an exposure. In therapy, prognosis, or harm studies the "exposure" is the intervention being studied.

External validity　　See *Applicability.*

False negative (FN)   Patients with disease who have a normal or negative test.

False positive (FP)   Patients without disease who have an abnormal or positive test.

FAR (false alarm rate)   Percentage of patients with a positive test who don't have disease and will be unnecessarily tested or treated based on the incorrect results of a test.

Filter   A process by which patients are entered into or excluded from a study. Inclusion and exclusion criteria when stated explicitly.

FNR (false negative rate)   One minus the sensitivity (1 – sens). Percentage of diseased patients with a negative or normal test.

FPR (false positive rate)   One minus the specificity (1 – spec). Percentage of non-diseased patients with a positive or abnormal test.

Framing effect   How a question is worded (or framed) will influence the answer to the question.

FRR (False reassurance rate)   Percentage of patients with a negative or normal test result who actually have disease and will lose benefits of treatment for the disease.

Functional status   An outcome which describes the ability of a person to interact in society and carry on with their daily living activities (e.g., Activities of Daily Living (ADL) or the Arthritis Activity Scale used in Rheumatoid Arthritis).

Gaussian   Typical bell-shaped frequency curve in which normal test values are 95% (± 2SD of all tests done) of all possible values.

Generalizability   See *Applicability*.

Gold standard   The reference standard for evaluation of a measurement or diagnostic test. The "gold-standard" test is assumed to correctly identify the presence or absence of disease 100% of the time.

Harm vs. benefit   An accounting of the positive and negative aspects of an exposure (positive or negative) on the outcomes of a study.

Heuristics   Models for the way people think.

Homogeneity   Whether the results from a set of independently performed studies on a particular question are similar enough to make statistical pooling valid.

Hypothesis   An educated guess on the nature of the patient's illness, usually obtained by selecting those diseases having the same history or physical examination characteristics as the patient.

Hypothetico-deductive strategy   A diagnosis is made by advancing a hypothesis and then deducing the correctness or incorrectness of that hypothesis through the use of statistical methods, specifically the characteristics of diagnostic tests.

Incidence   The rate at which an event occurs in a defined population over time. The number of new cases (or other events of interest) divided by the total population at risk.

Incorporation bias   The test being measured is part of the gold standard or inclusion criteria for entry into a study.

Incremental gain   Amount of increase in diagnostic certainty. The change in the pretest probability of a diagnosis as a result of performing a diagnostic test.

Independent variable(s)   The treatment or exposure variable that is presumed to cause some effect on the outcome or dependent variable.

Inferential statistics   Drawing conclusions about a population based on findings from a sample.

Instrumental rationality   Calculation of a treatment strategy which will produce the greatest benefit for the patient.

Instrumentation   The process of selecting or developing measuring devices.

Instruments (measuring devices)   Something that makes a measurement, e.g., thermometer, sphygmomanometer (blood pressure cuff and manometer), questionnaire, etc.

Intention-to-treat   Patients assigned to a particular treatment group by the study protocol are retained in that group for the purpose of analysis of the study results no matter what happens.

Internal validity   See *Validity*.

Inter-observer reliability   Consistency between two different observers' measurements.

Interval likelihood ratios (iLR)   Probability of a test result in the interval among diseased subjects divided by the probability of a test result within the interval among non-diseased subjects.

Intra-observer reliability   Ability of the same observer to reproduce a measure.

Intrinsic characteristics of a diagnostic test   See *Diagnostic test characteristics.*

Justice   Equal access to medical care for all patients who require it based only upon the severity of their disease.

Kappa statistic   A measure of inter- or intra-observer reliability.

Level of significance (confidence level)   Describes the probability of incorrectly rejecting the null hypothesis and concluding that there is a difference when in fact none exists (i.e., probability of Type I error). Many times this probability is 0.01, 0.05, or 0.10. For medical studies it is most commonly set at 0.05.

Likelihood ratio of a negative test (LR–)   The false negative rate divided by the true negative rate. The amount by which the pretest probability of disease is reduced in patients with a negative test.

Likelihood ratio of a positive test (LR+)   The true positive rate divided by the false positive rate. The amount by which the pretest probability is increased in patients with a positive test.

Likelihood ratio   A single number which summarizes test sensitivity and specificity and modifies the pretest probability of disease to give a post-test probability.

Linear rating scale   A scale from zero to one on which patients can place a mark to determine their value for a particular outcome.

Markov models   A method of decision analysis that considers all possible health states and their interactions at the same time.

Matching   An attempt in an experiment to create equivalence between the control and treatment groups. Control subjects are matched with experimental subjects based upon one or more variables.

Mean   A measure of central tendency; the arithmetic average.

Measurement   The application of an instrument or method to collect data systematically. What the use of the instrument tells us, e.g., temperature, blood pressure, results of dietary survey, etc.

Meta-analysis   A systematic review of a focused clinical question following rigorous methodological criteria and employing statistical techniques to combine data from multiple independently performed studies on that question.

Multiple-branching strategy   An algorithmic method used for making diagnoses.

N or *n*   Number of subjects in the sample or the number of observations made in a study.

Negative predictive value (NPV)   Probability of no disease after a negative test result.

Nodes   Junctures where something happens. The common ones are decision and probability nodes.

Non-inferiority trial   A study that seeks to show that one of two treatments is not worse than the other.

Normal   (1) A normal distribution or Gaussian distribution of variables, the bell-shaped curve. (2) A value of a diagnostic test which defines patients who are not diseased.

Null hypothesis   The assumption that there is no difference between groups or no association between predictor and outcome variables.

Number needed to follow (NNF)   Number of patients who must be followed before one additional bad outcome is noted. The lower this number, the worse the risk factor.

Number needed to treat to harm (NNTH)   Number of patients who must be treated or exposed to a risk factor to have one additional bad outcome. The lower this number the worse the exposure.

Number needed to treat to benefit (NNTB)   Number of patients who must be treated to have one additional successful outcome. The lower that number, the better the therapy.

Objective   Information observed by the physician from the patient examination and diagnostic tests.

Observational study   Any study of therapy, prevention, or harm in which the exposure is not assigned to the individual subject by the investigator(s). A synonym is "non-experimental" and examples are case–control and cohort studies.

Odds   The number of times an event occurred divided by the number of times it didn't.

Odds ratio   The ratio of the odds of an event in one group divided by the odds in another group.

One-tailed statistical test   Used when the alternative hypothesis is directional (i.e., specifies a particular direction of the difference between the groups.)

Operator-dependent   The results of a test are dependent on the skill of the person performing the test.

Outcome   Disease or final state of patient (e.g., alive or dead).

Outcomes study   The outcome of an intervention, exposure, or diagnosis measured over a period of time.

P value   The probability that the difference(s) observed between two or more groups in a study occurred by chance if there really was no difference between the groups.

Pathognomonic   The presence of signs or symptoms of disease which can lead to only one diagnosis (i.e. they are only characteristic of that one disease).

Patient satisfaction   A rating scale which measures the degree to which patients are happy with the care they received or feel that the care was appropriate.

Patient values   A number, generally from 0 (usually death) to 1 (usually complete recovery), which denotes the degree to which a patient is desirous of a particular outcome.

Pattern recognition   Recognizing a disease diagnosis based on a pattern of signs and symptoms.

Percentiles   Cutoffs between positive and negative test result chosen within preset percentiles of the patients tested.

Placebo   An inert substance given to a study subject who has been assigned to the control group to make them think they are getting the treatment under study.

Plan   What treatment or further diagnostic testing is required.

Point   On a decision tree, the outcome of possible decisions made by the patient and clinician.

Point estimate   The exact result that has been observed in a study. The confidence interval tells you the range within which the true value of the result is likely to lie with 95% confidence.

Point of indifference   The probability of an outcome of certain death at which a patient no longer can decide between that outcome and an uncertain outcome of partial disability.

Population   The group of people who meet the criteria for entry into a study (whether they actually participated in the study or not). The group of people to whom the study results can be generalized.

Positive predictive value   Probability of disease after the occurrence of a positive test result.

Post-test odds The odds of disease after a test has been done. Post-test odds = pretest odds × likelihood ratio.

Post-test probability The probability of disease after a test has been performed. This is calculated from post-test odds converted to probability. Also called *posterior* or *a-posteriori probability*.

Power The probability that an experimental study will correctly observe a statistically significant difference between the study groups when that difference actually exists.

Precision The measurement is nearly the same value each time it is measured. Measure of random variation or error, or a small standard deviation of the measurement across multiple measurements.

Predictive values The probability that a patient with a particular outcome on a diagnostic test (positive or negative) has or does not have the disease.

Predictor variable The variable that is going to predict the presence or absence of disease, or results of a test.

Pretest odds The odds of disease before a test is run.

Pretest probability The probability of disease before a test is run. This is converted to odds for use with Bayes' theorem. Also called *prior* or *a-priori probability*.

Prevalence The proportion of people in a defined group who have a disease, condition, or injury. The numbers affected by a condition divided by the population at risk. In the context of diagnosis, this is also called "pretest probability."

Probability node A point in the decision tree at which two or more events occur by chance.

Problem-oriented medical record (POMR) A format of keeping medical records by which one keeps track of and updates a patient's problems regularly.

Prognosis The possible outcomes for a given disease and the length of time to those outcomes.

Prospective study Any study done forward in time. Important in studies on therapy, prognosis, or harm, where retrospective studies make hidden biases more likely.

Publication bias The possibility that studies with conflicting results (most often negative studies) are less likely to be published.

Quality of life   A composite measure of the satisfaction of a patient with their life and their ability to function appropriately.

Quality-adjusted life years (QALYs)   Standardized measure of quality and life expectancy commonly used in decision analyses. Life expectancy times expected value or utility.

Random selection or assignment   Selection process of a sample of the population such that every subject in the population has an equal chance of being selected for each arm of the study.

Randomization   A technique that gives every patient an equal chance of winding up in any particular arm of a controlled clinical trial.

Randomized clinical trial or Randomized controlled trial (RCT)   An interventional study in which the patients are randomly selected or assigned either to a group which gets the intervention or to a control group.

Receiver operating characteristic (ROC) curve   A plot of sensitivity versus one minus specificity (true-positive rate versus false positive rate) can give the quality of a diagnostic test and determine which is the best cutoff point.

Referral bias   Patients entered into a study because they have been referred for a particular test or to a specialty provider.

Relative risk   The probability of outcome in the group with exposure divided by the probability of outcome in the group without the exposure.

Reliability   Loose synonym of precision, or the extent to which repeated measurements of the same phenomenon are consistent, reproducible, and dependable.

Representativeness heuristic   The ease with which a diagnosis is recalled depends on how closely the patient presentation fits the classical presentation of the disease.

Research question (hypothesis)   A question stating a general prediction of results which the researcher attempts to answer by conducting a study.

Retrospective study   Any study in which the outcomes have already occurred before the study and collection of data has begun.

Risk   Probability of an adverse event divided by all of the times one is exposed to that event.

Risk factor   Any aspect of an individual's life, behavior, or inheritance that could affect (increase or decrease) the likelihood of an outcome (disease, condition, or injury.)

Rule in   To effectively determine that a particular diagnosis is correct by either excluding all other diagnoses or making the probability of that diagnosis so high that other diagnoses are effectively excluded.

Rule out   To effectively exclude a diagnosis by making the probability of that disease so low that it effectively is so unlikely to occur or would be considered non-existent.

Sample   That part of the population selected to be studied. The group specifically included in the actual study.

Sampling bias   To select patients for study based on some criteria that could relate to the outcome.

Screening   Looking for disease among asymptomatic patients.

Sensitivity   The ability of a test to identify patients who have disease when it is present. True-positive rate.

Sensitivity analysis   An analytical procedure to determine how the results of a study would change if the input variables are changed.

Setting   The place in which the testing for a disease occurs, usually referring to level of care.

SOAP notes   Subjective, objective, assessment, and plan. The typical format for problem-oriented medical record notes.

Specificity   The ability of a test to identify patients without the disease when it is negative. True-negative rate.

Spectrum   In a diagnostic study, the range of clinical presentations and relevant disease advancement exhibited by the subjects included in the study.

Spectrum bias   The sensitivity of a test is higher in more severe or "well-developed" cases of a disease, and lower when patients present earlier in the course of disease, or when the disease is occult.

Standard gamble   A technique to determine patient values by which patients are given a choice between a known outcome and a hypothetical-probabilistic outcome.

Statistic   A number that describes some characteristic of a set of data.

Statistical power   See *Power.*

Statistical significance   A measure of how confidently an observed difference between two or more groups can be attributed to the study interventions rather than chance alone.

Stratified randomization   A way of ensuring that the different groups in an experimental trial are balanced with respect to some important factors that could affect the outcome.

Strategy of exhaustion   Listing all possible diseases which a patient could have and running every diagnostic test available and necessary to exclude all diseases on that list until only one is left.

Subjective   Information from the patient, the history which the patient gives you and which they are experiencing.

Surrogate marker   An outcome variable that is associated with the outcome of interest, but changes in this marker are not necessarily a direct measure of changes in the clinical outcome of interest.

Survival analysis   A mathematical analysis of outcome after some kind of therapy in which patients are followed for given a period of time to determine what percentage are still alive or disease-free after that time.

Systematic review   A formal review of a focused clinical question based on a comprehensive search strategy and structured critical appraisal of all relevant studies.

Testing threshold   Probability of disease above which we should test before initiating treatment for that disease, and below which we should neither treat nor test.

Threshold approach to decision making   Determining values of pretest probability below which neither testing nor treatment should be done and above which treatment should be begun without further testing.

Time trade-off   A method of determining patient utility using a simple question of how much time in perfect health a patient would trade for a given amount of time in imperfect health.

Treatment threshold   Probability of disease above which we should initiate treatment without first doing the test for the disease.

Triggering   A thought process which is initiated by recognition of a set of signs and symptoms leading the clinician to think of a particular disease.

Two-tailed statistical test   Used when alternative hypothesis is non-directional and there is no specification of the direction of differences between the groups.

Type I error   Error made by rejecting the null hypothesis when it is true and accepting the alternative hypothesis when it isn't true.

Type II error   Error made by not rejecting the null hypothesis when it is false and the alternative hypothesis is true.

Unadjusted life expectancy (life years)   The number of years a person is expected to live based solely on their age at the time. Adjusting would consider lifestyle factors such as smoking, risk-taking, cholesterol, weight, etc.

Uncertainty   The inability to determine precisely what an outcome would be for a disease or diagnostic test.

Utility   The measure of value of an outcome. Also whether a patient is truly better off as a result of a diagnostic test.

Validity   (1) The degree to which the results of a study are likely to be true, believable and free of bias. (2) The degree to which a measurement represents the phenomenon of interest.

Variable   Something that can take on different values such as a diagnostic test, risk factor, treatment, outcome, or characteristic of a group.

Variance   A measure of the spread of values around the mean.

Yule–Simpson paradox   A statistical paradox in which one group is superior overall while the other is superior for all of the subgroups.

Bibliography

Common medical journals

The following are the major peer-reviewed medical journals grouped by specialty. This is only a partial list. Many other peer-reviewed journals exist in all specialties.

General

New England Journal of Medicine
JAMA (Journal of the American Medical Association)
BMJ (British Medical Journal)
Lancet
Postgraduate Medicine

Emergency Medicine

Annals of Emergency Medicine
American Journal of Emergency Medicine
Journal of Emergency Medicine
Academic Emergency Medicine

Family Practice

Family Physician
Journal of Family Practice
Journal of the American Board of Family Practice
Archives of Family Practice

Internal Medicine

Annals of Internal Medicine
Journal of General Internal Medicine
Archives of Internal Medicine
American Journal of Medicine

Internal Medicine Specialties

American Journal of Cardiology
Circulation
Thorax

Annual Review of Respiratory Diseases
Gut
Gastroenterology
Nephron
Blood

Medical Education
Academic Medicine
Medical Teacher

Neurology and Neurosurgery
Annals of Neurology
Neurology
Stroke
Journal of Neurosurgery
Neurosurgery

Obstetrics and Gynecology
Obstetrics and Gynecology
American Journal of Obstetrics and Gynecology

Pediatrics
Pediatrics
Journal of Pediatrics
American Journal of Diseases of Children

Psychiatry
American Journal of Psychiatry
Journal of Clinical Psychiatry

Radiology
AJR (American Journal of Roentgenology)

Surgery
Annals of Surgery
American Journal of Surgery
Archives of Surgery
American Surgeon
Journal of the American College of Surgeons

Common non-peer-reviewed journals (also known as "throw-aways")
Hospital Physician
Resident and Physician

There has been a real explosion of books and articles that discuss EBM. This is just a brief selection.

Books

American National Standards Institute. *American National Standard for the Preparation of Scientific Papers for Written or Oral Presentation.* ANSI Z39.16. Washington, DC: American National Standards Institute, 1972.

Ball, C. M. & Phillips, R. S. *Evidence-Based on Call: Acute Medicine.* Edinburgh: Churchill Livingstone, 2001.

Bernstein, P. L. *Against the Gods: the Remarkable Story of Risk.* New York, NY: Wiley, 1998.

Bradford Hill, A. *A Short Textbook of Medical Statistics.* Oxford: Oxford University Press, 1977.

Cochrane, A. L. *Effectiveness & Efficiency: Random Reflections on Health Services.* London: Royal Society of Medicine, 1971.

Cohen, J. *Statistical Power Analysis for the Behavioral Sciences.* 2nd edn. Orlando, FL: Academic Press, 1988.

Daly, J. *Evidence-based medicine and the Search for a Science of Clinical Care.* Berkeley, CA: University of California Press, 2005.

Dawes, M., Davies, P., Gray, A., Mant, J., Seers, K. & Snowball, R. *Evidence-Based Practice: a Primer for Health Care Professionals.* Edinburgh: Churchill Livingstone, 1999.

Dixon, R. A., Munro, J. F. & Silcocks, P. B. *The Evidence Based Medicine Workbook: Critical Appraisal for Clinical Problem Solving.* Oxford: Oxford University Press, 1997.

Ebell, M. R. *Evidence-Based Diagnosis: a Handbook of Clinical Prediction Rules.* Berlin: Springer, 2001.

Eddy, D. *Clinical Decision Making.* Sudbury, MA: Jones & Bartlett, 1996.

Fletcher, R. H., Fletcher, S. W. & Wagner, E. H. *Clinical Epidemiology: the Essentials.* Baltimore, MD: Williams & Wilkins, 1995.

Friedland, D. J., Go, A. S., Davoren, J. B., Shlipak, M. G., Bent, S. W., Subak, L. L. & Mendelson, T. *Evidence-Based Medicine: A Framework for Clinical Practice.* Stamford, CT: Appleton & Lange, 1998.

Gelbach, S. H. *Interpreting the Medical Literature.* New York, NY: McGraw-Hill, 1993.

Geyman, J. P., Deyo, R. A. & Ramsey, S. D. *Evidence-Based Clinical Practice: Concepts and Approaches.* Boston, MA: Butterworth Heinemann, 1999.

Glasziou, P., Irwig, L., Bain, C. & Colditz, G. *Systematic Reviews in Health Care: a Practical Guide.* Cambridge: Cambridge University Press, 2001.

Glasziou, P., DelMar, C. & Salisbury, J. *Evidence-Based Practice Workbook.* 2nd edn. Blackwell Publishing 2007.

Greenhalgh, T. & Donald, A. *Evidence-Based Health Care Workbook.* London: BMJ Books, 2000.

Gray, J. A. M. *Evidence-Based Healthcare: How to Make Health Policy and Management Decisions.* Philadelphia, PA: Saunders, 2001.

Gross, R. *Making Medical Decisions: an Approach to Clinical Decision Making for Practicing Physicians.* Philadelphia, PA: American College of Physicians, 1999.

Decisions and Evidence in Medical Practice: Applying Evidence-Based Medicine to Clinical Decision Making. St Louis, MO: Mosby, 2001.

Guyatt, G. & Rennie, D. (eds.). *Users' Guides to the Medical Literature: a Manual for Evidence-Based Clinical Practice.* Chicago: AMA, 2002.

Hamer, S. & Collinson, G. *Achieving Evidence-Based Practice: A Handbook for Practitioners.* Edinburgh: Bailliere Tindall, 1999

Hulley, S. B. & Cummings, S. R. *Designing Clinical Research.* Baltimore, MD: Williams & Wilkins, 1988.

Matthews, J. R. *Quantification and the Quest for Medical Certainty.* Princeton, NJ: Princeton University Press, 1995.

McDowell, J. E. & Newell, C. *Measuring Health: a Guide to Rating Scales and Questionnaires.* New York, NY: Oxford University Press, 1987.

McGee, S. R. *Evidence-Based Physical Diagnosis.* Philadelphia, PA: Saunders, 2001.

McKibbon, A., Eady, A. & Marks, S. *PDQ Evidence-Based Principles and Practice.* Hamilton, BC: Decker Inc., 1999

Norman, G. & Streiner, D. *Biostatistics: the Bare Essentials.* Hamilton, BC: Decker Inc., 2000.

Riegelman, R. K. & Hirsch, D. S. *Studying a Study and Testing a Test. How to Read the Medical Literature.* 4th edn. Boston, MA: Little Brown, 2000.

Sackett, D. L., Haynes, R. B., Guyatt, G. H. & Tugwell, P. *Clinical Epidemiology: a Basic Science for Clinical Medicine.* 2nd edn. Boston, MA: Little Brown, 1991.

Sackett, D. L., Straus, S. E., Richardson, W. S., Rosenberg, W. & Haynes, R. B. *Evidence Based Medicine: How to Practice and Teach EBM.* 2nd edn. London: Churchill Livingstone, 2000.

Sox, H. C., Blatt, M. A., Higgins, M. C. & Marton, K. I. *Medical Decision Making.* Boston, MA: Butterworth Heinemann, 1988.

Spencer, J. W. & Jacobs, J. *Complementary and Alternative Medicine: an Evidence-Based Approach.* St Louis, MO: Mosby, 2003.

Straus, S. E., Hsu, S., Ball, C. M. & Phillips, R. S. *Evidence-Based Acute Medicine.* Edinburgh: Churchill Livingstone, 2001.

Straus, S. E., Richardson, W. S., Glasziou, P. & Haynes, R. B. *Evidence Based Medicine: How to Practice and Teach EBM.* 3rd edn. Edinburgh: Elsevier Churchill Livingstone, 2005.

Tufte, E. R. *The Visual Display of Quantitative Data.* Cheshire, CT: Graphics Press, 1983.

Velleman, P. *ActivStats.* Reading, MA: Addison-Wesley, 1999.

Wulff, H. R. & Gotzsche, P. C. *Rational Diagnosis and Treatment: Evidence-Based Clinical Decision-Making.* 3rd edn. London: Blackwell, 2000.

Journal articles

General

Ad Hoc Working Group for Critical Appraisal of the Medical Literature. A proposal for more informative abstracts of clinical articles. *Ann. Intern. Med.* 1987; **106**: 598–604.

Bradford Hill, A. Statistics in the medical curriculum? *Br. Med. J.* 1947; ii: 366.

Cuddy, P. G., Elenbaas, R. M. & Elenbaas, J. K. Evaluating the medical literature. Part I: abstract, introduction, methods. *Ann. Emerg. Med.* 1983; **12**: 549–555.

Day, R. A. The origins of the scientific paper: the IMRAD format. *AMWA J.* 1989; **4**: 16–18.

Department of Clinical Epidemiology and Biostatistics, McMaster University Health Sciences Centre. How to read clinical journals. I: why to read them and how to start reading them critically. *Can. Med. Assoc. J.* 1981; **124**: 555–558.

How to read clinical journals. V: to distinguish useful from useless or even harmful therapy. *Can. Med. Assoc. J.* 1981; **124**: 1156–1162.

Diamond, G. A. & Forrester, J. S. Clinical trials and statistical verdicts: probable grounds for appeal. *Ann. Intern. Med.* 1983; **98**: 385–394.

Elenbaas, R. M., Elenbaas, J. K., & Cuddy, P. G. Evaluating the medical literature. Part II: statistical analysis. *Ann. Emerg. Med.* 1983; **12**: 610–620.

Elenbaas, J. K., Cuddy, P. G. & Elenbaas, R. M. Evaluating the medical literature. Part III: results and discussion. *Ann. Emerg. Med.* 1983; **12**: 679–686.

Ernst, E. Evidence based complementary medicine: a contradiction in terms? *Ann. Rheum. Dis.* 1999; **58**: 69–70.

Greenhalgh, T. How to read a paper. The Medline database. *BMJ* 1997; **315**: 180–183.

Haynes, B., Glasziou, P. & Straus, S. Advances in evidence-based information resources for clinical practice. *ACP J. Club* 2000; **132**: A11–A14.

Haynes, R. B., Mulrow, C. D., Huth, E. J., Altman, D. G. & Gardner, M. J. More informative abstracts revisited. *Ann. Intern. Med.* 1990; **113**: 69–76.

Haynes, R. B., Wilczynski, N., McKibbon, K. A., Walker, C. J. & Sinclair, J. C. Developing optimal search strategies for detecting clinically sound studies in MEDLINE. *J. Am. Med. Inform. Assoc.* 1994; **1**: 447–458.

Isaacs, D. & Fitzgerald, D. Seven alternatives to evidence based medicine. *BMJ* 1999; **319**: 1618.

Mulrow, C. D., Thacker, S. B. & Pugh, J. A. A proposal for more informative abstracts of review articles. *Ann. Intern. Med.* 1988; **108**: 613–615.

Rennie, D. & Glass, R. M. Structuring abstracts to make them more informative. *JAMA* 1991; **266**: 116–117.

Sackett, D. L., Rosenberg, W. M., Gray, J. A., Haynes R. B. & Richardson W. S. Evidence based medicine: what it is and what it isn't. *BMJ* 1996; **312**: 71–72.

Sackett, D. L. & Straus, S. E. Finding and applying evidence during clinical rounds: the "evidence cart". *JAMA* 1998; **280**: 1336–1338.

Taddio, A., Pain, T., Fassos, F. F., Boon, H., Ilersich, A. L. & Einarson, T. R. Quality of non-structured and structured abstracts of original research articles in the British Medical Journal, the Canadian Medical Association Journal and the Journal of the American Medical Association. *CMAJ* 1994; **150**: 1611–1615.

Taplin, S., Galvin, M. S., Payne, T., Coole, D. & Wagner, E. Putting population-based care into practice: real option or rhetoric? *J. Am. Board Fam. Pract.* 1998; **11**: 116–126.

Woolf, S. H. The need for perspective in evidence-based medicine. *JAMA* 1999; **282**: 2358–2365.

Cause and effect

Department of Clinical Epidemiology and Biostatistics, McMaster University Health Sciences Centre. How to read clinical journals. IV: to determine etiology or causation. *Can. Med. Assoc. J.* 1981; **124**: 985–990.

Evans, A. S. Causation and disease: a chronological journey. The Thomas Parran Lecture. *Am. J. Epidemiol.* 1978; **108**: 249–258.

Weiss, N. S. Inferring causal relationships: elaboration of the criterion of "dose-response." *Am. J. Epidemiol.* 1981; **113**: 487–490.

Study design

Bogardus, S. T., Jr., Concato, J. & Feinstein, A. R. Clinical epidemiological quality in molecular genetic research: the need for methodological standards. *JAMA* 1999; **281**: 1919–1926.

Burkett, G. L. Classifying basic research designs. *Fam. Med.* 1990; **22**: 143–148.

Gilbert, E. H., Lowenstein, S. R., Koziol-McLain, J., Barta, D. C. & Steiner, J. Chart reviews in emergency medicine research: where are the methods? *Ann. Emerg. Med.* 1996; **27**: 305–308.

Hayden, G. F., Kramer, M. S. & Horwitz, R. I. The case-control study: a practical review for the clinician. *JAMA* 1982; **247**: 326–331.

Lavori, P. W., Louis, T. A., Bailar, J. C., III & Polansky, M. Designs for experiments – parallel comparisons of treatment. *N. Engl. J. Med.* 1983; **309**: 1291–1299.

Mantel, N. & Haenszel, W. Statistical aspects of the analysis of data from retrospective studies of disease. *J. Natl. Cancer Inst.* 1959; **22**: 719–748.

Measurement

Department of Clinical Epidemiology and Biostatistics, McMaster University Health Sciences Centre. Clinical disagreement. I: how often it occurs and why. *Can. Med. Assoc. J.* 1980; **123**: 499–504.

Clinical disagreement. II: how to avoid it and how to learn from one's mistakes. *Can. Med. Assoc. J.* 1980; **123**: 613–617.

Bias

Croskerry, P. Achieving quality in clinical decision making: cognitive strategies and detection of bias. *Acad. Emerg. Med.* 2002; **9**: 1184–1204.

Feinstein, A. R., Sosin, D. M. & Wells, C. K. The Will Rogers phenomenon. Stage migration and new diagnostic techniques as a source of misleading statistics for survival in cancer. *N. Engl. J. Med.* 1985; **312**: 1604–1608.

Sackett, D. L. Bias in analytic research. *J. Chronic Dis.* 1979; **32**: 51–63.

Sackett, D. L. & Gent, M. Controversy in counting and attributing events in clinical trials. *N. Engl. J. Med.* 1979; **301**: 1410–1412.

Schulz, K. F., Chalmers, I., Hayes, R. J. & Altman, D. G. Empirical evidence of bias. Dimensions of methodological quality associated with estimates of treatments effects in controlled trials. *JAMA* 1995; **273**: 408–412.

General biostatistics

Berwick, D. M. Experimental power: the other side of the coin. *Pediatrics* 1980; **65**: 1043–1045.

Moses, L. E. Statistical concepts fundamental to investigations. *N. Engl. J. Med.* 1985; **312**: 890–897.

Streiner, D. L. Maintaining standards: differences between the standard deviation and standard error, and when to use each. *Can. J. Psychiatry* 1996; **41**: 498–502.

Type I and II errors

Cook, R. J. & Sackett, D. L. The number needed to treat: a clinically useful measure of treatment effect. *BMJ* 1995; **310**: 452–454.

Cordell, W. H. Number needed to treat (NNT). *Ann. Emerg. Med.* 1999; **33**: 433–436.

Freiman, J. A., Chalmers, T. C., Smith, H. Jr. & Kuebler, R. R. The importance of beta, the type II error and sample size in the design and interpretation of the randomized control trial. Survey of 71 "negative" trials. *N. Engl. J. Med.* 1978; **299**: 690–694.

Todd, K. H. & Funk, J. P. The minimum clinically important difference in physician-assigned visual analog pain scores. *Acad. Emerg. Med.* 1996; **3**: 142–146.

Todd, K. H., Funk, K. G., Funk, J. P. & Bonacci, R. Clinical significance of reported changes in pain severity. *Ann. Emerg. Med.* 1996; **27**: 485–489.

Young, M., Bresnitz, E. A. & Strom, B. L. Sample size nomograms for interpreting negative clinical studies. *Ann. Intern. Med.* 1983; **99**: 248–251.

Risk

Concato, J., Feinstein, A. R. & Holford, T. R. The risk of determining risk with multivariable analysis. *Ann. Intern. Med.* 1993; **118**: 201–210.

Hanley, J. A. & Lippman-Hand, A. If nothing goes wrong, is everything all right? Integrating zero numerators. *JAMA* 1983; **249**: 1743–1745.

Schulman, K. A., Berlin, J. A., Harless, W., Kerner, J. F., Sistrunk, S., Gersh, B. J., Dubé, R., Taleghani, C. K., Burke, J. E., Williams, S., Eisenberg, J. M. & Escarce, J. J. The effect of race and sex on physicians' recommendations for cardiac catheterization. *N. Engl. J. Med.* 1999; **340**: 618–626.

Schwartz, L. M., Woloshin, S. & Welch, H. G. Misunderstandings about the effects of race and sex on physicians' referrals for cardiac catheterization. (Sounding Board.) *N. Engl. J. Med.* 1999; **341**: 279–283.

Clinical trials

Bailar, J. C., III, Louis, T. A., Lavori, P. W. & Polansky, M. Studies without internal controls. *N. Engl. J. Med.* 1984; **311**: 156–162.

Elwood, J. M. Interpreting clinical trial results: seven steps to understanding. *Can. Med. Assoc. J.* 1980; **123**: 343–345.

Ernst, E. & Resch, K. L. Concept of true and perceived placebo effects. *BMJ* 1995; **311**: 551–553.

Ernst, E. & White, A. R. Acupuncture for back pain: a meta-analysis of randomized controlled trials. *Arch. Intern. Med.* 1998; **158**: 2235–2241.

Hróbjartsson, A. & Gotzsche, P. C. Is the placebo powerless? An analysis of clinical trials comparing placebo with no treatment. *N. Engl. J. Med.* 2001; **344**: 1594–1602.

Louis, T. A., Lavori, P. W., Bailar, J. C. III & Polansky, M. Crossover and self-controlled designs in clinical research. *N. Engl. J. Med.* 1984; **310**: 24–31.

Standards of Reporting Trials Group. A proposal for structured reporting of randomized controlled trials. *JAMA* 1994; **272**: 1926–1931. Correction: *JAMA* 1995; **273**: 776.

Working Group on Recommendations for Reporting Clinical Trials in the Biomedical Literature. Call for comments on a proposal to improve reporting of clinical trials in the biomedical literature. *Ann. Intern. Med.* 1994; **121**: 894–895.

Communicating evidence to patients

Epstein, R. M., Alper, B. S., Quill, T. E. Communicating evidence for participatory decision making. *JAMA.* 2004; **291**: 2359–2366.

Halvorsen, P. A., Selmer, R. & Kristiansen, I. S. Different ways to describe the benefits of risk-reducing treatments: a randomized trial. *Ann. Intern. Med.* 2007; **146**: 848–856.

Gigerenzer, G. *Reckoning with Risk: Learning to Live with Uncertainty.* Harmondsworth: Penguin, 2002.

McNeil, B. J., Pauker, S. G., Sox, H. C. Jr., & Tversky, A. On the elicitation of preferences for alternative therapies. *N. Engl. J. Med.* 1982; **306**: 1259–1262.

Diagnostic tests

Mower, W. R. Evaluating bias and variability in diagnostic test reports. *Ann. Emerg. Med.* 1999; **33**: 85–91.

Patterson, R. E. & Horowitz, S. F. Importance of epidemiology and biostatistics in deciding clinical strategies for using diagnostic tests: a simplified approach using examples from coronary artery disease. *J. Am. Coll. Cardiol.* 1989; **13**: 1653–1665.

Miscellaneous

Department of Clinical Epidemiology and Biostatistics, McMaster University Health Sciences Centre. How to read clinical journals. III: to learn clinical course and prognosis of disease. *Can. Med. Assoc. J.* 1981; **124**: 869–872.

L'Abbé, K. A., Detsky, A. S. & O'Rourke, K. Meta-analysis in clinical research. *Ann. Intern. Med.* 1987; **107**: 224–233.

Olson, C. M. Consensus statements: applying structure. *JAMA* 1995; **273**: 72–73.

Sonnenberg, F. A. & Beck, J. R. Markov models in medical decision making: a practical guide. *Med. Decis. Making* 1993; **13**: 322–338.

Wasson, J. H., Sox, H. C., Neff, R. K. & Goldman, L. Clinical prediction rules: application and methodological standards. *N. Engl. J. Med.* 1985; **313**: 793–799.

Users' guides to the medical literature

Barratt, A., Irwig, L., Glasziou, P., Cumming, R. G., Raffle, A., Hicks, N., Gray, J. A. & Guyatt, G. H. Users' guides to the medical literature: XVII. How to use guidelines and recommendations about screening. Evidence-Based Medicine Working Group. *JAMA* 1999; **281**: 2029–2034.

Bucher, H. C., Guyatt, G. H., Cook, D. J., Holbrook, A. & McAlister, F. A. Users' guides to the medical literature: XIX. Applying clinical trial results. A. How to use an article measuring the effect of an intervention on surrogate end points. Evidence-Based Medicine Working Group. *JAMA* 1999; **282**: 771–778.

Dans, A. L., Dans, L. F., Guyatt, G. H. & Richardson, S. Users' guides to the medical literature: XIV. How to decide on the applicability of clinical trial results to your patient. Evidence-Based Medicine Working Group. *JAMA* 1998; **279**: 545–549.

Drummond, M. F., Richardson, W. S., O'Brien, B. J., Levine, M. & Heyland, D. Users' guides to the medical literature: XIII. How to use an article on economic analysis of clinical practice. A. Are the results of the study valid? Evidence-Based Medicine Working Group. *JAMA* 1997; **277**: 1552–1557.

Giacomini, M. K. & Cook, D. J. Users' guides to the medical literature: XXIII. Qualitative research in health care. A. Are the results of the study valid? Evidence-Based Medicine Working Group. *JAMA* 2000; **284**: 357–362.

Users' guides to the medical literature: XXIII. Qualitative research in health care. B. What are the results and how do they help me care for my patients? Evidence-Based Medicine Working Group. *JAMA* 2000; **284**: 478–482.

Guyatt, G. & Rennie, D. (eds.). *Users' Guides to the Medical Literature: a Manual for Evidence-Based Clinical Practice.* Chicago: AMA, 2002.

Guyatt, G. H., Sackett, D. L. & Cook, D. J. Users' guides to the medical literature: II. How to use an article about therapy or prevention. A. Are the results of the study valid? Evidence-Based Medicine Working Group. *JAMA* 1993; **270**: 2598–2601.

Users' guides to the medical literature: II. How to use an article about therapy or prevention. B. What were the results and will they help me in caring for my patients? Evidence-Based Medicine Working Group. *JAMA* 1994; **271**: 59–63.

Guyatt, G. H., Sackett, D. L., Sinclair, J. C., Hayward, R., Cook, D. J. & Cook, R. J. Users' guides to the medical literature: IX. A method for grading health care recommendations. Evidence-Based Medicine Working Group. *JAMA* 1995; **274**: 1800–1804.

Guyatt, G. H., Naylor, C. D., Juniper, E., Heyland, D. K., Jaeschke, R. & Cook, D. J. Users' guides to the medical literature: XII. How to use articles about health-related quality of life. Evidence-Based Medicine Working Group. *JAMA* 1997; **277**: 1232–1237.

Guyatt, G. H., Sinclair, J., Cook, D. J. & Glasziou, P. Users' guides to the medical literature: XVI. How to use a treatment recommendation. Evidence-Based Medicine Working Group and Cochrane Applicability Methods Working Group. *JAMA* 1999; **281**: 1836–1843.

Guyatt, G. H., Haynes, R. B., Jaeschke, R. Z., Cook, D. J., Green, L., Naylor, C. D., Wilson, M. C. & Richardson, W. S. Users' guides to the medical literature: XXV. Evidence-based medicine: principles for applying the Users' Guides to patient care. Evidence-Based Medicine Working Group. *JAMA* 2000; **284**: 1290–1296.

Hayward, R. S., Wilson, M. C., Tunis, S. R., Bass, E. B. & Guyatt, G. Users' guides to the medical literature: VIII. How to use clinical practice guidelines. A. Are the recommendations valid? Evidence-Based Medicine Working Group. *JAMA* 1995; **274**: 570–574.

Hunt, D. L., Jaeschke, R. & McKibbon, K. A. Users' guides to the medical literature: XXI. Using electronic health information resources in evidence-based practice. Evidence-Based Medicine Working Group. *JAMA* 2000; **283**: 1875–1879.

Jaeschke, R., Guyatt, G. H. & Sackett, D. L. Users' guides to the medical literature: III. How to use an article about a diagnostic test. A. Are the results of the study valid? Evidence-Based Medicine Working Group. *JAMA* 1994; **271**: 389–391.

Users' guides to the medical literature: III. How to use an article about a diagnostic test. B. What are the results and will they help me in caring for my patients? Evidence-Based Medicine Working Group. *JAMA* 1994; **271**: 703–707.

Laupacis, A., Wells, G., Richardson, W. S. & Tugwell, P. Users' guides to the medical literature: V. How to use an article about prognosis. Evidence-Based Medicine Working Group. *JAMA* 1994; **272**: 234–237.

Levine, M., Walter, S., Lee, H., Haines, T., Holbrook, A. & Moyer, V. Users' guides to the medical literature: IV. How to use an article about harm. Evidence-Based Medicine Working Group. *JAMA* 1994; **271**: 1615–1619.

McAlister, F. A., Laupacis, A., Wells, G. A. & Sackett, D. L. Users' guides to the medical literature: XIX. Applying clinical trial results. B. Guidelines for determining whether a drug is exerting (more than) a class effect. *JAMA* 1999; **282**: 1371–1377.

McAlister, F. A., Straus, S. E., Guyatt, G. H. & Haynes, R. B. Users' guides to the medical literature: XX. Integrating research evidence with the care of the individual patient. Evidence-Based Medicine Working Group. *JAMA* 2000; **283**: 2829–2836.

McGinn, T. G., Guyatt, G. H., Wyer, P. C., Naylor, C. D., Stiell, I. G. & Richardson, W. S. Users' guides to the medical literature: XXII. How to use articles about clinical decision rules. Evidence-Based Medicine Working Group. *JAMA* 2000; **284**: 79–84.

Naylor, C. D. & Guyatt, G. H. Users' guides to the medical literature: X. How to use an article reporting variations in the outcomes of health services. The Evidence-Based Medicine Working Group. *JAMA* 1996; **275**: 554–558.

Users' guides to the medical literature: XI. How to use an article about a clinical utilization review. Evidence-Based Medicine Working Group. *JAMA* 1996; **275**: 1435–1439.

O'Brien, B. J., Heyland, D., Richardson, W. S., Levine, M. & Drummond, M. F. Users' guides to the medical literature: XIII. How to use an article on economic analysis of clinical practice. B. What are the results and will they help me in caring for my patients? Evidence-Based Medicine Working Group. *JAMA* 1997; **277**: 1802–1806.

Oxman, A. D., Sackett, D. L. & Guyatt, G. H. Users' guides to the medical literature: I. How to get started. The Evidence-Based Medicine Working Group. *JAMA* 1993; **270**: 2093–2095.

Oxman, A. D., Cook, D. J., Guyatt, G. H. Users' guides to the medical literature: VI. How to use an overview. Evidence-Based Medicine Working Group. *JAMA* 1994; **272**: 1367–1371.

Randolph, A. G., Haynes, R. B., Wyatt, J. C., Cook, D. J. & Guyatt, G. H. Users' guides to the medical literature: XVIII. How to use an article evaluating the clinical impact of a computer-based clinical decision support system. *JAMA* 1999; **282**: 67–74.

Richardson, W. S. & Detsky, A. S. Users' guides to the medical literature: VII. How to use a clinical decision analysis. A. Are the results of the study valid? Evidence-Based Medicine Working Group. *JAMA* 1995; **273**: 1292–1295.

Users' guides to the medical literature: VII. How to use a clinical decision analysis. B. What are the results and will they help me in caring for my patients? Evidence-Based Medicine Working Group. *JAMA* 1995; **273**: 1610–1613.

Richardson, W. S., Wilson, M. C., Guyatt, G. H., Cook, D. J. & Nishikawa, J. Users' guides to the medical literature: XV. How to use an article about disease probability for differential diagnosis. Evidence-Based Medicine Working Group. *JAMA* 1999; **281**: 1214–1219.

Richardson, W. S., Wilson, M. C., Williams, J.W. Jr, Moyer, V. A. & Naylor, C. D. Users' guides to the medical literature: XXIV. How to use an article on the clinical manifestations of disease. Evidence-Based Medicine Working Group. *JAMA* 2000; **284**: 869–875.

Wilson, M. C., Hayward, R. S., Tunis, S. R., Bass, E. B. & Guyatt, G. Users' guides to the medical literature: VIII. How to use clinical practice guidelines. B. What are the recommendations and will they help you in caring for your patients? The Evidence-Based Medicine Working Group. *JAMA* 1995; **274**: 1630–1632.

Web sites

The classic sites

Centre for Evidence-Based Medicine, Oxford University   This is the one of the oldest and best EBM sites, with many features including a toolbox, Critically Appraised Topics (CAT) maker, a glossary, and links to other sites. There is also a CAT-bank of previously prepared critical analyses. The toolbox has an all-purpose four-fold calculator, which requires Macromedia Shockwave Player.
www.cebm.net

Bandolier   This is an excellent site for getting quick information about a given topic. They do very brief summary reviews of the current literature. Sponsored by the Centre for Evidence-Based Medicine.
www.medicine.ox.ac.uk/bandolier

Evidence Based Emergency Medicine at the New York Academy of Medicine   This is an excellent site with many features including a Journal Club Bank, critical review forms, glossary, the Users' Guides to the Medical Literature, and links to other sites.
www.ebem.org/cgi-bin/index.php

University of British Columbia   Written by Martin Schechter, this is an excellent site for online calculations of NNT, likelihood ratios, and confidence intervals. Select links, then go to Calculators and select either the Bayesian or Clinical Significance Calculators. Must have data in dichotomous form.
www.spph.ubc.ca

Evidence Based Medicine Tool Kit, University of Alberta   An excellent site to do the Users' Guides to the Medical Literature. This site has worksheets for all the guides and links to text versions of the original articles, made available by the Canadian Centres for Health Evidence.
www.ebm.med.ualberta.ca/

Best evidence compilations

Evidence Updates from the BMJ   Sponsored by the BMJ Group and McMaster University's Health Information Research Unit, this site is a great place to look for evaluation of recent studies and reviews. Very much up to date with a searchable database and email alert service, this is a free service of BMJ. Citations are all pre-rated for quality, clinical relevance and interest by practicing physicians.

http://bmjupdates.mcmaster.ca/index.asp

Evidence-Based On-Call   This is a wonderful site for Critically Appraised Topics (CATs). Tends to favor acute care medicine, but you never know if you'll find the answer to your query very quickly. Professional team writes and reviews all CATs. There are 39 topic areas with a total of hundreds of CATs.

http://www.eboncall.org

Agency for Health Research and Quality   This US government agency is responsible for evaluating the evidence behind new and upcoming technologies and improvements in the practice of health care in the United States. They have an excellent list of topics with an evaluation of the strength of the evidence behind them.

http://www.ahrq.gov

BestBETs   is a free site that contains CATs, many of which are related to acute-care topics. There are also unfinished CATS and topics needing CATS, and the site developers hope that others will input their information into the site.

www.bestbets.org

Ganfyd (Get a note from your doctor)   This is a medical wiki that catalogues medical knowledge and can be edited by any registered medical practitioner and tries to be evidence based with many of the citations graded for quality of the evidence. Some of the evidence is better than other with no consistency, but that is the fun of wikis.

www.ganfyd.org

Trip Answers   This is a spin off from the Trip Data Base search engine. Questions can be posed to the site and will be answered quickly using the best evidence available.

www.tripanswers.org/

   The following websites contain excellent links and other resources for learning and practicing EBM

Evidence-Based Health Informatics   Health Information Research Unit, McMaster University.

http://hiru.mcmaster.ca/hiru

Netting the Evidence.

www.shef.ac.uk/scharr/ir/netting

New York Academy of Medicine EBM Resource Center.

www.ebmny.org

Mount Sinai School of Medicine.

www.mssm.edu/medicine/general-medicine/ebm

Cochrane Collaboration abstracts   The abstracts of the Cochrane reviews can all be accessed here and no subscription is required to view the abstracts. The full Cochrane Library is free in many countries, but not in the United States. Many libraries have subscriptions. The abstracts are good if you want only the bottom line, but you won't get any of the details and be able to decide for yourself if the review is valid or potentially biased.

www.update-software.com/abstracts/crgindex.htm

Golden Hour   is an Israeli site with many features, including links and evidence-based medical information.

www.goldenhour.co.il

NHS Centre for Reviews and Dissemination   at the University of York is the sponsoring site for the Database of Abstracts of Reviews of Effects (DARE)
www.york.ac.uk/inst/crd

Sites requiring subscription

InfoPOEMs   Now called Essential Evidence Plus, this is the website for family-practice-related CATs (called POEMs, or Patient-Oriented Evidence that Matters). The site has a free trial period, but requires subscription after that.
www.essentialevidenceplus.com
Cochrane Collaboration   main site. It contains a collection of the best and most uniformly performed systematic reviews publications.
www.update-software.com/cochrane
Clinical Evidence from the *British Medical Journal* (*BMJ*).   This is mainly geared to internal medicine and has an accompanying book and CD-ROM.
www.clinicalevidence.com

Searching sites

TRIP Database   contains a free set of critically appraised topics and evidence-based references.
www.tripdatabase.com
University of Virginia – Health Sciences Library   Excellent access to evidence based sites, which appears to be free to the public.
http://www.hsl.virginia.edu/internet/library/collections/ebm/index.cfm

Position statements

The AGREE Research Trust   This is the home of the AGREE instrument for the evaluation of Clinical Practice Guidelines. The instrument and training manual are free downloads from the site.
http://www.agreetrust.org/
The Consort Group   The CONSORT Group stands for Consolidated Standards of Reporting Trials. Their site has the CONSORT statement for reporting RCTs with its associated check list and flow diagram.
http://www.consort-statement.org/

Learning EBM

JAMAevidence   A new feature of the JAMA site will have the User's Guides to the Medical Literature and the Rational Clinical Examination series available without cost. Look for it to open to the general public early in 2009.
http://jamaevidence.com/
Evidence-Based Knowledge Portal   The Vanderbilt University (Tennessee, United States) has a series of very nice and simple to use tutorials introducing EBM. There are also some

virtual cases that can be used to learn and practice the principles of EBM. Passwords required but open to the general public.

http://www.mc.vanderbilt.edu/biolib/ebmportal/login.html

Delfini Group　This consulting group has put together some nice resources to use in critical appraisal of the medical literature. There are also some slide shows, which are excellent for EBM education. They are free.

http://www.delfini.org

Michigan State University. Introduction to EBM Course　This is an excellent interactive introduction to EBM. The seven modules covering Information Mastery, Critical Appraisal and Knowledge Transfer can be done in a total of about 14–20 hours total.

http://www.poems.msu.edu/InfoMastery/

Anesthetist.com – Interactive Receiver Operating Characteristic Curves　This is an excellent way to learn about the use of diagnostic tests through the use of interactive ROC curves. Other interesting stuff can be found on the Anesthetist.com website.

http://www.anaesthetist.com/mnm/stats/roc/Findex.htm

Contacts within EBM

CHAIN　Contact, Help, Advice, and Information Networks are a free networking tool for health care workers and others. Specific areas of interest relevant to EBM include knowledge transfer and life long learning. It is a way of connecting with others in the field and exchanging ideas. It is free to join. CHAIN Canada is found at

http://www.epoc.uottawa.ca/CHAINCanada.

http://chain.ulcc.ac.uk/chain/index.html

Centre for Evidence-Based Child Health　This is a main link in child health EBM in the United Kingdom. The website has an excellent list of links for physicians and non-physicians who are interested in child health.

http://www.ich.ucl.ac.uk/ich/academicunits/Centre_for_evidence_based_child_health/Homepage

Teachers and Developers of EBM International　A worldwide group of interested parties meet every 2 years to discuss the teaching and practice of Evidence Based Medicine. Their activities are chronicled on this site.

http://www.ebhc.org/

Create your own EBM sites

EBM Page Generator　This shareware created by Yale and Dartmouth Universities (United States) allows anyone to set up an interactive site to link to any EBM sources. It is easy to adapt to most interactive educational web platforms.

http://www.ebmpyramid.org/home.php

Index

Locators in *italic* refer to figures and tables
Locators in **bold** refer to major entries
Locators for headings with subheadings refer to general aspects of that topic

α error 29
a-posteriori probability *see* post-test
    probability
a-priori probability *see* pre-test probability
AAR (absolute attributable risk) 147
abdication 165
absolute attributable risk (AAR) 147
absolute rate reduction (ARR) 114,
    396
absolute risk 142, *143*, *144*, **143–4**,
    396
absolute risk increase (ARI) 147, 151
absolute risk reduction (ARR) 136, 147,
    205
abstracts 28, *28*, **28**
acronyms, mnemonic 221, *221*, **222–3**, 223,
    257, *257*; *see also* mnemonics
accuracy 73, **75–6**, 233, 272, 396
accuracy criteria 245–7
ACP (American College of Physicians) 12, 13
ACP Journal Club 13
Activities of Daily Living (ADL) Scale 346
ActivStats 108
actuarial-life tables 366
adjustment *231*, 396
adjustment heuristic 230–1
ADL (Activities of Daily Living) Scale 346
Agency for Healthcare Research and Quality
    318
AGREE criteria 322
AHRQ, US 357
AIDS 57, 313
Alcohol Use Disorders Identification Test
    (AUDIT) 72
algebra 4
algorithms, definition 396

all-or-none case series 58, 190, 396
alternative hypotheses 28, 110, 140, 396
American College of Physicians (ACP)
    12, 13
American Society of Internal Medicine 13
analogy, reasoning by **196**
anchoring *231*, 396
anchoring heuristic 230–1
ancient history of medicine **2–3**
ANCOVA *387*
AND (Boolean operator) *36*, 35–7
animal research studies 25–7
Annals of Internal Medicine 13
ANOVA (analysis of variance) *387*
applicability **187–8**, **306–7**, 332, 396; *see also*
    strength of evidence/applicability
appropriate tests **241**; *see also* diagnostic tests
Arabic numerals 4
area under the curve (AUC) 277–9, 397
ARI (absolute risk increase) 147, 151
arm, decision tree 397
ARR *see* absolute rate reduction; absolute risk
    reduction; attributable risk reduction
Ars magna (The Great Art) 5
art of medicine **16–18**, 187, *225*, 288, 291,
    377
assessment 397
association (between cause and effect) 59
asterisk truncation function 50
attack rates *107*
attributable risk *148*, **147–8**
attributable risk reduction (ARR) 354
attrition, patient 63, **88–9**, 171, *361*, 360–1
AUC (area under the curve) 277–9, 397
AUDIT (Alcohol Use Disorders Identification
    Test) 72

author bias 368
availability heuristic 230, 397

β errors 29, **135–6**; *see also* Type II errors
background questions *14*, **13–14**
Bacon, Francis 109, **110–11**
Bacon, Roger 109
balance sheets 394–5
Bandolier 12, 50
bar graphs *97*, 98
baseline variables 169
Bayes' theorem 251, *251*, **262–3**, **264–6**, 294, 330
    definition 397
    formulas 391
    proof 392, *393*
bell-shaped curve *104*, **103–4**, 198
beneficence, principle of 185
Berkerson's bias 85, 169
Bernard, Claude 6
Bernoulli, Daniel 6, 334
Bernoulli, Jacob 5
Best Bets 54
best case/worst case strategies 88, 172–3
bias 15, 27, 31, **90–2**, 235; *see also* diagnostic tests, critical appraisal; error; precision; Type I errors
bibliography, medical literature *28*, **31**, 413–14; *see also* journals
biological plausibility **195**
biological variability
    patient **237**
    physician **235**
biomedical research, recent history **7–8**
biopsy 305
blinding 29, 65, **170**
    and bias 85, 86, 361, 362
    clinical prediction rules development 328
    definition 397
    error reduction 242
    gold standard comparisons 304
    unobtrusive measurements 75
bloodletting 4, 6, 7
BMJ (*British Medical Journal*) 16, 18, 25, 31, 52, 54
body mass index (BMI) 73, 195
bone marrow transplantation 177
Bonferroni correction 123
Boolean operators *36*, 35–7, 39, 50
Boots Pharmaceuticals 91
box-and-whisker plots 98, *100*
Bradford Hill, Austin 8, 16, 188
Breslow-Day test 370

British Medical Journal (BMJ) 16, 18, 25, 31, 52, 54
Broad Street Pump study 6, 193
burden of proof 311

CA *see* critical appraisal
CAGE questionnaire for alcoholism 72, 74, *280*, *280*, 279–81
CAM (complementary and alternative medicines) 167
CAPRIE trial 362–3
Cardano, Girolamo 5, 333–4
cardiopulmonary resuscitation (CPR) 335
CART analysis 329
Case Records journal feature 229
case-control studies 22, 23, *61*, **60–2**
    definition 397
    measures of risk 142
    odds ratios/relative risk 146–7
    overview 385
    recall bias 83
    research design strength 189
case-mix bias **297**
case reports 57, **57–8**, 189–90, 397
case series 57, **57–8**, 189–90, 397
case studies 7, 25
cases 60
CAT (critically appraised topic) 12, 399
causation/cause-and-effect 19–20, 59, 61
    bibliography 415–16
    clinical question **21–3**
    cohort studies 62
    contributory cause 62
    learning objectives 19
    multiple 194
    proving 189
    quotation 19
    randomized clinical trials 168
    strength of 188, *188*
    temporal **194**
    types 20–1
CDSR (Cochrane Database of Systematic Reviews) 48, 54
censored data 364, *365*
censoring bias 364, *365*
CENTRAL (Cochrane Central Register of Controlled Trials) 49, 54, 369
central limit theorem 116
central tendency measures 30, 94, 98–100
Centre for Evidence-Based Medicine 12, 190, 369, 378–81
centripetal bias 360
CER (control event rate) 114
chakras 2, *2*

chance nodes 336, *336*
children, examining **240**
Chinese belief systems 2, *2*, 2–3
chi-squared analysis **363**
chi-squared test 370
CI *see* confidence intervals
CINAHL 34
circulation of blood 4
classification and regression trees (CART)
     analysis 329
clinical consistency **217–20, 233–4**
Clinical Decision Making journal feature 229
Clinical Evidence database 50, 52, 54
clinical examination *220, 221*, **220–2**
clinical guidelines *see* guidelines
clinical prediction rules 325, *327*, **327–32**; *see
     also* guidelines; Ottawa ankle rules
Clinical Queries search function 38, **38–9**, 47,
     50
clinical question **15–16, 21–3**
clinical research studies **27–8**
clinical reviews 27, **27**, 30, 188; *see also*
     meta-analyses
clinical significance **124–5**, 173, 397–8; *see also*
     significance
clinical trials 46, *65*, **64–6**, 128–9, 417–18; *see
     also* controlled clinical trials; randomized
     clinical trials
clinical uncertainty 112
clinically significant effect size 114
clipboard function **42**
CME (continuing medical education) 197, 323
Cochrane, Archie 8
Cochrane Central Register of Controlled Trials
     49, 54, 369
Cochrane Collaboration 8, 47, 48, 53, 54, 189
     definition 398
     GRADE scheme 369
     levels of evidence 191
     meta-analyses/systematic reviews 375–6
Cochrane databases 50, 55
Cochrane Library 13, 34, *49*, **47–50**
Cochrane Methodology Register 49
Code of Hammurabi 2
coding 213, 376
coffee 131, 142
cohort studies 22, 23, **62–4**
     definition 398
     measures of risk 142
     odds ratios to estimate relative risk 146–7
     overview 384–5
     research design strength 189
cointervention 88, 398
colorectal screening *35*

common sense **196–7**, 367, 377
common themes, identifying 212
communication with patients *200*, 377
     bibliography 205
     checking for understanding/agreement
          207
     converting numbers to words 204, 206
     decision making, shared 200
     framing bias 205–6
     learning objectives 199
     natural frequencies 205, 206
     patient experience/expectations **200, 202**
     patient scenario **199–200**, 200, 201, 202,
          203
     presenting information **203–4**
     presenting recommendations **206–7**
     providing evidence **203**, 204–6
     quotation 199
     rapport, building **202–3**
     steps toward **200**
     too much information 204, 206
comparison groups *see* controls/control
     groups
comparisons, PICO/PICOT model 15–16, 21,
     35
competing hypothesis heuristic 230, 398
complementary and alternative medicines
     (CAM) 167
Complete Metabolic Profile 106
compliance bias 315–16
compliance rates 173
composite endpoints/outcomes 72, 90, **122–3**,
     128, 171, 362–3
computer software 212
computerization 342
conclusions *28*, **31**, **173**, **374–6**
concomitance 161
conditional probability 106
confabulation **238, 240**
confidence formula 132
confidence intervals (CI) 30, *116*, 173, 398
     calculator 291
     formulas 389, 390
     hypothesis testing **116**
     meta-analyses/systematic reviews 371,
          376
     negative studies, evaluating **136–7**
     relative risk *391*
     results strength 192–3
     risk assessment 149, *154*
     rules of thumb *124*
     Type I errors **123–4**
confidence levels *see* significance
conflicts of interest 177, *183*, **182–4**

confounding bias **87**, 318
confounding variables 59, 76, 145, 156, 169,
   170; *see also* multivariate analysis
   cohort studies 63
   prognosis 362
   research design strength 189
   specificity 194
consistency of evidence **193**
consistency of evidence over time **195–6**
Consolidating Standards of Reporting Trials
   Group (CONSORT) statement *177*, **176–7**
construct validity 73
contamination bias **88**
contamination of results 76
content analysis 213
context bias **300**
continuing medical education (CME) 197,
   323
continuous data 69
continuous test results 251–2, 398
continuous variables *139*, **138–40**
contradictory answers **238**
contributory cause 21, *22*, 62
control event rate (CER) 114
controlled clinical trials *63*, 398; *see also*
   randomized clinical trials
controls/control groups 58, 60, 65, 70, 114,
   178, 398
cookbook medicine 18
cost-benefit analysis 323, 398; *see also*
   cost-effectiveness
cost-effectiveness 216, 398
   accurate cost measurement **353**
   baseline variables **356–7**
   clinical effectiveness, establishing **353**
   clinical prediction rules development
      331
   comparison of relevant alternatives **352–3**
   costs per unit of health gained **354–6**
   deciding if a test/treatment is worth it
      350–2
   differing perspectives **352**
   discounting **356**
   ethics **357–8**
   guidelines for assessing economic analysis
      352–7
   learning objectives 350
   quotation 350
   screening 319
cost-minimization analysis 398
costs, medical tests 227, *228*, 246, 248, **307**
Cox proportional hazard model 160, 366, *387*
Cox regression 158
criterion-based validity 73, 246, 398

critical appraisal 10, **12–13**, 377, 384–6, 399
critical value 399
critically appraised topic (CAT) 12, 399
cross-reactivity, diagnostic tests 246
cross-sectional studies 22, 23, 57, **59–60**, 142
CT scanning 245, 295
   intra-observer consistency 234
   screening 311–12
   technological improvement of tests **301–2**
cumulative frequency polygons 98, *99*
cumulative meta-analysis 374–6
cutoff points *258*

DARE (Database of Abstracts of Reviews of
   Effects) 48–9, 54
data acquisition 29
data analysis **212–13**, 370–1, 377
data collection, qualitative research **211–12**
data display *see* graphing techniques
data dredging 122–3, 168
Database of Abstracts of Reviews of Effects
   (DARE) 48–9, 54
database studies *see* non-concurrent cohort
   studies
databases 34, **51–2**
death
   certificates 71
   guidelines 322
   outcome criteria 361
   outcome measure 72
   probability 349
   rates 37
   from unrelated causes 364
decimal system 4
decision making 215–16, *219*, **333–4**
   clinical consistency/physician
      disagreement **217–20**
   clinical examination *220*, *221*, **220–2**
   decision trees *336*, 335–6, *337*, *338*, **336–8**
   definition 399
   differential diagnosis 216, *224*, *225*, *225*,
      223–5, 226, *227*
   ethics **345–6**, *347*
   exhaustion strategy 229
   expected-values 334, **334–6**
   expert vs. evidence-based **11–12**
   guidelines/automation 218, *219*
   heuristics **231**
   hypothesis generation 221, **222–3**
   hypothetico-deductive strategy 229
   learning objectives 215, 333
   Markov models *345*, **345**
   multiple branching strategy 229
   patient/physician shared 200, *200*

pattern recognition 228–9, 231
physician **165–6**
premature closure 229, **231–2**
pre-test probability *225*, 224–5, 226
quotation 215, 333
reality checks **341–3**
refining the options **226–8**
risk, attitudes to **348–9**
sensitivity analysis *339, 340*, **339–40**, *341, 342*
threshold approach **343–5**
uncertainty/incomplete information 218, *219*
values, patient **346–8**
decision nodes 336, *336*, 399, 404
decision theory 363
decision trees 216, *337, 338*, 397
  methods of construction *336*, **336–8**
  thrombolytic therapy example *337, 338*, **336–8**
deduction 165
de-facto rationing 351
degenerative diseases 21, 26
degrees of freedom 399
denial, patient **239**
dependent events 105
dependent tests 293
dependent variables 20, 68, 399
depreciation 356
depression 59, 69, 72, 81–2, 235, 247
derivation sets 62, 123, 158
descriptive research 399
descriptive statistics **94**, *387*, **389**, 399
descriptive studies 56, **57–60**, 189–90
detection bias 83
diagnosis, consistency 217; *see also* decision making
diagnosis, study type 22, *22*, 23, 38, 385–6
diagnostic classification schemes **234–5**
diagnostic review bias 299–300
diagnostic tests **303–4, 309**; *see also* probability of disease; utility
  absence of definitive tests **299**
  accuracy criteria 245–7
  applicability **306–7**
  bibliography 418
  characteristics 216, 399
  comparison 276, *278, 280, 280*, **277–81**
  context bias **300**
  costs/applicability **307**
  definition 399
  diagnostic thinking 247
  filter bias **296–7**
  formulas 391

gold standard comparisons **304, 305–6**
ideal research study **302–3**
incorporation bias **298**
indeterminate/uninterpretable results **300**
learning objectives 244, 276, 295
observer bias **299–300**
overview of studies of diagnostic tests **295–6**
patient outcome criteria 248; *see also* decision trees; values, patient
post-hoc selection of positivity criteria **301**
post-test probability and patient management **308–9**
pretest probability **307–8**
publication bias **302**
quotations 244, 276, 295
reproducibility **301**
results impact **306**
review/interpretation bias **299–300**
ROC curves **276–7**, *278, 280*
sampling bias **305**
selection bias **296–8**
social outcome criteria 248
spectrum/subgroup bias **297**, 305
study description/methods **304–5**
technical criteria 245–6
technological improvement of tests **301–2**
therapeutic effectiveness criteria 247–8
two by two tables *391*
uses/applications **244–5**
validity of results **304–6**
verification bias **298**
diagnostic thinking 247
diagnostic-suspicion bias 361, 362
dichotomous data 69
dichotomous outcomes 399
dichotomous test results 251, 400
dichotomous variables **138**, *139*
diet 65
differential diagnosis 216, *224, 225, 225*, **223–5**, 226, *227*, **282**, 400
difficult patients **240**
digitalis 4
disability 322, 337, 347, 349
discounting **356**
discrete data 69
discriminant function analysis 158, *387*
discussions *28*, **30–1**, **173**; *see also* IMRAD style
disease-free interval 205
disease oriented evidence (DOE) 12, 13
disease-oriented outcomes 72
dispersion measures 30, **94**, 100–1
distribution of values 101–2

doctor–patient relationship 3, **202–3**
doctrine of clinical equipoise 185
DOE (disease oriented evidence) 12, 13
dogmatists, Ancient Greek 3
doing/doers 11
dose-response gradients **194–5**
Double, Francois 7
double-blinded studies 29, 76; *see also*
    blinding
drop-out, patient (attrition) 63, **88–9**, 171, *361*,
    360–1
DynaMed database 34, 51

early detection 37
early termination of clinical trials 128–9,
    165
EBCP (evidence-based clinical practice) 10
EBHC *see* evidence-based health care
Economic Evaluation Database 49
editorials 27
educational prescription 14
EER (experimental event rate) 114
effect size 30, **113–14**, **133**, *134*, 400
    meta-analyses/systematic reviews 371, 376
    results strength 192–3
effectiveness 400
Effectiveness and Efficiency (Cochrane) 8, 47
effects 19
efficacy 400
eligibility requirements 29
embarrassment, patient **239**
EMBASE records 54
empowerment, patient 18
empiricists, Ancient Greek 3
energy balance beliefs *2*, 2–3, 4
Entrez dates 40
environmental sources of error **240–1**
epidemiology 6, *107*, **107–8**, 193
equation, evidence usefulness 53
equivalence studies **140**
Erlich, Paul 6
error **69–70**; *see also* bias; precision; Type I-IV
    errors
    appropriate tests 241; *see also* diagnostic
        tests
    biological variations 235, 237
    chance 90
    clinical consistency, measuring 233–4
    confabulation **238**
    contradictory answers **238**
    denial, patient **239**
    diagnostic classification schemes 234–5
    diagnostic tools malfunction 241, 242
    difficult patients **240**

    disruptive examination environments **240**,
        241
    embarrassment, patient **239**
    environmental sources of error **240–1**
    examinee sources **240**
    examiner sources **234–7**
    expectations, physician **235**
    hypothesis testing **111–13**
    inference and evidence **234**, 242
    language barriers **239**
    learning objectives 233
    lying, patient **240**
    medical 217
    medication effects **237**
    mimimization strategies **241–3**
    patient ignorance **238**
    physician ignorance **236**
    physician off-days **237**
    problem-oriented medical record *242*
    questioning patients **235–6**
    quotation 233
    recall bias **237–8**
    research conduct/misconduct 181
    risk maximization/minimization **236–7**,
        239
    staff non-cooperation **240–1**
    validity 74
Essential Evidence Plus database 34, 51–2
ethics 66; *see also* responsible conduct of
    research
    cost-effectiveness 351, **357–8**
    decision making **345–6**, *347*
    randomized clinical trials **177–8**
etiology, study type 22, *22*, 22–3, 38
event rates 104, **114**, *115*, *389*, *390*, 400
evidence, consistency 193
evidence, strength of *see* strength of
    evidence/applicability
evidence-based clinical practice (EBCP) 10
Evidence Based Emergency Medicine Group
    12
Evidence Based Health Care (EBHC)
    university course ix, 218–19
evidence-based health care *10*
    art of medicine **16–18**
    background/foreground questions *14*,
        13–14
    clinical question structure **15–16**
    critical appraisal 10, **12–13**
    definition 10
    expert vs. evidence-based decision making
        11–12
    importance of evidence **9–10**, *188*
    learning objectives 9

quotation 9
steps in practicing **14–15**
Evidence-Based Interest Group, ACP 12
Evidence Based On Call 54
evidence carts 13
evidence-and-outcomes-based approach
    324
examiner error **234–7**
executive tests 244–5, 311; *see also* screening
exclusion criteria 29, **168–9**, **369–70**, 376
exercise 119
exhaustion strategy 229, 409
expectation bias 361, 362
expectations, patient **200**, **202**, 218, *219*; *see
    also* placebo effect
expectations, physician **235**
expected-values decision making 334, **334–6**,
    352, 355, 400
experimental event rate (EER) 114
experimental group 114, 400
experimental settings 29, 329, 408
expert based randomization 167
expert bias 27
expert opinion 54
expert reviews 25
expert vs. evidence-based decision making
    11–12
explanatory research 400
explicit reviews 61
exploratory studies 59
exposure 400
exposure suspicion bias 84
external validity 74, **89–90**, **168–9**, 396; *see also*
    applicability

fabrication of results 181–2; *see also*
    responsible conduct of research
face validity 74
fail-safe N method 374
false alarm rates (FARs) 262, 289, 401
false labeling 313, 319
false negative 401
false negative rates (FNR) 257, 401
false negative test results 112, 130, 246, 253,
    253
false positive 401
false positive rates (FPR) 205, 256, 401
false positive test results 112, 120, 246, 253,
    253
false reassurance rates (FRRs) 262, 265, 401
falsification of results 181–2; *see also*
    responsible conduct of research
FARs (false alarm rates) 262, 289, 401
fatal flaws 81, 173

Fibonacci 4
field searching **47**
file-drawer effect 374
filter bias **296–7**, 360
filtering 85
filters 401
filters, literature search **38–9**, **46–7**
financial incentives 183, **302**
Fisher, Sir Ronald 8, 111, 263
five S schema 53
fixed-effects model 371
Florence Nightingale 6
FNR (false negative rates) 257, 401
focus-group interviews 210
follow-up, patient 171, 247, 330, *361*, 360–1
foreground questions *14*, **13–14**
Forest plot 372
FPR (false positive rates) 205, 256, 401
framing bias 205–6
framing effects **348–9**, 401
fraud, research 180; *see also* responsible
    conduct of research
frequency polygons 98, *99*
frequency tables **363**
Freud, Sigmund 6
FRRs (false reassurance rates) 262, 265, 401
functional status 401
funnel plot *374*, 373–4

Galen 3
gambling odds 263–4
Ganfyd 34
Gaussian distribution *104*, **103–4**, 106, 401
    gold standard comparisons 304
    strength of evidence/applicability 198
    test results 252, *252*
gender 150, **195**
generalizability 396; *see also* applicability
generalizability of population 101
germ theory 6
gold-standard tests 59, 76, 234, 245
    comparing with other tests 252–3, **305–6**
    comparisons **304**
    definition 401
    diagnostic tests, comparison 279
    diagnostic tests, critical appraisal 309
    examples 246–7
    ideal research study 303
    interpretation bias 299–300
    post-test probability/patient management
        308
    pulmonary angiograms 295
    strep throat 290
    tarnished **299**

gold-standard tests (*cont.*)
    threshold values 288
    verification bias **298**
Google/Google Scholar 54
GRADE (Grading of Recommendations
    Assessment, Development and
    Evaluation) scheme 191, *192*, 325, 369,
    382
grades of evidence 190–1, 378–81; *see also*
    levels of evidence
grades of recommendation *382*
graphing techniques
    bar graphs *97*, 98
    box-and-whisker plots **98**, *100*
    deceptive **94–5**
    frequency polygons 98, *99*
    histograms 98, *98*
    meta-analyses/systematic reviews 372–4
    presenting information to patients 203
    stem-and-leaf plots *97*, **96–7**
Graunt, John 5
grounded theory 213
Guide to Clinical Preventive Services (USPHS)
    317
guidelines 218, 219, *322*, 397; *see also* clinical
    prediction rules
    critical appraisal **324–5**
    development **322–4**
    learning objectives 320
    nature of/role in medicine **320–2**
    quotation 320

handwriting, legible **243**
harm vs. benefit 401
Hawthorne effect 75, 86
hazard ratios 363
health literacy 201
Health Technology Assessment Database 49
heterogeneity 370, 371–2, 373, 376
heuristics **231**, 401
hierarchies of research studies **190–1**
Hippocratic principle 3
histograms 98, *98*
history and physical (H & P) *220*, *221*, 220–2,
    241, 268; *see also* medical history-taking
history function *41*, **41**
history of medicine
    ancient history **2–3**
    learning objectives 1
    modern biomedical research **7–8**
    quotation 1
    recent history **6–7**
    Renaissance **3–4**
    statistics **4–6**

homeopathy 4
homogeneity 401
hospital bed management 321
human participants in research **184–5**
humours 2, *2*
hypothesis **167–8**, 402; *see also* research
    question
hypothesis generation 221, **222–3**
hypothesis testing *110*, **109–10**, *112*; *see also*
    statistics
    confidence intervals **116**
    effect size **113–14**
    error **111–13**
    event rates 104, **114**
    hypothesis, nature of 109, **110–11**
    learning objectives 109
    placebo effect **118–19**
    quotation 109
    signal-to-noise ratio **115–16**
    statistical tests **116–18**, 387
hypothetico-deductive strategy 229, *231*, 402

ignorance, patient/physician **236**, **238**
iLR (interval likelihood ratios) *272*, *275*, **272–5**,
    402
IM *see* information mastery
implicit reviews 61
IMRAD style (introduction, methods, results,
    discussion) 27
inception cohort *361*, **359–61**
incidence 59, 62, *107*, 108, 402
incidence bias 59, 360
inclusion criteria 29, **168–9**, **369–70**, 376
incorporation bias **298**, 402
incremental gain *286*, *287*, **285–7**, 402
    learning objectives 282
    likelihood ratios **283**
    multiple tests *292*, **291–3**
    quotation 282
    real-life applications **293–4**
    sensitivity/specificity **282**, *283*, *284*, **283–5**
    threshold values *289*, **287–91**, 395
    two by two tables *283*, *284*, **283–5**
independent events 105
independent tests 292
independent variables 20, 67, 160, 161, 402
in-depth interviews *210*
indeterminate/uninterpretable results **300**
Indian belief systems 2, *2*, 3
indication creep 307
induction 165
inductive reasoning 7
industrial revolution **3–4**
inference and evidence **234**

inferential statistics 94, *387*, 402
inflation 356
InfoPOEMS 50; *see also* Essential Evidence
    Plus database
information, patient 18; *see also* medical
    records
information mastery 10, 12, 53
information presentation to patients 206; *see
    also* communication with patients
information retrieval strategies **35–7**
informed consent 177, 185
initial exploratory studies 59
Institutional Review Boards (IRBs) 66, 177,
    185
instrumental rationality 334, 402
instruments/instrument selection 29, **70–2**,
    241, 242, 402; *see also*
    measurements/instruments
insurance, medical 351, 352
integrating 213
integrity, scientific *see* responsible conduct of
    research
intention-to-treat 89, 172, 402
interference, test results 246
inter-observer consistency 76, 78, 234, 246,
    328, 374
inter-observer reliability **76–7**, 370, 402
internal validity 74; *see also* validity
interpretation bias **299–300**
interquartile range 101
interval data 68, 363, *387*
interval likelihood ratios (iLR) *272, 275*, **272–5**,
    402
intervention criteria **361**
intervention studies 214; *see also* clinical trials
interventions, PICO/PICOT model 15, 35
interviews *210*
intra-observer consistency 76, 78, 234, 246
intra-observer reliability 402
intra-rater agreement 76
intrinsic characteristics, test 399
introductions, medical literature *28*, **28**; *see
    also* IMRAD style
intuition 377

JCB (journal club bank) 12
Jones criteria 247
journal club bank (JCB) 12
*Journal of the American Medical Association
    (JAMA)* 25, 31, 91, 151
journals 411–13
jumping to conclusions **234–5**; *see also*
    premature closure
justice, principle of 185, 403

Kaplan-Meier curve *365*, 366
Kaposi's sarcoma 57
kappa statistic *77, 78*, 212, 234, 403
    clinical prediction rules development
        328
    meta-analyses/systematic reviews 376
    precision/validity 76–7, *78*, **78–9**
Kelvin, Lord 19
key words 35
knowledge transfer model **197–8**
Koch, Robert 6
Koch's postulates 20–1, *22*
KT (knowledge translation) 10

L'Abbé plots 174, *373*, 373
lack of proportionality 94, *96*
The Lancet 25, 31
language barriers **239**
Laplace, Pierre 7, 263
law of large numbers 5
laws, professional conduct 184; *see also*
    malpractice suits; responsible conduct of
    research
lead-time bias *315*, 314–15, 360
legal cases, professional misconduct 180; *see
    also* malpractice suits; responsible
    conduct of research
length-time bias 315, *316*, 360
level of significance 120, *134*, **133–5**, 376, 403
levels of evidence **188–90**, 378–81; *see also*
    grades of evidence
Liber abaci (Book of the Abacus) 4
Liber de ludo aleae (Book on Games of
    Chance) 5
librarians, health science 55
life years 410
likelihood ratios 216, 251, **283**, 403; *see also*
    interval likelihood ratios
    positive/negative *254, 255, 255*, 254–5, 403
    pretest probability *265*, **264–6**
Likert Scales 68, 71–2
limits function *40*, **39–40**
Lind, James 7, 164–5
linearity *160*, 160
linear-rating scales 347, *347*, 403
Lister, Joseph 6
literature *see* medical literature
literature searching *see* medical literature
    searching
Lloyd, Edward 5
local variations in healthcare provision 9
logistic analysis **363–4**
log-rank test 366
longitudinal studies 56–7, **60–4**

Louis, Pierre 6, 7
lying, patient **238**, **240**

MAGIC study 368
malpractice suits 218, *219*, 308; *see also*
    responsible conduct of research
mammography *77*, 76–7, *78*, 244, 245
    framing bias 206
    intra-observer consistency 234
    screening 316
managed care organizations (MCOs) 321, 351
Mantel-Cox curve 366
Mantel-Haentszel chi-squared test 370
Markov models *345*, **345**, 403
Massachusetts General Hospital 229
MAST (Michigan Alcohol Screening Test) 72,
    74
matching 403
mathematics and medicine ix
McMaster University, Canada 11
MCOs (managed care organizations) 321, 351
mean 94, 99–100, 403; *see also* regression to
    the mean; standard error of the mean
measurements/instruments 29
    attributes **72–3**
    bibliography 416
    definition 403
    error **69–70**
    evaluating 171
    improving precision/accuracy **75–6**
    instruments/instrument selection **70–2**
    inter/intra-rater reliability tests **76–7**
    kappa statistic *77*, 76–7, *78*, *78*, **78–9**
    learning objectives 67
    quotation 67
    types of data/variables **67–9**
    validity 73, **73–5**
measures of central tendency 30, 94, 98–100
measures of dispersion 30, 94, 100–1
median 94, 100
Medicaid 351
medical history-taking *220*, *221*, **220–2**, 241;
    see also history and physical (H & P)
medical literature 25, *28*, **31–2**
    abstracts *28*, *28*, **28**
    basic science research **25–7**
    bibliography/references *28*, **31**, 414–16, 421;
        see also journals
    clinical research studies **27–8**
    clinical reviews 27
    conclusions *28*, **31**
    discussion *28*, **30–1**
    editorials **27**
    explosion 367

introductions *28*, **28**
journals **24–5**
learning objectives 24
meta-analyses/clinical reviews **27**
methods *28*, **29**
quotation 24
results *28*, **29–30**
searching *see* medical literature searching
medical literature searching 15, **33–4**, **54–5**;
    see also MEDLINE; PUBMED website
    clipboard function **42**
    Cochrane Library *49*, **47–50**
    databases 34
    field searching 47
    history function **39–40**, *41*
    information retrieval strategies **35–7**
    learning objectives 33
    limits function *40*, **39–40**
    MeSH search terms *44*, *44*, *45*, *46*, **43–6**
    methodological terms/filters **46–7**
    point of care databases *53*, **51–4**
    printing/saving **42**
    quotation 33
    responsible **180–1**
    synonyms/wildcard symbol **37**
    TRIP database **50–1**
medical records *242*, 406
medication 154, 167, **237**
medicine
    art/science of **16–18**, 187, *225*, 288, 291, 377
    and mathematics ix
MEDLINE 34, **37–8**, 54; *see also* PUBMED
    website
    clipboard function **42**
    field searching **47**
    general searching **42**, *43*
    history function *41*, **41**
    limits function *40*, **39–40**
    MeSH search terms *44*, *44*, *45*, *46*, **43–6**
    methodological terms/filters **46–7**
    saving/printing functions **42**
member checking 213
membership bias **84–5**
memoing 213
MeSH database 38, 39
MeSH search terms *44*, *44*, *45*, *46*, **43–6**, 50
meta-analyses 27, *372*, 403; *see also* clinical
    reviews; systematic reviews
    additional guidelines **376–7**
    guidelines for evaluating **368–76**
    inclusion criteria **369–70**, 376
    learning objectives 367
    quotation 367
    rationale **367–8**

methods *28*, **29**, **171**, **304–5**, **368–9**, 370
microscope, invention 3
Middle Ages 3
'Mikey liked it' phenomenon 58
milk pasteurization 194
mining, data 122–3
misclassification bias 64, **86–7**
misconduct, scientific *see* ethics; responsible
    conduct of research
mnemonics 224, *225*, 257, *257*; *see also*
    acronyms, mnemonic
mode 94, 100
Modified Rankin Scale 337
Moivre, Abraham de 103
monitoring therapy 245
mortality rates *107*, 108, 202
    cardiovascular disease 168
    colon cancer 36, 37
    measles 142
    pneumonia 74
Morton, William 6
multiple branching strategy 229, 403
multiple causation 194
multiple linear regression analysis 158, *387*
multiple logistic regression analysis 158, *387*
multiple outcomes **122–3**, 362–3
multiple regression 158, 364, *387*; *see also*
    CART analysis
multiple tests use *292*, **291–3**
multiplication tables 4
multivariate analysis 87, 161
    applications 157–9
    concomitance **161**
    independent variables – coding **161**
    interactions between independent
      variables **160**
    learning objectives 156
    linearity *160*, **160**
    nature of 156–7
    outliers to the mean **161**
    overfitting **159**
    prognosis 362
    propensity scores **162–3**
    quotation 156
    research design strength 189
    risk determination **157**, *158*, *159*
    underfitting **160**
    Yule–Simpson paradox *162*, **163**
mutually exclusive events 105–6

n-of-1 trial **175**, 189
National Institutes of Health 186, 369
National Research Act (1974) 184
Native American belief systems 2, *2*

natural frequencies 205, 206
Nazi atrocities 179
NCBI accounts 42, 50
negative in health (NIH) test result 256, *257*
negative likelihood ratios *254*, *255*, *255*, 254–5,
    403
negative predictive values (NPVs) 262, 265,
    404
negative studies, evaluating **130–1**, **135–6**; *see*
    also Type II errors
    confidence intervals **136–7**
    continuous variables *139*, **138–40**
    dichotomous variables **138**, *139*
    nomograms *138*, *139*, **137–40**
New England Journal of Medicine 25, 31, 150,
    229
new tests **301–2**
New York Academy of Medicine 12
NHS (National Health Service) 13, 48, 49
NICE, UK 357
Nightingale, Florence 6
NIH (negative in health) test result 256, *257*
NLM (National Library of Medicine), US 47,
    369
NNEH (number needed to expose to harm)
    127
NNF (number needed to follow) 404
NNSB (number needed to screen to benefit)
    127, *317*, 316–17, 318
NNSH (number needed to screen to harm)
    319
NNTB (number needed to treat to benefit)
    125, 125, 205, 346, 354, 404
NNTH (number needed to treat to harm)
    125–7, 148, *148*, 151, 404
nodes 404; *see also* decision nodes;
    probability nodes
noise **115–16**, 276, 277–81; *see also* ROC curves
nominal data 68, 363, *387*
nomograms *138*, *139*, **137–40**, *267*, **267**, *268*
non peer-reviewed journals 25
non-concurrent cohort studies 62, 64, 83
non-inferiority trial **140**, 404
non-respondent bias **84**
non-steroidal anti-inflammatory drugs
    (NSAIDs) 26, 183
normal distribution *103*, *104*, **103–4**, 106,
    404
    gold standard comparisons 304
    strength of evidence/applicability 198
    test results 252, *253*
NOT (Boolean operator) *36*, 35–7
NPVs (negative predictive values) 262, 265,
    404

NSAIDs (non-steroidal anti-inflammatory
    drugs) 26, 183
null hypothesis 28, 110–11, 140, 404
null point 136
numbering systems 4

objective information 404
objectivity, research 185, 186
observational studies 65, 189, *210*, 404
observer bias **85–6**, **299–300**, 328
odds *264*, **263–4**, 404
odds ratios 142, *146*, *147*, **145–7**, **150**, 363
    definition 404
    formulas *390*, **389–90**
    meta-analyses/systematic reviews 371
    results strength 192–3
    two by two tables *390*
off-days, physician **237**
OLDCARTS acronym 221, *221*, 222–3
one-tailed tests *121*, **121–2**, 132, 140, 404
operator dependence 246, 404
opportunity costs 351, 353
OPQRSTAAAA acronym 221, *222–3*
OR (Boolean operator) *36*, 35–7
ordinal data 68, 363, *387*
outcome criteria 248, **361–3**; *see also* decision
    trees; values, patient
outcome measurement bias **85–7**
outcome misclassification 87
outcomes 64, 328, 404
    PICO/PICOT model 16, 21, 35
outcomes study 405
outliers to the mean 99, 376
overfitting **159**
Oxford Database of Perinatal Trials 48
Oxford University, UK 11, 12, 190

P value 30, 405
P4P (Pay for Performance) 321
Paccioli, Luca 4
pain
    confidence intervals 136
    contradictory answers **238**
    guidelines 322
    measurement 71–2
    placebo effect 119
    relief **240**
    scales 70
Paracelsus 3
particularizability 396
Pascal, Blaise 5, 333–4
passive smoking 127, 183
Pasteur, Louis 6, 56
Pathman's pipeline analogy *197*, **197–8**

pathognomonic 405
pathological specimens 246
patient attrition 63, **88–9**, 171, *361*, 360–1
patient inception cohort *361*, **359–61**
patient satisfaction 405
patient values *see* values, patient
patient-oriented evidence that matters
    (POEMS) 12, 13; *see also* Essential
    Evidence Plus database
patient-oriented outcomes 72
patients, PICO/PICOT model 15, 22
pattern recognition 228–9, 231, 405
Pay for Performance (P4P) 321
Pay-Per-View 50
peer pressure 218, *219*
peer review **186**
peer-review guidelines 324
peer-reviewed journals 24
percent of a percent 104
percentages **104–5**
percentages of small numbers 105
percentiles 94, 100, 405
performance criteria 321
persistent vegetative states 335
perspectives, patient 201; *see also* values,
    patient
phototherapy 368
physician behavior, changing 323–4
physician ignorance **236**
PICO/PICOT model 14, 15–16, 35, 295–6
PID (positive in disease) test result 256,
    i257
Pisano, Leonardo 4
placebo 405
placebo controls *see* controls/control groups
placebo drugs 113
placebo effect **118–19**, 167, *219*
plagiarism 181–2
plans 405
podcasts 55
POEMS (patient-oriented evidence that
    matters) 12, 13; *see also* Essential
    Evidence Plus database
PogoFrog 54
point estimate 405
point of care databases *53*, **51–4**
point of indifference 405
points, decision tree 405
POMR (problem-oriented medical record)
    242, 406
popularity bias 360
population, patient 22, 35, 101, 405
Port Royal text on logic 334
positive in disease (PID) test result 256, *257*

positive likelihood ratios *254, 255, 255*, 254–5, 403

positive predictive values (PPVs) 262, 265, 405

possession by demons 2

posterior probability *see* post-test probability

post-hoc subgroup analysis 128, 171

post-test odds 406

post-test probability *225*, 251, 262, **267–8**, *269*, 286, **308–9**, 406

potential bias 31

power, statistical 29, 30, 112, 131, 406
   determining **131–5**
   effect size **133**, *134*
   level of significance *134*, **133–5**
   sample size *133*, **132–3**
   standard deviation *135*, **135**

PPVs (positive predictive values) 262, 265, 405

practice guidelines *see* guidelines

precision 30, 72–3, 233, 406
   diagnostic tests 245
   improving **75–6**, 76
   kappa statistic 78

prediction rules *see* clinical prediction rules

predictive validity 74

predictive values **262**, *270*, **268–72**, 406

predictor variables 328, 406

prehistory of medicine **2–3**

premature closure 229, **231–2**

pretest odds 406

pretest probability *224, 225*, 224–5, 226, 250, 406
   diagnostic tests, critical appraisal **307–8**
   incremental gain 285–7
   and likelihood ratios *265*, **264–6**
   multiple tests 293

prevalence 59, 62, *107*, 108, 311, 406

prevalence bias 59, 360

prevention studies 23

primary analysis 367

principle of beneficence 185

principle of justice 185

principle of respect for persons 185

printing/saving functions **42**

prior probability *see* pre-test probability

probability **105–7**, *264*, **263–4**, 334, **334–6**

probability of disease, diagnostic tests **261–2**
   Bayes' theorem **262–3**, **264–6**, **392**
   interval likelihood ratios *272, 275*, **272–5**
   learning objectives 261
   likelihood ratios/pretest probability *265*, **264–6**
   nomograms *267*, **267**, *268*
   odds/probability *264*, **263–4**

post-test probability calculation *225*, **267–8**, *269*

predictive values **262**

predictive values calculation *270*, **268–72**

quotation 261

probability nodes 336, *336*, 404, 406

probability of survival, historical comparisons *6*

probability theory **5–6**, 389

procedures, experimental 29

professional misconduct *see* ethics; responsible conduct of research

prognosis 406
   frequency tables **363**
   inception cohort *361*, **359–61**
   intervention criteria **361**
   learning objectives 359
   logistic analysis **363–4**
   outcome criteria **361–3**
   quotation 359
   study type 22, *22*, 23, 38
   survival analysis **364**, *365*, 409
   survival curves *365*, **364–6**

prognostics 245

propensity scores **162–3**

proportional hazards regression analysis 158, 160, 366, *387*

proportionality 94, *96*

prospective studies 57, 406

PsycINFO 34

publication bias 90, **302**, 369, 374, 406

publish or perish 177

PUBMED website **37–8**, *39*, **38–9**, 53, 55
   Clinical Queries search function 50, 51
   clipboard function **42**
   field searching **47**
   general searching **42**, *43*
   history function *41*, **41**
   limits function *40*, **39–40**
   MeSH search terms *44, 44, 45, 46*, **43–6**
   methodological terms/filters **46–7**
   saving/printing functions **42**

purposive sampling 211

Q statistic 370

QALYs (quality-adjusted life years) 348, 351, 355–6, 357, 407

qi 2, *2*, 2–3

qualitative research
   applications **209**
   applying results **214**
   data analysis **212–13**
   data collection **211–12**
   learning objectives 208

qualitative research (*cont.*)
  methods **209**
  quotation 208
  sampling **211**
  study objectives **210–11**
  study types **209**, *210*
qualitative reviews 367, 376
quality-of-life 202, 340, 346, 407
quantitative systematic review *see*
      meta-analyses; systematic reviews
quartiles 94, 100
question, research 369, 407; *see also*
      hypothesis
questioning patients **235–6**
questionnaires 70

race 150
random error 69–70
random selection/assignment 407
random-effects model 371–2
randomization 29, 65, **169–70**, 407
randomized clinical trials (RCTs) 8, 23, 47,
      164–5, **166–7**, **173–4**
  blinding **170**
  CONSORT statement *177*, **176–7**
  definition 407
  discussions/conclusions **173**
  early termination 165
  ethics **177–8**
  evaluating *166*, 166
  hypothesis **167–8**
  inclusion/exclusion criteria **168–9**
  learning objectives 164
  measures of risk 142
  methods, description **171**
  methodological terms/filters 46
  n-of-1 trial **175**
  overview 384
  physician decision making **165–6**, **176**
  quotation 164
  randomization **169–70**
  research design strength 189
  results **176**
  results, analysis **172–3**
  user's guide **175–6**
  validity **175–6**
range 94, 100
ratio data 68–9, *387*
recall bias 61, 62, **83–4**, **237–8**
receiver operating characteristic (ROC) curves
      216, **276–7**, *278*, *280*, 306, 407
recursive partitioning 329
reference standards *see* gold-standard tests
references, medical literature *28*, **31**

referral bias 61, **82–3**, 150, 329, 360, 407
registry of clinical trials 178
regression to the mean 118
relative rate reduction (RRR) 114
relative risk (RR) *145*, **144–5**, *147*, **146–7**, **150**,
      363
  communication with patients 205
  confidence intervals (CI) *391*
  definition 407
  formulas *390*, **389–90**
  meta-analyses/systematic reviews 371
  results strength 192–3
  two by two tables *390*
relevance 396
reliability 73, 245, 407
removing patients from study 172
Renaissance **3–4**
repeat observations 241
replication 54
replicators 11
reporting bias 61, **83–4**, 150
representativeness heuristic 230, 407
reproducibility **301**
research conduct/misconduct *see* responsible
      conduct of research
research design strength **188–90**
Research and Development Programme, NHS
      48
research question 369, 407; *see also* hypothesis
respect for persons, principle of 185
responsible conduct of research; *see also*
      ethics
  conflicts of interest *183*, **182–4**
  definitions of misconduct 181–2
  human participants in research **184–5**
  learning objectives 179
  managing conflicts of interest 184
  motives for misconduct 182, 183
  objectivity 185, 186
  peer-review **186**
  quotation 179
  research conduct/misconduct **179–82**
results *28*, **29–30**, 176; *see also* IMRAD style
  applicability **187–8**, 332
  case–control studies 385
  clinical prediction rules 331–2
  cohort studies 384–5
  diagnosis – study type 385–6
  impact **306**
  meta-analyses/systematic reviews **370–4**
  randomized clinical trials (RCTs) **172–3**, 384
  risk assessment 151
  specificity **193–4**
  strength **191–3**

retrospective bias 368
retrospective studies 57, 83, 407; *see also* case-control studies; non-concurrent cohort studies
review bias **299–300**
risk 407, 417
risk assessment
    absolute risk *143, 144,* **143–4**
    attributable risk *148,* **147–8**
    confidence intervals 149, *154*
    learning objectives 141
    measures of risk *143,* **142–3**
    nature of risk **153–5**
    number needed to treat to harm (NNTH) 148, *148*
    odds ratios 142, *146, 147,* **145–7, 150**
    perspectives on risk **148–9**
    quotation 141
    relative risk *145,* **144–5,** *147,* **146–7, 150**
    reporting bias **150**
    user's guide **151**
    zero numerator *153,* **152–3,** *154*
risk, attitudes to 334, 348, **348–9**
risk determination 157, *158, 159*
risk factors 62, 63, 407
    decision making 333–4; *see also* decision making
    estrogen therapy **83**
    multiple 156; *see also* multivariate analysis
    and study design 64
risk maximization/minimization **236–7**
robust results 173
ROC (receiver operating characteristics) curves 216, **276–7,** *278, 280,* 306, 407
Roentgen, William 6
Roman numerals 4
RRR (relative rate reduction) 114
RR *see* relative risk
RSS feeds 55
rule in/out 408
rules *see* clinical prediction rules
Rush, Benjamin 4

sample selection/assignment 29
sample size 30, *133,* **132–3,** *137*
samples 29, 94, 101–2, 408
sampling **211**
sampling bias 61, 81–2, **305,** 408
sampling theory *see* statistical sampling
sampling to redundancy 211
sanitary engineering 6, 20
saving/printing functions **42**
schizophrenia 321

School of Health, University of British Columbia 291
science of medicine **16–18;** *see also* art of medicine
scientific misconduct *see* responsible conduct of research
Scopus 34, 54
screening *311,* **310–12,** 408
    compliance bias 315–16
    criteria for screening *312,* **312–14**
    critical appraisal of studies **318–19**
    effectiveness 318
    executive tests 244–5, 311
    lead-time bias *315,* 314–15
    learning objectives 310
    length-time bias 315, *316*
    medical literature searching 36, 37
    pitfalls **314–16**
    quotation 310
    spectrum/subgroup bias 297
scurvy 7, 164–5
secondary analysis 367
second-guessing 218
sedation **240**
selection bias **81–2,** 86, **296–8,** 328–9
self-assessment learning exercises (SALES) 13
SEM (standard error of the mean) 94, 101, *115,* 115–16, **389**
Semmelweis, Ignatz 6
senses, biological variations **235**
sensitive results 172
sensitivity 38, *258,* 408
    analysis *339, 340,* **339–40,** *341, 342,* 374, 376, 408
    cost-effectiveness 356
    diagnostic tests 256
    differential diagnosis **282**
    guidelines 325
    incremental gain *284,* **283–5**
    mnemonics 257, *257*
    physician senses **235**
    post-test probability and patient management 309
    screening 311, 313
    spectrum/subgroup bias 297
settings, experimental 29, 329, 408
side effects, medication 154
signal-to-noise ratio **115–16**
significance, statistical 30, *117,* **124–5,** 173, 346, 408
    levels of 120, *134,* **133–5,** 376, 403
single-blinded studies 29, 76
size of study 193
SK (streptokinase) 126–7, 375, *375*

skewed distributions 101, *102, 103*
smallpox vaccine 4
snooping 122–3
SnOut (sensitive tests rule out disease)
    acronym *257*
Snow, John 6, 193
snowballing 55
SOAP formats 242, *242*, 408
social context of medicine 242–3
social desirability bias 211
social outcome criteria 248
software, computer 212
SORT (standards of reporting trials) 28
specificity 38, **193–4**, *258*, 408
    diagnostic tests 256
    differential diagnosis **282**
    incremental gain *284*, **283–5**
    mnemonics 257, *257*
    post-test probability/patient management
        309
    screening 313
    spectrum/subgroup bias 297
spectrum 408
spectrum bias **83**, **297**, **305**, 408
spin 357
SpIn (specific tests rule in disease) acronym
    257, *257*
spirits 2
SRs (systematic reviews) 54, 188, 409; *see also*
    clinical reviews; meta-analyses
staff non-cooperation **240–1**
standard deviation 94, 101, *135*, **135**
standard gamble *348*, 408
standardized therapy groups *see*
    controls/control groups
stationary nodes 336, *336*
statistical analysis 29, 362
statistical power *see* power, statistical
statistical sampling 5, *6*, 7
statistical significance *see* significance,
    statistical
statistical tests **116–18**, 387
statistically significant effect size 114
statistics 408; *see also* hypothesis testing
    bibliography 416–17
    descriptive **94**, *387*, **389**, 399
    distribution of values 101–2
    epidemiology *107*, **107–8**
    formulas 389–91
    history of **4–6**, 16
    inferential **94**, *387*, 402
    learning objectives 93
    measures of central tendency 30, 94,
        98–100
measures of dispersion 30, 94, 100–1
nature of/role in medicine **93**
normal distribution *104*, **103–4**, 106
percentages **104–5**
populations 101
probability **105–7**
quotation 93
samples 101–2
visual display *see* graphing techniques
StatSoft 108
stem-and-leaf plots **97**, *96–7*
stepwise regression analysis 364
strategy of exhaustion *see* exhaustion
    strategy
stratified randomization 409
strength of evidence/applicability *383*
    analogy, reasoning by **196**
    applicability of results *188*, **187–8**
    biological plausibility **195**
    common sense **196–7**
    consistency of evidence **193**
    consistency of evidence over time **195–6**
    dose-response gradients **194–5**
    hierarchies of research studies **190–1**
    learning objectives 187
    levels of evidence **188–90**
    Pathman's pipeline analogy *197*, **197–8**
    quotation 187
    research design strength **188–90**
    results strength **191–3**
    specificity of results **193–4**
    temporal relationships **194**
strong recommendations *383*
study design
    bibliography 416
    case reports/series 57, **57–8**
    case–control studies *61*, **60–2**
    clinical trials *65*, **64–6**
    cohort studies **62–4**
    cross-sectional studies **59–60**
    descriptive studies 56, **57–60**
    learning objectives 56
    longitudinal studies 56–7, **60–4**
    prospective studies 57
    quotation 56
    retrospective studies 57
    strengths/weaknesses 61, 63, 64, 66
    types 56–7
study size 193
subgroup analysis 90, 171
subgroup bias **297**
subject bias **85**
subjective information 409
surgery 3, 7, 154, 170

surrogate markers 20, 59, 72, **89–90**, 145, 194, 409
survival analysis **364**, *365*, 409; *see also* prognosis
survival curves *365*, **364–6**
survival rates 37
symmetrical distributions 101, *102*, 103
synonyms 37, *44*
systematic error 70

technical criteria 245–6
technological improvement of tests **301–2**
temporal relationships, cause-and-effect **194**
terminology, non-medical 238
test minimizers **236–7**
test review bias 299
testing thresholds 216, 288, 409
tests, diagnostic *see* diagnostic tests
theoretical saturation 211
therapeutic relationship 3, **202–3**
therapy studies 22, *22*, 23, 38
threshold approach to decision making **343–5**, 409
threshold values *289*, **287–91**, 394–5; *see also* incremental gain
time, PICO/PICOT model 16
time trade-offs 409
timelines, disease *311*
tissue samples 234, 245, 305
TNRs (true negative rates) 256
TPRs (true positive rates) 205, 256
translation services **239**
treatment thresholds 216, 274, 275, 288, 409
trephination 2
triangulation 213
triggering 409
TRIP database 34, **50–1**
triple-blinded studies 29, 76
true negative rates (TNRs) 256
true negative test results 130, 253, *253*
true positive rates (TPRs) 205, 256
true positive test results 253, *253*
trust 180; *see also* responsible conduct of research
truth 74
Tuskeegee syphilis studies 179
two alternative-forced choice problem 279, 396
two by two tables *224*, 257, *258*, *259*, 269, *275*
  diagnostic tests *391*
  incremental gain *283*, *284*, **283–5**
two-tailed tests *121*, **121–2**, 132, 140, 409
Type I errors 90, 112, **120–1**, 173, 409

bibliography 417
clinical prediction rules development 329
confidence intervals *124*, **123–4**
learning objectives 120
meta-analyses/systematic reviews 368
multiple outcomes **122–3**
number needed to treat **125–7**
one-tailed/two-tailed tests *121*, **121–2**
other sources of error **127–9**
quotation 120
randomized clinical trials 171
statistical/clinical significance **124–5**
Type II errors 112–13, **131**, 173, 410; *see also* negative studies, evaluating
bibliography 417
clinical prediction rules development 329
determining power **131–5**
effect size **133**, *134*
learning objectives 130
level of significance *134*, **133–5**
meta-analyses/systematic reviews 368, 370, 375
non-inferiority/equivalence studies **140**
prognosis 362
quotation 130
sample size *133*, **132–3**
standard deviation *135*, **135**
Type III errors 113, 133
Type IV errors 113, 133

unadjusted life expectancy 410
uncertainty 410
underfitting **160**
University of British Columbia 291
unobtrusive measurements 75–6
users 11, 53
Users' Guides to the Medical Literature 151, 318, 366, 384–6
bibliography 418–21
randomized clinical trials **175–6**
risk assessment **151**
website 175
USPHS (United States Public Health Service) 317
utility, diagnostic tests **306**
  cutoff points *258*
  definition 410
  function **250–1**
  indications **250**
  learning objectives 249–50
  normal test results **252–3**
  quotation 249
  sample problem *259*, **258–60**
  sensitivity/specificity 256

utility, diagnostic tests (*cont.*)
  sensitivity/specificity, using *225, 257, 258, 259*, **257–60, 267–8**, *269*
  strength of tests **253**
  two by two tables *254*, 253–4
  types of test result **251–2**
utility theory 6, 334, **334–6**

validation samples 362
validation sets 62
validation studies 158
validity 175–6, 410
  case–control studies 385
  clinical prediction rules 331
  cohort studies 384–5
  diagnosis – study type 385–6
  diagnostic tests 246
  diagnostic tests, critical appraisal b304–6
  guidelines 324–5
  measurements/instruments 73
  randomized clinical trials (RCTs) 384
  risk assessment 151
  screening studies 318
  types **73–5**
values, patient *10*, 319, 335, 349, 356, 405
  and decision making **346–8**
variables 410; *see also* confounding variables
  continuous *139*, **138–40**
  dependent 68
  dichotomous **138**, *139*
  independent 67
variance 101, 410
VAS (visual analog scale) 71, 136, 347, *347*
Venn diagrams *35*, 35
verification bias **298**

Vesalius 3
VINDICATE mnemonic 224, *225*
visual analog scale (VAS) 71, 136, 347, *347*
vitamins 4, 87, 164–5, 195, 196
V/Q (ventilation-perfusion) scan 296

water treatment engineering 6, 20
weak recommendations *383*
Web of Science 34, 54
websites 12, 34, **421–4**
  Clinical Evidence database 52
  clinical trials 369
  Cochrane Collaboration 49
  confidence intervals calculator for Bayes Theorem 291
  GRADE scheme 369
  levels of evidence 191
  number needed to treat 127
  PogoFrog 54
  PUBMED **37–8**, *39*, **38–9**
  registry of clinical trials 178
  risk assessment 151
  Users' Guides to the Medical Literature 175
weight 73
weighted outcomes 371
whistle-blowers 180, 182
wildcard symbol **37**, 39
Wiley InterScience interface 49, *49*
World Health Organization (WHO) 52
writing, legible 243

Yule–Simpson paradox *162*, **163**, 410

zero numerator *153*, **152–3**, *154*
zero points 94, *95*